D1065957

Multicultural Approaches to Health and Wellness in America

Multicultural Approaches to Health and Wellness in America

Volume 2: Mental Health and Mind–Body Connections

Regan A. R. Gurung, Editor

Foreword by Michael Winkelman

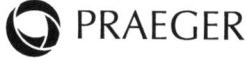 PRAEGER

AN IMPRINT OF ABC-CLIO, LLC
Santa Barbara, California • Denver, Colorado • Oxford, England

Library of Congress Cataloging-in-Publication Data

Multicultural approaches to health and wellness in America / Regan A.R. Gurung, editor ; foreword by Michael Winkelman.
     pages cm
  ISBN 978-1-4408-0349-9 (pbk. : alk. paper) — ISBN 978-1-4408-0350-5 (ebook)
1. Health attitudes—United States—Cross-cultural studies. 2. Health behavior—United States—Cross-cultural studies. 3. Transcultural medical care—United States. I. Gurung, Regan A. R.
  RA776.9.M85 2014
  362.1—dc23   2013031733

ISBN: 978-1-4408-0349-9
EISBN: 978-1-4408-0350-5

18 17 16 15   2 3 4 5

This book is also available on the World Wide Web as an eBook.
Visit www.abc-clio.com for details.

Praeger
An Imprint of ABC-CLIO, LLC

ABC-CLIO, LLC
130 Cremona Drive, P.O. Box 1911
Santa Barbara, California 93116-1911

This book is printed on acid-free paper ∞
Manufactured in the United States of America

To my father, Douglas Narendra Raj Gurung,
for inspiring me to always consider the extraordinary
and think beyond the bounds of the normally accepted.

Contents

Chapter One — Understanding International Perspectives: Implications for U.S. Health and Wellness — 1
P. S. D. V. Prasadarao

Chapter Two — Mental Health Assessment among Ethnic Minorities in the United States — 35
Sussie Eshun and Donna Hodge

Chapter Three — The Mental Health of Latina/os: A Cultural Focus — 59
Rocío Rosales Meza and Leticia Arellano-Morales

Chapter Four — Stress and Culture — 89
Angela R. Wendorf, Amanda M. Brouwer, and Katie E. Mosack

Chapter Five — Mood and Anxiety Disorders across Ethnic Minority Groups in the United States — 115
Sussie Eshun

Chapter Six — Religion and Health: Ideological Contexts and Their Influences on Health-Associated Behaviors — 137
Dean D. VonDras

Chapter Seven — Islamic Healing Approaches, Beliefs, and Health-Related Behaviors — 167
Sujata R. Swaroop, Chanté D. DeLoach, and Fyeqa Sheikh

Chapter Eight   The Health and Wellness of Sexual
                        and Gender Minorities   195
                        David W. Pantalone, John E. Pachankis,
                        Brian A. Rood, and Sarah M. Bankoff

Chapter Nine   Childhood Obesity and Cultural Influences   225
                        Jacqueline Woods, Stephen K. Trapp,
                        and Marilyn Stern

Chapter Ten   Suicide across Cultures   253
                        Kristin M. Vespia and Kaitlyn J. Florer

Afterword   285

About the Editor and Contributors   287

Index   293

Understanding International Perspectives: Implications for U.S. Health and Wellness

P.S.D.V. Prasadarao

The United States of America (U.S.) is a country with widespread racial and ethnic diversity. According to the 2010 Census, 308.7 million people resided in the United States on April 1, 2010—an increase of 27.3 million people (9.7 percent) between 2000 and 2010. The vast majority of the growth in the population came from a rise in those who reported their race(s) as something other than White alone and those who reported their ethnicity as Hispanic or Latino (Humes, Jones and Ramirez 2011), thus multiculturalism and cultural diversity have become integral parts of the United States. In this chapter I describe mental health issues from a cultural perspective. I also explore specific aspects such as cultural conceptualizations and belief systems, and indigenous mental health models across some cultures with a particular focus on how health beliefs around the world can shed light on multicultural approaches to health in the United States.

Mental Health Issues in America: A Multicultural Perspective

Mental disorders are common, often serious, and treatable disorders that have a major impact on the U.S. population. Mental illness and its associated impairment may impose a substantial burden on individuals and families that could potentially be reduced by effective treatment approaches. Expenditure on mental health treatment in America was about $113 billion in 2005, about 6.1 percent of the total U.S. expenditure on all types of health care. Serious mental illness (SMI) is of particular concern to policy makers and health care providers because having diagnosable mental illness involves serious functional impairment impacting a person's quality of life (Substance Abuse and Mental Health Services Administration 2012).

Approximately 11 million U.S. adults aged 18 or older (4.8 percent) had severe mental illness in 2009. Similarly, in the same year, more than one in eight U.S. adults received some type of mental health treatment in the past year. In 2009, 40 percent of adults with SMI reported not receiving any treatment. In 2009, 19.9 percent of the U.S. adult population experienced a mental illness (AMI) (excluding substance use disorders) in the past year. Prevalence of AMI was higher for females (23.8 percent) than males (15.6 percent). In 2009, 6.5 percent of U.S. adults had experienced a major depressive episode in the past year (Substance Abuse and Mental Health Services Administration 2012).

In 2009, 3.2 percent of U.S. adults experienced serious psychological distress in the past 30 days. The percentage of adults with past year severe mental illness was highest among adults aged 18 to 25 (7.3 percent) and lowest among adults aged 50 or older (2.8 percent). SMI was particularly prevalent among adults living in poverty (9.1 percent) and among those covered by Medicaid/children's health insurance programmes (10.7 percent) (Substance Abuse and Mental Health Services Administration 2012). Presence of mental and substance use disorders is a major risk factor for suicide (Goldsmith et al. 2002).

It is estimated that one out of eight American children has had some form of emotional or behavioral disorder in the past year (Merikangas et al. 2010). Based on the combined data from 2001 through 2004, prevalence of diagnosable mental disorders with severe impairment was 11.3 percent for children aged 8–15. During 2001–2004, more than half of all children with mental disorders received treatment in a hospital, clinic, or office within the previous year (Substance Abuse and Mental Health Services Administration 2012).

People in America receive mental health treatment in a wide range of settings, including specialty outpatient and inpatient settings; general medical clinics; non-specialty settings such as schools, nursing homes, or correctional facilities; and through prescription medication. Approximately one in eight adults in America received some type of specialty mental health treatment in the past year. In 2009, 13.3 percent of all U.S.

adults (over 30 million) used outpatient, inpatient, or prescription medication treatment for a mental health problem in the past year. Over 11 percent—about 85 percent of the 13 percent—used prescription medication. Among adults with any mental illness (AMI), 21.2 percent received outpatient mental health treatment, 3.1 percent received inpatient treatment, and 32.4 percent received a prescription medication for mental health. For adults with SMI, the corresponding proportions were 38.0 percent (outpatient), 6.8 percent (inpatient), and 54.0 percent (medication). In 2009, individuals with SMI were more likely to receive mental health treatment than individuals with AMI, but both groups were often unlikely to receive any treatment. Among those with AMI in the past year, 62.1 percent (or an estimated 27.9 million people) did not receive treatment. Among those with SMI, 39.8 percent (or an estimated 4.3 million people) did not receive treatment (Substance Abuse and Mental Health Services Administration 2012). This illustrates how mental health is an important component in a multicultural/multiethnic society such as America, where cultural aspects play a pivotal role in health, development, and quality of life of the people.

Barriers to Mental Health Practices in America

In America progress in mental health service development seems to be rather slow. Barriers to such development include a shortage of qualified mental health professionals, challenges in implementing mental health care in primary-care settings, the prevailing public-health priority agenda and its effect on funding, and problems in decentralization of mental health services (Saraceno et al. 2007). In line with the international trends, the increasing racial and ethnic diversity of the United States presents a formidable challenge to the delivery of effective, culturally appropriate health and mental health care (Kavanaugh and Kennedy 1992).

Currently, the reasons for low utilization of mental health services by Hispanics are relatively unexplored. Little attention has been given to patients' perspectives on illness, including their conceptions of illness, expectations and preferences for care, and the impact of these factors on the course of mental disorder. Understanding these factors might help in designing culturally-sensitive mental health treatments and service delivery systems (Berkman et al. 2005).

African Americans are significantly less likely than White Americans to seek mental health treatment (Brown and Palenchar 2004, Snowden 1999), attend fewer sessions when they do seek treatment, and are more likely than their White counterparts to terminate treatment prematurely (Kessler et al. 1994, Neighbors 1988). Despite numerous information sources, African Americans attribute illness to bad luck, fate or chance. Good health is equated with social entities such as luck or success. Home remedies are often the initial attempt in addressing an illness and the health care provider is consulted only after a failed attempt with such home remedies (Giger, Davidhizar, and Turner 1992, cited in Revell 2012). Rao, Feinglass, and Corrigan (2007) found that African Americans perceived people with mental illness as more dangerous and wanted separation from them more than their White counterparts. These findings highlight the importance of examining the impact of stigma on attitudes toward mental health treatment. Specific barriers have been identified for African Americans, including lack of access to services, transportation, racial/ethnic mismatch, mistrust of providers, and stigma (Conner et al. 2009, Diala et al. 2000). Similarly, social attitudes and perceptions of mental health treatment seem to impact help-seeking behaviors in African Americans. Conner, Koeske and Brown (2009) found that African Americans endorsed significantly more negative attitudes about mental health services than Whites. These attitudes may become a significant barrier to seeking mental health treatment when an individual internalizes these negative beliefs. These authors recommend the need to address stigma as an important barrier to the utilization of mental health services among older African Americans. Utilizing a nationally representative sample, Diala and colleagues (2000) found that African Americans and White Americans with negative attitudes toward treatment were five times less likely to seek mental health services than individuals with more positive attitudes. Recognizing the importance of attitudes toward treatment as a significant predictor of service utilization, it is imperative to understand what factors influence these attitudes and perceptions.

Asian Americans have lower rates of utilization of mental health services than the general U.S. population. Only 34.1 percent of Asian Americans who had a probable DSM-IV diagnosis according to the American Psychiatric Association's *Diagnostic and Statistical Manual of Disorders* and 8.6 percent of the general Asian American population sought any mental health-related services during a 12-month period compared with 41.1 percent of all individuals who had a probable *DSM-IV* diagnosis and 17.9 percent of the general U.S. population (Abe-Kim et al. 2007, Wang et al. 2005).

To avoid stigma, Asians often report physical signs and symptoms which are in fact a reflection of mental problems (Hsu et al. 2008). In Asian cultures, families feel ashamed and guilty when there is mental illness in a member, and they often blame themselves (Lam et al. 2010, Ting and

Hwang 2009). Health care providers' lack of understanding of cultural beliefs held by Asian people toward mental illness might lead to misdiagnosis. Various factors seem to have an influential role on the underutilisation of mental health services. These include cultural barriers (e.g., beliefs about causes of mental illness, stigma, unfamiliarity with mental health services, acculturation, communication, etc.), lack of knowledge about available services, problems accessing health care, lack of health insurance, and low income (Abe-Kim et al. 2007, Chen 2005, Choi and Kim 2010, Lam et al. 2010, Ting and Hwang 2009, Tung 2011 Wong et al. 2010, Yeung and Kung 2004).

Explanatory Models across Cultures and Their Importance in Health Care

It has been of interest to both clinicians and researchers, in the area of health in general and mental health specifically, to understand how illness is conceived by people from different cultures. These explanatory models describe how illness is understood from their own framework and how people attribute meaning to the illness (Coleman, Koffman, and Daniels 2007). The concept of explanatory models has been studied in mental health and they vary across cultures (Aidoo and Harpham 2001, Carpenter-Song et al. 2010). Such models focus on "cultural construction" and "specificity" of mental disorders in persons with specific cultural roots. It is also known that how an individual responds to his/her illness is dependent on the conceptualization and the explanatory model unique to the individual and his/her culture (Carpenter-Song et al. 2010, Coleman et al. 2007). For example, Euro-Americans conceptualize severe mental illness from a contemporary biomedical perspective, whereas African-Americans attribute mental health problems to supernatural or demonological forces (Carpenter-Song et al. 2010). In India, patients who attributed epilepsy to supernatural causes initially consulted traditional healers, whereas those who attributed it to biomedical causes sought modern medical treatment (Banerjee and Banerjee 1995); similar trends were observed in persons with schizophrenia (Banerjee and Roy 1998). These conceptualizations of mental health across cultures need to be understood appropriately in order to appreciate the illness in its own perspective (Durie 2004, 2011). Developing insights into these explanatory models aids health care professionals in formulating culturally appropriate communication paradigms and diagnostic tools, and culturally sensitive intervention programmes (Coleman et al. 2007). Furthermore, comprehensive understanding of such models can influence the mental health policy planning and developing culturally appropriate mental health care models (Aidoo and Harpham 2001).

Cultural conceptions are defined as the culturally-patterned classification of symptoms into illness categories that shape and constrain how patients perceive, express, explain, and evaluate health and illness (Ell and Castaneda 1998, Angel and Thoits 1987). As the cultural beliefs and help-seeking from faith healing are common across cultures, it is important to understand the culturally based explanatory models of mental health and illness, and how various healing practices impact mental health. There is also a need to understand cultural expressions of psychiatric distress (Guarnaccia, Good, and Kleinman 1990). Such an understanding will help mental health professionals to have better cultural competency in managing mental disorders in people from diverse cultures (Kar 2008). Non-medical explanatory models for mental illness are more commonly seen in developing countries compared to Western countries (McCabe and Priebe 2004). Cultural conceptions are the source of cognitive attributions that patients make about the meaning of a symptom; whether or not a symptom is perceived as a problem or as a condition requiring action; about the social acceptability or shamefulness of a symptom, and about the perceived cultural pathways for treatment. These cultural conceptions provide the labels people use to define and describe their pain and the explanations they give for their distress. There are indications, for example, that Hispanics are more likely to somatize psychological disorders or psychosocial distress (Guarnaccia, Good, and Kleinman 1990, Hulme 1996, Guarnaccia 1991, Guarnaccia, Angel, and Worobey 1989). Cultural conceptions of illness are thought to be critical antecedents of health seeking behaviour (Ell and Castaneda 1998). Awareness of, and sensitivity to, these belief systems and faith healing practices in different cultures are important for practising mental health professionals (Kar 2008).

These cultural explanatory models may need to be considered in the modern health care system if treatment is to be accepted by people. For example, taking western medication may not make sense to patients who perceive their problems to be a consequence of "religious misdemeanour" (Dein 1997). However, views regarding the role and utilisation of faith healing methods alongside medical models of understanding and treatment are far from any consensus. Debates in this area have highlighted the need for a comprehensive and systematic conceptualization of actual practices, the methods and processes employed, and their implications to health and wellness of people across the globe.

In many parts of the Third World, explanations of mental illness take into account broader social and religious factors. These include such phenomena as witchcraft, spirit possession, the capture of the soul by a spirit, breaking of religious taboos, and divine retribution (Dein 1997).

engraved words, drawings or incantations, considered to have supernatural or magical powers to bring good luck and repel evil or bad luck), administering compounds (e.g., plant derivatives, chemical compounds of unknown origin, etc.), oil baths, exposure to fumes, recitation of religious scriptures, etc. (Kar 2008, Prasadarao 2009).

Kar (2008) explored help seeking from faith-healers among patients with severe mental illness in India. He studied belief systems, psychopathology, and socio-cultural factors and their impact on faith healing. Kar observed that a considerable proportion (66.7 percent) of patients sought help from faith healers and they believed that black magic, sorcery and the planetary influences were the causes of mental illness. Perception of abnormal behavior as a manifestation of 'mental illness' was associated with discomfort and possible long-term negative consequences. The subjects believed that a person with an abnormal mental state is a victim of external factors, without any focus on body or mind, hence faith healing is an appropriate approach for cure. Most patients suffering from major psychiatric disorders were found to seek help from faith healers prior to medical treatment. Factors which led to consulting a faith healer included trust, easy availability and accessibility, and recommendation by significant others, besides belief in supernatural causes. A considerable proportion of patients and families reported faith healing to be supportive, reassuring, and more acceptable in the community. In most cases, an immediate family member suggested faith healing (71.9 percent) as a treatment approach. Educational background of family members didn't seem to have significant impact on consulting faith healers (28.1 percent of these subjects had formal school education, 24.6 percent had college education, and 5.3 percent had university education). About one in five (21.2 percent) consulted faith healers for special prayers or offerings (Kar 2008). It was also noted that 75 percent of patients who attended faith healing at some point also sought medical treatment; many of them continued using the advice provided by the faith healers while receiving modern psychiatric treatment.

Mental Health Beliefs and Practices in Sub-Saharan Africa

Shizha and Charema (2012) in their seminal work explored the application of traditional beliefs and practices in African traditional medicine and health. In South Africa, several tribes such as the Zulu, Xhosa, Ndabele and Swazi, maintain ancestral worshipping traditions (Bae 2007). In Africa, people believe that the problem or illness originates from outside themselves in the environment, including the actions of malevolent people, spirits or acts of witchcraft and that divination will reveal the true cause of their lack of well-being. Since the causation of wellness or ill health is explained in metaphysical terms, healers and clients practice a "directive" approach using "external oriented" techniques (e.g., ritual cleaning, enactment, sacrifices). "Health care" is provided by indigenous healers who are often the first choice, although most Africans may also consult the modern health system for some types of illness or when they do not respond to traditional healing (Mpofu, Peltzer, and Bojuwoye 2011, Sabuni 2007).

In South Africa, traditional healers are called *Sangomas,* who practice a form of traditional medicine called *ngoma.* It is believed that the *Sangomas* bind with their ancestors who have chosen them for healing work. These *Sangomas* are a) diviners (they often determine the cause of an illness) and b) healers (herbalists). In the management of an illness, the diviner provides a diagnosis and the healer then applies a remedy appropriate to a specific diagnosis (Jolles and Jolles 2000). A "diviner" is considered as a person skilled in "holding a key to the secrets of life-lines, having knowledge of the underworld, and possessing the ability to see things and transmit that knowledge to others in need" (Malidoma 1993, cited in Shizha and Charema 2012). The *Sangomas* not only provide physiological healing but also employ strategies aimed at restoring spiritual and social balance. These practitioners prepare and apply herbal medicines, do divination with bones, and invoke spirits to heal both physical and spiritual illness (Bae 2007). In various regions of sub-Saharan Africa such as Malawi, Lesotho, South Africa, Swaziland, Zimbabwe, and Zambia, people associate traditional medicine with application of herbs and remedies (*Mishonga*), advice imparted by *Sangomas* or *Inyangas,* and with strong spiritual components. According to the WHO traditional medicine strategy (WHOTMS) 2000 to 2005 statistics, traditional practitioners outnumber modern health care practitioners and they are culturally accepted and respected (Simwaka, Peltzer, and Maluwa-Banda 2007). According to UNAIDS, in 2000, there were approximately 45,000 traditional healers in Zimbabwe and only 1,400 medical doctors (UNAIDS 2000).

It is estimated that 80–85 percent of the population of sub-Saharan Africa receives health education and health care from traditional medicine practitioners (WHO 2002). Up to 80 percent of South Africa's people consult traditional healers as their first contact for the treatment of health concerns (Felhaber 1997, cited in Berg 2003); about 90 percent of people in Zimbabwe utilize services of the traditional healers. Similarly, in Mozambique, one in every 200 people visits traditional healers whereas only one in 50,000 visits a medical doctor. Over 60 percent of the population in rural South Africa seek advice and treatment from traditional

traditional values of marriage, honesty, good behaviour, respect towards elders, cooperation with others, and group responsibility. Men play the role of authority figures within the family and the oldest men act as decision-makers. The eldest son holds an important position within the family. The family is expected to care for aging persons or ill members (Scuglik et al. 2007).

Somalis generally present with somatic symptoms such as headaches, stomach or muscle aches, heart palpitations, and tiredness rather than with psychological symptoms. From a religious point of view, expressing suicidal thoughts or a passive death wish is considered a sin. They adopt a fatalistic stance attributing problems to God's will and belief that it should not be questioned (Jimale et al. 2002, Lennon 2000). Attributing illness to supernatural causes is common; mental illness is often attributed to a curse, possession by *Satan,* or as a consequence of wrong doings. When they need help, Somalis seek assistance from a *Sheik* (an Islamic clergyman) who provides guidance based on the *Qur'an* (Islamic religious scripture). Somalis attribute illness to spirit possession (*waddado*) and the illness is treated by a traditional healer known as *waddad*. The *Waddad* is a person who recovered from an illness and practices a wide range of rituals such as prayers, bathing the patient in special perfumes, animal sacrifice, dancing, and interpreting visions, in order to exorcise the spirit. Somalis also believe in the "*evil eye*" directed at them by others, either purposefully or inadvertently, as a cause for illness. Sometimes it is believed that an illness in the husband might have been caused by the disgruntled wife, as an expression of her hostility, without involving in a verbal altercation with him. One of the healing rituals practiced by Somalis is 'fire-burning,' in which wood from a special tree is burned and applied over a person's body parts (e.g., wrist, abdomen, or head) in order to cure such conditions as pneumonia, hepatitis, and malnutrition. The rapidly growing Somali population in the United States presents a challenge to the mental health caregivers, especially in a situation where mental health problems are rarely acknowledged by Somalis and their families, leading to poor help seeking behaviour. (Scuglik et al. 2007).

Whittaker, Hardy, Lewis, and Buchan (2005) studied the individual and collective understandings of psychological well-being among young Somali asylum seekers or refugee women growing-up in northern England. Three themes emerged which included "resilience and protection," "identity and beliefs," and "concealment, secrets and distancing." Spirit possession was explored in relation to culture and religion, mental health, protection and treatment. In Somalis, spirit (*jinn* and *zar*) possession was a key concept and the women described *jinn* possession, grounded in the Islamic teachings of the *Qur'an,* and *zar* spirit, derived from a traditional African concept. Prayer, rituals, reciting and reading the *Qur'an* were ways that the women protected themselves from *zar* and *jinn* spirits, and it was believed that *zar possession* could be a punishment for not observing religious practices. It was interesting to note that the women who had been in England for longer (and were more acculturated to western ideologies) were sceptical about the existence of *zar* and of cultural methods for dealing with problems such as possession, and they were more likely to feel that spirit possession was "freaky," "weird," and "silly." Although they were less frightened and less aware of the phenomenon, they acknowledged it was "scary." Findings from this study highlight how understanding of mental health can be influenced by religious beliefs, and the importance of spirit possession and spirituality in clinical presentations among Somali people.

Simmerlink, Lightfoot, Dube, Blevins, and Lum (2013) studied the health beliefs and practices of East African refugees living in the United States. It was found that they have strong traditional practices to prevent and cope with physical and mental health problems. Three aspects of their traditional culture seem to help people to cope with illness and disease, namely, a) religion and religious practices (religious leaders assist in recovery and prevention of illness); b) social support from family, friends and neighbors within the community; and c) traditional medicines and practices.

Culture and Mental Health: An Indian Perspective

India is a multicultural society and people practice several religions. In India, approximately 83 percent of the population practice Hinduism, 13 percent Islam, and 2.5 percent Christianity. Other religions practiced include Sikhism, Jainism, and Buddhism among many others. Thus, India is described as the country of "unity in diversity" (Khandelwal et al. 2004, Prasadarao and Sudhir 2001). India is characterized by a range of diverse cultural and philosophical systems, which have in recent years mixed with western modes of thinking, making it difficult to identify a uniform Indian paradigm of mind and mental health (Wig 1999). Consequently, many explanations for mental disorders exist. Some understand and explain mental distress using a western biomedical framework, while many others believe in traditional concepts such as Ayurveda, which attributes illness, including mental illness, to an imbalance of humors. Supernatural, astrological, and religious explanations are also common, including karma, evil eye, and spirit possession (Chowdhury, Chakraborty, and Weiss 2001, Halliburton 2003, Kapur 2008, Khandelwal et al. 2004, Miovic 2008,

Padmavati, Thara, and Corin 2005, Raguram et al. 2002, Ramakrishna Rao and Paranjpe 2008, Saravanan et al. 2007). It was also found that economic and relational factors, such as poverty and family conflicts, are commonly identified as causes of mental disorders (Kermode et al. 2007, Srinivasan and Thara 2001; Thara, Islam, and Padmavati 1998). The situation in India is complex because many people adopt a pluralist approach to healthcare and are willing to access a range of services, some of which may not be congruent with their conceptualization of the health problem—for example, people might seek biomedical solutions for problems perceived to have social (or even supernatural) causes (Charles et al. 2007, Saravanan et al. 2008).

Those families who do seek treatment will often turn to non-allopathic providers, including practitioners of Indian traditional medicine, religious healers, faith healers and astrologers. Religious healing in particular is well described in the literature and can be Hindu, Islamic, or Christian. Some religious centers provide residential care for people with severe mental illness (Chowdhury et al. 2001; Halliburton 2003; Khandelwal et al. 2004; Padmavati et al. 2005; Raguram et al. 2002; Thara, Padmavati and Srinivasan 2004). Family makes important decisions if and when help-seeking for mental distress is warranted, and from where help is to be sought. Care of the mentally ill is primarily the responsibility of the family; the family may tolerate, protect and shield or reject the mentally ill family member. Patients are usually accompanied by their family members when they seek mental health consultation (Khandelwal et al., 2004). Beliefs about causes of mental illness tend to influence the nature of help-seeking, i.e., those who subscribe to supernatural causes are more likely to consult traditional or religious healers (Banerjee and Roy 1998, Padmavati et al. 2005, Sheikh and Furnham 2000).

An Indian Hindu Perspective

Hinduism, one of the world's oldest religions, made significant contributions to the understanding of mental health and illness in India. The roots of Indian psychology can be traced back to the religious scriptures such as *Vedas, Yoga Sutras,* and *Bhagavad Gita.* Systematic attempts have been made to understand human behavior based on the insights gained from ancient Indian scriptures and folklore (Balodhi 1990, 1991, Balodhi and Keshavan 2011, Reddy 2012). There have also been attempts to understand the concept of positive mental health. In Indian psychology, personality is a composition of three basic human qualities (*gunas*), namely, *sattva* (clarity, light), *rajas* (passion, desire), and *tamas* (dullness, darkness). According to this Indian concept, human beings are endowed with a combination of these *gunas* from the time they were born, and it is determined by their actions in past lives (Hodge 2004, Kakar 1978). This is also explained in terms of the person's state of mind. The ideal state of mind is called *sattvik*, where there is equipoise and harmony among all three attributes. However, when the mind is under stress, agitated or frustrated, this equilibrium is believed to be disturbed. Such a state is called *rajasik* (equated with the sympathetic activity of the autonomic nervous system). When the mind is in a state of lethargy and gloominess, it is considered *tamasik* (corresponding to the parasympathetic activity of the autonomic nervous system) (see Antony 2001, Juthani 2001). Kakar (1978) explained the Hindu world view in three core concepts, namely, *dharma* (righteousness that determines one's own behavior), *moksha* (self-realization, transcendence, salvation, and release from worldly affairs), and *karma* (course of one's life in terms of fate and cycles of birth and death) (see Braud 2008, Dalal and Misra 2010, Hodge 2004, Jha 2008).

In Indian culture, mental illness is explained by a wide range of models. It is commonly believed that *karma* (one's actions in a past life) determines one's present life's successes, failures and illnesses (Hodge 2004). *Karma* is defined as "the sum of a person's actions in this and previous states of existence, viewed as affecting their future fate" (Oxford Dictionary, 10th ed. 1999, 772). Thus, illness is perceived as a punishment for the wrongdoings in one's past life. Other common explanations, especially in the rural cultures, include supernatural visitation and environmental shock (Khandelwal et al. 2004).

The Role of Traditional Healers in India

Kapur (1975, 1979) conducted studies in an Indian rural village to explore preference for type of healer by people and the conceptual framework of the healers. Besides modern medical practitioners, three types of traditional healers, namely, *vaids* (healers practising indigenous system of medicine), *mantarwadis* (healers using astrology and charms for cure), and *patris* (healers who act as mediums for spirits and demons), offer treatment to physical and mental illness in rural villages of India. The *vaids* practice Ayurveda—the traditional Indian medicine system, and they offer treatment predominantly by administering "medications." These *vaids* believe that illness is due to "an imbalance between the natural elements" brought forth by environmental factors, certain diets, uninhibited sexual indulgence, and by the influence of demons. These factors cause "excess heat, cold, bile, wind or fluid secretions," leading to the development of physical and mental illness. Mental illness (*unmada*) is caused by the exaggerated activity of any of the three humors and three types of "madness," namely, *vatounmada* (due to wind), *pittounmada* (due to bile) and *kaphounmada* (due to water), are possible. According to these *vaids*, certain food substances cause excess heat, leading to excitement whereas some others cause excess cold, contributing to the development of depression. The centre for heat in man is considered to be in the head and he loses heat through an excessive seminal discharge. The centre for heat in woman is in the vagina and the heat is lost as a consequence of childbirth. For both physical and mental illness, *vaids* provide treatment using various substances, namely, herbal medications, oils, decoctions, and by prescribing certain dietary restrictions (Kapur 1975, 1979). Both *mantarwadis* and *patris* also believe that illness is due to misdeeds either in the past or present life. These misdeeds are punished by Lord Shiva, by affecting an individual through spirits and demons or by influencing the malign conjunction of stars. Accordingly, the symptoms of a particular "illness" are dependent on the constellation of stars and the nature of specific demons/spirits acting on the individual. These *mantarwadis* treat by chanting mystical verses, offering a *talisman,* sacred threads, and by suggesting a specific penance for the individual's "misdeeds." The *patris* act as a medium for the spirits and demons and they don't claim any special abilities. Since illness is conceptualized as the negative effect of the demons and spirits, interventions are carried out through 'negotiations' with these demons/spirits who affected the individual. In this complex process, specific offerings (e.g., an animal sacrifice, a feast, or offering a "house" for the demon's use) are negotiated with the demon/spirit. The client is expected to obey and perform these agreed upon rituals and practices. Kapur (1975, 1979) also found that a large majority (59 percent) consult one or more of these healers. The selection of a specific healer was determined by the severity of illness rather than by the sociodemographic factors (e.g., age, educational level, and financial status) of the affected person. Interestingly, most people consulted both traditional healers and modern practitioners despite the presence of a clear contradiction in their operating frameworks.

Mental Illness and Temple Healing in India

Raguram et al. (2002) conducted a study at a south Indian temple, a popular healing place for people with severe psychiatric problems. Mentally ill patients are brought by their family members to stay in this temple. The person with psychiatric problems takes part in a wide range of daily rituals of the temple (e.g., cleaning and watering). During the study period, 31 people sought help and stayed at the temple. The severity of psychopathology in subjects was assessed by a psychiatrist using the Brief Psychiatric Rating Scale (BPRS) (Overall and Gorham 1962) on the first day of their stay in the temple. Subjects' impressions, caregivers' perceptions of change over the course at the temple, and their level of satisfaction were assessed. Caregivers rated satisfaction with their experience at the temple and the change they noted in their mentally ill family member. A significant reduction in scores on the BPRS was evident in these subjects at the time of their departure from the temple. As rated by the family caregivers, 22 subjects "improved" and three had "total recovery." These researchers pointed out that the "help" received at this temple served as an alternative to modern psychiatric treatment for people with severe mental illness. They noted significant improvement in the symptoms in people who received no formal psychiatric treatment during their stay in the temple. Raguram et al. opined that the "cultural power" of residing in the temple known for its "healing potency," may have contributed to such a change in psychopathology among these subjects; improvement may also be attributed to the "supportive, non-threatening, and reassuring" environment of the temple. Raguram et al. concluded that healing temples may constitute a community resource for people with psychiatric problems in settings where they are recognized and valued. These researchers suggest that the role of such healing places in local community settings needs to be understood and acknowledged when making policies and planning for mental health services; they highlighted the need to consider an alliance with such indigenous resources. Kapur (1975, 1979) and Raguram et al. (2002), through their seminal work, highlight the role that traditional indigenous resources may play in providing care to mentally ill persons at a community level.

Culture and Mental Health: A Chinese Perspective

Various philosophical and religious views influence Chinese people and their health-related beliefs (Lai and Surood 2009). The Chinese culture, as a way of thinking, appears to affect the state of mind and body, social relationships, and help-seeking behaviours. Harmony is believed to be the most important social value. Traditionally, the Chinese have their unique way of conceptualizing the causes of illness, its prevention, and its treatment (Wu and Tseng 1985). Ancient Chinese medicine has influences from the principles of Confucianism, Taoism, and Buddhism. These major perspectives have also formed the philosophical bases for understanding health beliefs in Chinese culture (Lai and Surood 2009, Torsch and Ma 2000, Wu and Tseng 1985).

In Chinese traditional literature there is no phrase equivalent to mental health. Words such as *fa lok* (happiness), *wor* (harmony), *sim on* (internal sense of security), and *tin yu* (relaxed) have been used in a manner that is similar to western concepts of mental health. The phrase *jing shum geen hong* is sometimes considered equivalent to the term "mental health" (Yip 2005). The traditional Chinese mental health model is influenced by three major ancient schools of thought, namely, (a) traditional Chinese medicine, (b) Confucianism, and (c) Taoism. From the Chinese traditional medicine perspective, mental health is the balance of *yin* and *yang*, and the mutual equilibrium of the five elements (see chapter 9, volume 1). Thus, mental health is conceptualized as a harmony between nature and the individual.

From the Confucian perspective, there are specific internal and external requirements on the part of the individual to maintain positive mental health. The internal requirements include aspects such as self-cultivation, practicing paths to achieve collective harmony and restraining from expression of intense emotions. The external requirements involve maintaining moral standards in everyday interpersonal relationships. Confucius described principles, which are considered important in life, including being kind, humane, and considerate towards others (*yen*), righteousness and equality (*yin*), being faithful towards country, family and friends (*chung*), and forgiving faults and shortcomings of others (*shu*). These principles need to be practiced as per the social norms in a culture. In Taoism, mental health is considered as ultimate peace of mind and absolute happiness in relating to the universe. One can achieve such "absolute happiness" through a state of nothingness (infinite Tao), and when one allows events such as life, death, and calamity to happen naturally (see Lai and Surood 2009, Yip 2005).

Torsch and Ma (2000) examined health perceptions, concerns, and coping strategies among elders in two Asian and Pacific Islander American communities. They compared the elder Chamorros of Guam with elder Chinese of the United States. The authors identified two basic themes in their health perceptions: (a) a sense of holism among body, mind, and spirit, and (b) an orientation toward others. The health concerns of these two communities include universal experiences of aging, structural elements within the American health care system, and cultural changes impacting health. Torsch and Ma (2000) found that the Chinese Elders in America, in line with their traditional belief system, focused on the concept of the *yin* and *yang* or hot and cold balance.

They also believed that practices such as Chinese massage ("*tai ji quan*") and Chinese health exercises ("*qi gong*") were useful for promoting the free circulation of "*qi*" and blood through the body, which helps to prevent diseases and maintain a healthy status. The Chinese tended not to trust Western doctors, believing that they (western doctors) did not truly understand the Chinese physiology, which is based on the *yin-yang* principles. Many Chinese continue to hold unique cultural health beliefs and values (Lai and Surood 2009).

In Chinese culture, parental factors seem to play a role in the onset of mental health problems. For example, Xia and Qian (2001) studied 127 adolescents (16–22 yrs) from two Chinese sub-cultures—*Han* and *Kejia*—to assess the relationship between parenting styles and self-rated mental health problems. The authors found that a high degree of psychosomatic symptoms and poor general mental health, in both genders, were associated with parental factors such as rejection and denial, high punitive tendencies, overprotection, over-involvement and poor emotional warmth and understanding.

Conclusion

Every culture has its own health belief system, which determines how its members respond to an illness, when they seek help, and the expected treatment outcomes (Wynaden et al. 2005). Culture defines not only what causes illness, but also how illness is manifested and interpreted. Causal explanations are linked to beliefs concerning appropriateness of treatments (Cole, Stevenson, and Rodgers 2009). With the growing ethnic diversity of the United States health care professionals are constantly exposed to clients whose spiritual and cultural values and beliefs differ from their own (Johnson et al. 2005). Meeting the health care needs of people from diverse cultures requires a comprehensive understanding of the diversity of people, their health beliefs, and practices. As Kleinman (1975) put it, culturally constructed health and health beliefs result in a wide range of unique patterns in health-seeking and maintenance behaviors in different societies and illness and health care are directly woven into the cultural fabric. Consideration of explanatory models of health and illness is increasingly becoming important in various clinical settings from both consumers and health care providers' points of view. It is essential that the health care providers are sensitive to these belief systems and practices and acknowledge their importance so that attempts can be made to improve their competency while offering services to people from multiple cultures. Increased awareness of these belief systems and cultural differences may lead to better communication with clients from these diverse ethnic backgrounds. Further, this can have significant impact on addressing the barriers in providing health care facilities. It is time that the health care system takes appropriate steps to provide culturally appropriate and culturally sensitive mental health care facilities to the people of America. It is also important that the health care providers in the United States focus on the "*emic*" and "*etic*" approaches to understanding the people, their cultural practices, their causal explanations and belief systems.

Acknowledgments

Portions of this chapter are reprinted from Prasadarao, P.S.D.V. 2009. "International Perspectives on Culture and Mental Health," *Culture and Mental Health: Sociocultural Influences, Theory and Practice,* edited by Eshun, S. and Gurung R.A.R. Chapter 8. Boston, MA: Wiley-Blackwell.

The author would like to gratefully acknowledge the support and assistance of the following persons: Dr. Colin Patrick, clinical director, and Fran Marsh, Team leader, Mental Health Service for Older People, Waikato DHB, Hamilton, New Zealand.

References

Abe-Kim, J., D. T. Takeuchi, H. Seunghye, H. Appel, E. Nicdao, N. Zane, and M. Alegría. 2007. "Use of Mental Health-Related Services among Immigrant and U.S.-Born Asian Americans: Results from the National Latino and Asian American Study." *American Journal of Public Health* 97: 91–98.

Aidoo, M., and T. Harpham. 2001. "The Explanatory Models of Mental Health amongst Low-Income Women and Health Care Practitioners in Lusaka, Zambia." *Health Policy and Planning* 16: 206–213.

American Psychiatric Association. 1994. *Diagnostic and Statistical Manual of Mental Disorders* (4th Ed.). Washington, DC: Author.

Angel, R. and P. Thoits. 1987. "The Impact of Culture on the Cognitive Structure of Illness." *Culture, Medicine, and Psychiatry* 11: 465–494.

Antony, P. A. 2001. "The Concept of Mind in Ayurveda." Paper presented at the National Seminar on Psychology in India: Past, Present and Future. 12th Annual Conference of NAOP, 22–24 October 2001, Kollam, India.

Bae, C. S. 2007. "Ancestor Worship and the Challenges it Poses to the Christian Mission and Ministry." PhD Thesis, University of Pretoria, Pretoria. http://upetd.up.ac.za/thesis/available/etd-05272008–141650/

Balodhi, J. P. 1990. "Psychotherapy Based on Hindu Philosophy." *Journal of Personality and Clinical Studies* 6: 51–56.

Balodhi, J. P. 1991. "Holistic Approach in Psychiatry: Indian View." *NIMHANS Journal* 9: 101–104.

Balodhi, J. P. and M. S. Keshavan. 2011. "Bhagavadgita and Psychotherapy." *Asian J Psychiat.* 4: 300–302.

Banerjee, G., and S. Roy. 1998. "Determinants of Help-Seeking Behaviour of Families of Schizophrenic Patients Attending a Teaching Hospital in India: An Indigenous Explanatory Model." *International Journal of Social Psychiatry* 44: 199–214.

Banerjee, T. and G. Banerjee. 1995. "Determinants of Help-Seeking Behaviour in Cases of Epilepsy Attending a Teaching Hospital in India: an Indigenous Explanatory Model." *International Journal of Social Psychiatry* 41: 217–230.

Berg, A. 2003. "Ancestor Reverence and Mental Health in South Africa." *Transcultural Psychiatry* 40: 194–207.

Berkman, C. S., P. J. Guarnaccia, N. Diaz, L. W. Badge, and G. J. Kennedy. 2005. "Concepts of Mental Health and Mental Illness in Older Hispanics." *Journal of Immigrant and Refugee Services* 3: 59–85.

Bonsi, S. K. 1982. "Traditional African Ideas and Medical Practices." *Contact* 66: 18–25.

Braud, W. G. 2008. "Patanjali Yoga and Siddhis: Their Relevance to Parapsychological Theory and Research." In *Handbook of Indian Psychology,* edited by K. Ramakrishna Rao, A. C. Paranjpe, and A. K. Dalal, 217–243. New Delhi: Cambridge: University Press.

Brown, C., and D. R. Palenchar. 2004. "Treatment of Depression in African American Primary Care Patients." *African American Research Perspectives* 10: 55–65.

Callan, V. J., J. Wilks, and S. Forsyth. 1983. "Cultural Perceptions of the Mentally Ill: Australian and Papua New Guinean High School Youth." *Australian and New Zealand Journal of Psychiatry* 17: 280–285.

Campion, J. and D. Bhugra. 1998. "Religious and Indigenous Treatment of Mental Illness in South India—A Descriptive Study." *Mental Health, Religion, and Culture* 1: 21–29.

Carpenter-Song, E., E. Chu, R. E. Drake, M. Ritsema, B. Smith, and H. Alverson. 2010. "Ethno-Cultural Variations in the Experience and Meaning of Mental Illness and Treatment: Implications for Actions and Utilization." *Transcultural Psychiatry* 47: 224–251.

Chadda, R. K., V. Agarwal, M. C. Singh, and D. Raheja. 2001. "Help Seeking Behaviour of Psychiatric Patients before Seeking Care at a Mental Hospital." *International Journal of Social Psychiatry* 47: 71–78.

Charema, J., and E. Shizha. 2008. "Counselling Indigenous Shona People in Zimbabwe: Traditional Practices versus Western Eurocentric Perspectives." *AlterNative: An International Journal of Indigenous Peoples* 4: 124–141.

Charles, H., S. D. Manoranjitham, and K. S. Jacob. 2007. "Stigma and Explanatory Models among People with Schizophrenia and Their Relatives in Vellore, South India." *International Journal of Social Psychiatry* 53: 325–332.

Chavunduka, G. L. 1978. *Traditional Healers and the Shona Patient.* Gweru: Mambo Press.

Chen, H. J. 2005. "Mental Illness and Principal Physical Diagnoses among Asian American and Pacific Islander Users of Emergency Services." *Issues in Mental Health Nursing* 26: 1061–1079.

Choi, N. G. and J. Kim. 2010. "Utilization of Complementary and Alternative Medicines for Mental Health Problems among Asian Americans." *Community Mental Health Journal* 46: 570–78.

Chowdhury, A. N., A. K. Chakraborty, and M. G. Weiss. 2001. "Community Mental Health and Concepts of Mental Illness in the Sundarban Delta of West Bengal, India." *Anthropology and Medicine* 8: 109–129.

Coakley, D. V. and G. W. McKenna. 1986. "Safety of Faith Healing." *Lancet* 22: 327 (8478): 444.

Cole, E., M. Stevenson, and B. Rodgers. 2009. "The Influence of Cultural Health Beliefs on Self-Reported Mental Health Status and Mental Health Service Utilization in an Ethnically Diverse Sample of Older Adults." *Journal of Feminist Family Therapy* 21: 1–17.

Coleman, K., J. Koffman, and C. Daniels. 2007. "Why is This Happening to Me? Illness Beliefs Held by Haredi Jewish Breast Cancer Patients: An Exploratory Study." *Spirituality and Health International* 8: 121–134.

Conner, K. O., G. Koeske, and C. Brown. 2009. "Racial Differences in Attitudes toward Professional Mental Health Treatment: The Mediating Effect of Stigma." *Journal of Gerontological Social Work* 52: 695–712.

Cuéllar, I. and F. A. Paniagua, eds. 2000. *Handbook of Multicultural Mental Health: Assessment and Treatment of Diverse Populations.* San Diego: Academic Press.

Dalal, A. K. and G. Misra. 2010. "The Core and Context of Indian Psychology." *Psychology and Developing Societies* 22: 121–155.

Dein, S. 1997. "A.B.C of Mental Health: Mental Health in a Multiethnic Society." *British Medical Journal* 315: 473–476.

Department of Health and Human Services. 2001. *Mental Health: Culture, Race, and Ethnicity—A Supplement to Mental Health: A Report of the Surgeon General.* Rockville, MD: Author.

Diala, C., C. Muntaner, C. Walrath, K. J. Nickerson, T. A. LaVeist, and P. J. Leaf. 2000. "Racial Differences in Attitudes toward Professional Mental Health Care and in the Use of Services." *American Journal of Orthopsychiatry* 70: 455–464.

Durie, M. 2004. "Understanding Health and Illness: Research at the Interface Between Science and Indigenous Knowledge." *International Journal of Epidemiology* 33: 1138–1143.

Durie, M. 2011. "Indigenizing Mental Health Services : New Zealand Experience." *Transcultural Psychiatry* 48: 24–36.

Ell, K. and I. Castaneda. 1998. "Health Care Seeking Behavior." In *Handbook of Immigrant Health,* edited by S. Loue. New York: Plenum Press.

Fabrega, H. and H. Nutini. 1993. "Witchcraft-Explained Childhood Tragedies in Tlaxcala, and Their Medical Sequelae." *Social Science and Medicine* 36: 793–805.

Felhaber, T. 1997. *Southern African Primary Health Care Handbook*. Cape Town: South Africa: Copy Cat Communications in conjunction with Kagiso.

Friedson, S. M. 1996. *Dancing Prophets: Musical Experience in Tumbuka Healing*. Chicago, IL: University of Chicago Press.

Furnham, A. and S. Pereira. 2008. "Beliefs about the Cause, Manifestation, and Cure of Schizophrenia: A Cross-Cultural Comparison." *Mental Health, Religion and Culture 11*: 173–191.

Giger, J. N., R. E. Davidhizar, and G. Turner. 1992. "Black American Folk Medicine Health Care Beliefs: Implication for Nursing Plans of Care." *Association of Black Nursing Faculty Journal 3*: 42–46.

Goldsmith, S. K., T. C. Pellmar, A. M. Kleinman, and W. E. Bunney, eds. 2002. *Reducing Suicide: A National Imperative*. Washington, DC: The National Academies Press.

Guarnaccia, P. J. 1991. "The Role of Culture in Psychiatric Epidemiology: An Examination of Research on Latin American Mental Health (Abstract)." *Sante Ment Que 16*: 27–43.

Guarnaccia, P. J., R. Angel, and J. L. Worobey. 1989. "The Factor Structure of the CES-D in the Hispanic Health and Nutrition Examination Survey: The Influences of Ethncity, Gender, and Language." *Social Science and Medicine 29*: 85–94.

Guarnaccia, P. J., B. J. Good, and A. Kleinman. 1990. "A Critical Review of Epidemiological Studies of Puerto Rican Mental Health." *American Journal of Psychiatry 147*: 1449–1456.

Halliburton, M. 2003. "The Importance of a Pleasant Process of Treatment: Lessons on Healing from South India." *Culture Medicine and Psychiatry 27*: 161–186.

Hodge, D. R. 2004. "Working with Hindu Clients in a Spiritually Sensitive Manner." *Social Work 49*: 27–38.

Hsu, L. K. G., Y. M. Wan, H. Chang, P. Summergrad, B. Y. P. Tsang, and H. Chen. 2008. "Stigma of Depression is More Severe in Chinese Americans than Caucasian Americans." *Psychiatry 71*: 210–218.

Hulme, P. A., 1996. "Somatization in Hispanics." *Journal of Psychosocial Nursing Mental Health Services 34*: 33–37.

Humes, K. R., N.A. Jones, and R. R.Ramirez. 2011. "Overview of Race and Hispanic Origin: 2010." *2010 Census Briefs*. U.S. Census Bureau.

Hussain, F., R. Cochrane. 2004. "Depression in South Asian Women Living in the U.K.: A Review of the Literature with Implications for Service Provision." *Transcultural Psychiatry 41*: 253–270.

Jacob, K. S., P. Sharan, I. Mirza, M. Garrido-Cumbrera, S. Seedat, J. J. Mari, et al. 2007. "Mental Health Systems in Countries: Where are We Now?" *Lancet 370*: 1061–1077.

Jha, A. K. 2008. "Personality in Indian Psychology". *Handbook of Indian Psychology*, edited by K. Ramakrishna Rao, A. C. Paranjpe, and A. K. Dalal, 348–361. New Delhi: Cambridge University Press.

Jimale, M., B. Ahmed, M. Hamud, S. Leinonen, H. Mohamed, and J. Hughes. 2002. "Cultural Awareness: The Somali Culture." Paper presented at the Mayo Clinic Foundation Education, Mayo Clinic Foundation, Rochester, MN.

Johnson, K. S., K. I. Elbert-Avila, and J. A. Tulsky. 2005. "The Influence of Spiritual Beliefs and Practices on the Treatment Preferences of African Americans: a Review of the Literature." *J Am Geriatric Soc.* 53: 711–719.

Jolles, F. and S. Jolles. 2000. "Zulu Ritual Immunisation in Perspective." *Africa: Journal of the International African Institute* 70: 229–248.

Juthani, N. V. 2001. "Psychiatric Treatment of Hindus." *International Review of Psychiatry* 13: 125–130.

Kakar, S. 1978. *The Inner World: A Psychoanalytic Study of Childhood and Society in India.* New Delhi: Oxford University Press.

Kapur, M. 2008. "Psychological Theories and Practices in Ayurveda. In *Handbook of Indian Psychology,* edited by K. Ramakrishna Rao, A. C. Paranjpe, and A. K. Dalal, 299–313. New Delhi: Cambridge University Press.

Kapur, R. L. 1975. "Mental Health Care in Rural India: A Study of Existing Patterns and Their Implications for Future Policy." *British Journal of Psychiatry* 127: 286–293.

Kapur, R. L. 1979. "The Role of Traditional Healers in Mental Health Care in Rural India." In *Social Sciences and Medicine 13B*: 27–31.

Kar, N. 2008. "Resort to Faith-Healing Practices in the Pathway to Care for Mental Illness: A Study on Psychiatric Inpatients in Orissa." *Mental Health, Religion and Culture 11*: 720–740.

Kasoro, S., S. Sebudde, G. Kabagambe-Rugumba, E. Ovuga, and A. Boardman. 2002. "Mental Illness in One District of Uganda." *International Journal of Social Psychiatry 48*: 29–37.

Kavanaugh, K., and P. Kennedy. 1992. *Promoting Cultural Diversity: Strategies for Health Care Professionals.* Newbury Park, CA: Sage.

Kermode, K., K. Bowen, S. Arole, K. Joag, and A. F. Jorm. 2010. "Community Beliefs about Causes and Risks for Mental Disorders: A Mental Health Literacy Survey in a Rural Area of Maharashtra, India." *International Journal of Social Psychiatry 56*: 606–622.

Kermode, M., H. Herrman, R. Arole, J. White, R. Premkumar, and V. Patel. 2007. "Empowerment of Women as a Strategy for Mental Health Promotion in Developing Countries: A Qualitative Study from Rural Maharashtra." *BMC Public Health 7*: 225.

Kessler, R. C., K. A. McGonagle, S. Zhao, C. B. Nelson, M. Hughes, S. Eshleman, et al. 1994. "Lifetime and 12-Month Prevalence of DSM-III-R Psychiatric Disorders in the United States. Results from the National Comorbidity Survey." *Archives of General Psychiatry 51*: 8–19.

Khandelwal, S. K., H. P. Jhingan, S. Ramesh, R. K. Gupta, and V. K. Srivastava. 2004. "India Mental Health Country Profile." *International Review of Psychiatry 16*: 126–141.

Kiima, D. M., F. G. Njenga, M. M. O. Okonji, and P. A. Kigamwa. 2004. "Kenya Mental Health Country Profile." *International Review of Psychiatry 16*: 48–53.

Kleinman, A. 1975. *Medicine in Chinese Cultures: Comparative Studies of Health Care in Chinese and Other Societies.* Washington, DC: Department of Health, Education, and Welfare.

Kleinman, A. 1980. *Patients and Healers in the Context of Culture: An Exploration of the Borderland between Anthropology, Medicine, and Psychiatry.* Berkeley: University of California Press.

Lai, D. W. L. and S. Surood. 2009. "Chinese Health Beliefs of Older Chinese in Canada." *Journal of Aging and Health 21*: 38–62.

Lam, C. S., H. W. H. Tsang, P. W. Corrigan, Y. T. Lee, B. Angell, K. Shi, and J. E. Larson. 2010. "Chinese Lay Theory and Mental Illness Stigma: Implications for Research and Practices." *Journal of Rehabilitation 76*: 35–40.

Lennon, E. 2000. *Strengthening Lives, Rebuilding Communities: Somalis Recover from War.* Minneapolis, MN: Center for Victims of Torture.

Luongo, K. 2008. "Witches, Westerners, and HIV: AIDS and Cultures of Blame in Africa (review)." *Magic, Ritual, and Witchcraft 3*: 101–104.

Malidoma, P. S. 1993. *Ritual: Power, Healing, and Community.* Oregon: Swan Raven and Company.

Marsella, A. J. and A. M. Yamada. 2000. "Culture and Mental Health: An Introduction and Overview of Foundations, Concepts, and Issues." In *Handbook of Multicultural Mental Health,* edited by I. Cuéllar and F. A. Paniagua, 3–24. San Diego, USA: Academic.

Mayeya, J., R. Chazulwa, P. N. Mayeya, et al. 2004. "Zambia Mental Health Country Profile." *International Review of Psychiatry 16*: 63–72.

McCabe, R., and S. Priebe. 2004. "Explanatory Models of Illness in Schizophrenia: Comparison of Four Ethnic Groups." *British Journal of Psychiatry 185*: 25–30.

Merikangas, K. R., J. P. He, D. Brody, P. W. Fisher, K. Bourdon, and D. S. Koretz. 2010. "Prevalence and Treatment of Mental Disorders among U.S. Children in the 2001–2004 NHANES." *Pediatrics 125*: 75–81.

Miovic, M. 2008. "Therapeutic Psychology and Indian Yoga." In *Handbook of Indian Psychology,* edited by K. Ramakrishna Rao, A. C. Paranjpe, and A. K. Dalal, 449–470. New Delhi: Cambridge University Press.

Mpofu, E., K. Peltzer, and O. Bojuwoye. 2011. "Indigenous Healing Practices in Sub-Saharan Africa." In *Counseling People of African Ancestry,* edited by E. Mpofu, 3–21. New York: Cambridge University Press.

Murguia, A., M. C. Zea, C. A. Reisen, and R. A. Peterson. 2000. "The Development of the Cultural Health Attributions Questionnaire (CHAQ)." *Cultural Diversity and Ethnic Minority Psychology 6*: 268–283.

Ndyanabangi, S., D. Basangwa, J. Lutakome, and C. Mubiru. 2004. "Uganda Mental Health Country Profile." *International Review of Psychiatry 16*: 54–62.

Neighbors, H. W. 1988. "Help-Seeking Behavior of Black Americans: A Summary of Findings from the National Survey of Black Americans." *Journal of the National Medical Association 80*: 1009–1012.

Otieno, L. S., S. O. McLigeyo, and M. Luta. 1991. "Acute Renal Failure following the Use of Herbal Remedies." *East African Medical Journal* 68: 993–998.

Overall, J. and D. Gorham. 1962. "Brief Psychiatric Rating Scale." *Psychological Reports* 10: 799.

Oxford Dictionary. 1999. (10th ed.) New York: Oxford University Press.

Padmavati, R., R. Thara. and E. Corin. 2005. "A Qualitative Study of Religious Practices by Chronic Mentally Ill and Their Caregivers in South India." *International Journal of Social Psychiatry 51*: 139–149.

Patel, V. 2007. "Mental Health in Low- and Middle-Income Countries." *British Medical Bulletin 81 & 82*: 81–96.

Patel, V., T. Musara, T. Butau, P. Maramba, and S. Fuyane. 1995. "Concepts of Mental Illness and Medical Pluralism in Harare." *Psychological Medicine* 25: 485–493.

Patel, V., C. Todd, M. Winston, F. Gwanzura, E. Simunyu, W. Acuda, et al. 1997. "Common Mental Disorders in Primary Care in Harare, Zimbabwe: Associations and Risk Factors." *British Journal of Psychiatry* 171: 60–64.

Peltzer, K. 1988. "The Role of Traditional and Faith Healers in Primary Mental Health Care: A Southern African Perspective." *Curare 11*: 207–210.

Pesek, T. J., L. R. Helton, and M. Nair. 2006. "Healing across Cultures: Learning from Traditions." *EcoHealth 3*: 114–118.

Prasadarao, P. S. D. V. 2009. "International Perspectives on Culture and Mental Health." In *Culture and Mental Health: Sociocultural Influences Theory, and Practice,* edited by S. Eshun and R. A. R. Gurung, 149–177. Malden, MA: Wiley.

Prasadarao, P. S. D. V. and P. M. Sudhir. 2001. "Clinical Psychology in India." *Journal of Clinical Psychology in Medical Settings 8*: 31–38.

Puckree, T., M. Mkhize, Z. Mgobhozi, and J. Lin. 2002. "African Traditional Healers: What Health Care Professionals Need to Know." *International Journal of Rehabilitation Research 25*: 247–251.

Raguram, R., A. Venkateswaran, J. Ramakrishna, and M. G. Weiss. 2002. "Traditional Community Resources for Mental Health: A Report of Temple Healing from India." *British Medical Journal 325*: 38–40.

Ramakrishna Rao, K., and A. C. Paranjpe. 2008. "Yoga Psychology: Theory and Application." In *Handbook of Indian Psychology,* edited by K. Ramakrishna Rao, A. C. Paranjpe, and A. K. Dalal, 186–216. New Delhi: Cambridge University Press.

Rao, D., J. Feinglass, and P. Corrigan. 2007. "Racial and Ethnic Disparities in Mental Illness Stigma." *Journal of Nervous and Mental Disease* 195: 1020–1023.

Razali, S. M., U. A. Khan, and C. I. Hasanah. 1996. "Belief in Supernatural Causes of Mental Illness among Malay Patients: Impact on Treatment." *Acta Psychiatrica Scandinavica* 94: 229–233.

Reddy, M.S. 2012. "Psychotherapy: Insights from Bhagavad Gita." *Indian J. Psychol. Med. 34*: 100–104.

Revell, M. 2012. "Use of Complementary and Alternative Medicine in the African American Culture." *International Journal of Childbirth Education 27*: 55–59.

Reynolds, P. 1990. "Zezuru Turn of the Screw. On Children's Exposure to Evil." *Culture, Medicine and Psychiatry* 14: 313–37.

Roy, L. C., D. Torrez,, and J. C. Dale. 2004. "Ethnicity, Traditional Health Beliefs, and Health Seeking Behavior : Guardians' Attitudes Regarding their Children's Medical Treatment." *Journal of Pediatric Health Care* 18: 22–29.

Sabuni, L. P. 2007. "Dilemma with the Local Perception of Causes of Illnesses in Central Africa: Muted Concept but Prevalent in Everyday Life." *Qualitative Health Research* 17: 1280–1291.

Saraceno, B., M. van Ommeren, R. Batniji, A. Cohen, O. Gureje, J. Mahoney, et al. 2007. "Barriers to Improvement of Mental Health Services in Low-Income and Middle-Income Countries." *Lancet* 370: 1164–1174.

Saravanan, B., K. S. Jacob, M. G. Deepak, M. Prince, A. David, and D. Bhugra. 2008. "Perceptions about Psychosis and Psychiatric Services: A Qualitative Study from Vellore, India." *Social Psychiatry and Psychiatric Epidemiology* 43: 231–238.

Saravanan, B., S. Johnson, M. Prince, and D. Bhugra. 2007. "Belief Models in First Episode Schizophrenia in South India." *Social Psychiatry and Psychiatric Epidemiology* 42: 446–451.

Scuglik, D. L., R. D. Alarcón, A. C. Lapeyre III, M. D. Williams, and K. M. Logan. 2007. "When the Poetry No Longer Rhymes: Mental Health Issues Among Somali Immigrants in the USA." *Transcultural Psychiatry* 44: 581–595.

Shankar, B. R., B. Saravanan, and K. S. Jacob. 2006. "Explanatory Models of Common Mental Disorders among Traditional Healers and Their Patients in Rural South India." *International Journal of Social Psychiatry* 52: 221–233.

Sharp, P. T. 1982. "Ghosts, Witches, Sickness and Death: The Traditional Interpretation of Injury and Disease in a Rural Area of Papua New Guinea." *Papua and New Guinea Medical Journal* 25: 108–115.

Sheikh, S. and A. Furnham. 2000. "A Cross-Cultural Study of Mental Health Beliefs and Attitudes towards Seeking Professional Help." *Soc Psychiatry Psychiatr Epidemiol* 35: 326–34.

Shizha, E. and J. Charema. 2012. "Health and Wellness in Southern Africa: Incorporating Indigenous and Western Healing Practices." *International Journal of Psychology and Counselling* 4: 59–67.

Simmerlink, J., E. Lightfoot, A. Dube, J. Blevins, and T. Lum. 2013. "Understanding the Health Beliefs and Practices of East African Refugees." *A J Health Behav.* 37: 155–161.

Simwaka, A., K. Peltzer, and, D. Maluwa-Banda. 2007. "Indigenous Healing Practices in Malawi." *J. Psychol. Afr.* 17: 155–162.

Snowden, L. 1999. "African American Service Use for Mental Health Problems." *Journal of Community Psychology* 27: 303–313.

Srinivasan, T.N., and R. Thara. 2001. "Beliefs about Causation of Schizophrenia: Do Indian Families Believe in Supernatural Causes?" *Social Psychiatry and Psychiatric Epidemiology* 36: 134–140.

Stekelenburg, J., B. E. Jager, P. R. Kolk, E. H. M. N. Westen, A. van der Kwaak, and I. N. Wolffers. 2005. "Health Care Seeking Behaviour and Utilization of Traditional Healers in Kalabo, Zambia." *Health Policy* 71: 67–81.

Substance Abuse and Mental Health Services Administration. 2012. *Mental Health United States, 2010*. HHS Publication No. (SMA) 12–4681. Rockville, MD: Substance Abuse and Mental Health Services Administration.

Thacore, V. R. and S. C. Gupta. 1978. "Faith Healing in a North Indian City." *International Journal of Social Psychiatry 24*: 235–240.

Thara, R., A. Islam, and R. Padmavati. 1998. "Belief about Mental Illness: A Study of a Rural South Indian Community." *International J Mental Health 27*: 70–85.

Thara, R., R. Padmavati, and T. Srinivasan. 2004. "Focus on Psychiatry in India." *British Journal of Psychiatry 184*: 366–373.

Ting, J. Y. and W. C. Hwang. 2009. "Cultural Influences on Help Seeking Attitudes in Asian American Students." *American Journal of Orthopsychiatry 79*: 125–132.

Torsch, V. L. and G. X. Ma. 2000. "Cross-Cultural Comparison of Health Perceptions, Concerns, and Coping Strategies among Asian and Pacific Islander American Elders." *Qual Health Res 10*: 471–489.

Tung, W. C. 2011. "Cultural Barriers to Mental Health Services among Asian Americans." *Home Health Care Management and Practice 23*: 303–5

UNAIDS. 2000. *Report of the Inter-regional Workshop on Intellectual Property Rights in the Context of Traditional Medicine*. Bangkok, Thailand: Author.

U.S. Department of Health and Human Services. 2001. *Mental Health: Culture, Race, and Ethnicity—A Supplement to Mental Health: A Report of the Surgeon General*. Rockville, MD: U.S. Department of Health and Human Services, Substance Abuse and Mental Health Services Administration, Center for Mental Health Services.

Wang, P., M. Lane, M. Olfson, H. A. Pincus, K. B. Wells, and R. C. Kessler. 2005. "Twelve-Month use of Mental Health Services in the United States: Results from the National Comorbidity Survey Replication." *Archives of General Psychiatry 62*: 629–640.

Wardwell, W. I. 1994. "Alternative Medicine in the United States." *Social Science and Medicine 38*: 1061–1068.

Whittaker, S., G. Hardy, K. Lewis, and L. Buchan. 2005. "An Exploration of Psychological Wellbeing with Young Somali Refugee and Asylum-Seeker Women." *Clin Child Psychol Psychiatry 10*: 177–196.

Wig, N. N. 1999. "Mental Health and Spiritual Values: A View from the East." *International Review of Psychiatry 11*: 92–96.

Wong, Y. J., K. K. Tran, S. H. Kim, V. V. H. Kerne, and N. A. Calfa. 2010. "Asian Americans' Lay Beliefs about Depression and Professional Help Seeking." *Journal of Clinical Psychology 66*: 317–332.

World Health Organization. 2001. "Indigenous Knowledge Initiatives in Sub-Saharan Africa, IK Notes, Indigenous Knowledge and HIV/AIDS, Ghana and Zambia." Geneva: Author.

World Health Organization. 2002. *Traditional Medicine Strategy 2002–2005*. Geneva: Author.

World Health Organization. 2003. *Investing in Mental Health*. Geneva: Author.

World Health Organization. 2005. *Mental Health Atlas, 2005*. Geneva: Author.

Wu, D., and W. S. Tseng. 1985. *Chinese Culture and Mental Health.* Orlando, FL: Academic Press.

Wynaden, D., R. Chapman, A. Orb, S. McGowan, Z. Zeeman, and S. H. Yeak. 2005. "Factors that Influence Asian Communities' Access to Mental Health Care." *International Journal of Mental Health Nursing* 14: 88–95.

Xia, G., and M. Qian. 2001. "The Relationship of Parenting Style to Self-Reported Mental Health among Two Subcultures of Chinese." *Journal of Adolescence* 24: 251–260.

Yeung, A., and W. W. Kung. 2004. "How Culture Impacts on the Treatment of Mental Illnesses among Asian-Americans." *Psychiatric Times* 21: 34–36.

Yip, K. 2005. "Chinese Concepts of Mental Health: Cultural Implications for Social Work Practice." *International Social Work* 48: 391–407.

CHAPTER TWO

Mental Health Assessment among Ethnic Minorities in the United States

Sussie Eshun and Donna Hodge

Culture is essential in shaping various aspects of mental illness, including the prevalence and presentation of various disorders, as well as referent meaning systems in the societies in which they occur (Eshun and Gurung 2009, Hwang et al. 2008, Kirmayer and Santhanam 2001). It should therefore be one of the key factors to be considered in assessing mental illness (American Psychological Association 2003). In spite of the acknowledgment of sociocultural influences on psychopathology, many health practitioners, including primary care physicians, psychologists, and counselors seem to lag behind with keeping sociocultural factors in mind, in their endeavor to select the right tools, administer selected tools appropriately, interpret patient responses, and ultimately develop an appropriate and effective treatment plan. In general, the failure to include assessment tools that consider relevant sociocultural factors such as gender, religion, and ethnic norms or values is even more prevalent for ethnic minority patients, mostly because of a lack of research-derived information and trained professionals. In this chapter we review some basic principles of psychometrics as they apply to assessment of psychopathology and also provide practical insights and suggestions pertaining to evaluating psychopathology in ethnic minorities.

Given that our chapter focuses on assessment among ethnic minorities groups within the United States (Hispanic Americans, African Americans, Asian Americans, and Native Americans), it is important to provide a general historic/background overview (see chapters in volume 1 for more details on each group).

Basic Demographics

If you've had to complete forms in a hospital or doctor's office, you probably remember answering a question about your ethnic background. Most clients, patients, or consumers of healthcare services wonder why that question is relevant and they may be right in questioning this because there is often a response option that allows you to opt out of responding (e.g., "Choose not to answer"). An even more important question is, "What is the purpose of the question about ethnic background?" In this section we review basic demographic statistics for the major ethnic minority groups in the United States as pertinent background information for the entire chapter.

Hispanic Americans make up approximately 16.3 percent (about 50.5 million people), which is the largest minority group in the United States (U.S. Census Bureau, 2009a, 2010a). A significant proportion of the rapid increase in the Hispanic population is from continued immigration from Latin America, which often means they may be confronted by issues pertaining to lack of English proficiency. Although many tend to group Latinos together as one homogenous cultural group, it is more of a complex, heterogeneous, group with unique characteristics and values based on their country of origin and whether they are U.S.-born (Guarnaccia et al. 2007).

African Americans constitute the second largest ethnic minority group in the United States (Seccombe 2007), making up approximately 13.6 percent of the population or 41.8 million (U.S. Census Bureau 2009b). Historically the impact of slavery and continued, persistent experiences of prejudice and discrimination, have somehow influenced their view of the health system and negatively influenced their perceptions about mental illness as well as their health-seeking behaviors (Ayalon and Young 2005, Mills and Edwards 2002).

Asian Americans are the third largest ethnic minority group in the United States According to data from the 2010 Census (U.S. Census Bureau 2010b), they consist of 5.6 percent of the U.S. population and constitute about 17.3 million people. Asian Americans consist of individuals from several countries, with the largest being Chinese, followed by Filipinos,

Indians, Koreans, Vietnamese, Japanese, and Cambodians in order (U.S. Census Bureau 2002).

Last but equally important are Native Americans/Alaskian Natives, who constitute 1.7 percent of the U.S. population, an estimated 5.2 million people (U.S. Census Bureau 2010c). There are more than 560 federally recognized Native tribes or nations, with approximately 40 percent of them in Alaska (Russell 2004). A large proportion of the Native American population lives in urban regions and the remainder either live in rural areas or on federal and state recognized reservations. Given the great diversity among Native American tribes and nations, effective work and intervention requires assessment of individuals' level of acculturation to mainstream American norms and values. Issues pertaining to acculturation and assessment are discussed later in this chapter. Compared to other ethnic groups, Native American Indians have been reported to live in poverty (Urban Indian Health Institute 2009) and lack some basic resources, especially access to healthcare.

With the background demographic information of ethnic minorities provided so far, it could be argued that together, they make up a crucial portion of the U.S. population and therefore must be included in any effort to develop assessment instruments. However, as argued earlier in this section, although relevant demographic data or information is collected in hospitals and clinics, there is little evidence that such information is really used in developing an appropriate treatment plan. It is worth exploring this argument, because in the era of rapid technological development, most offices have scanning devices for identification cards and some even take photograph of new patients (mostly for billing and other legal purposes), but patients have very little information as to why. In this chapter we emphasize that proper test selection is integral to any meaningful evaluation, and thus, argue that ethnic minority identification be used as an essential fact in determining appropriateness of psychological tests and treatment planning. But, before proceeding any further, it is imperative that we discuss the construct or condition to be measured, mental health.

Definition of Mental Illness

What is mental health? Is it the presence of tangible somatic symptoms? Or is it the absence or presence of dysfunctional behavior? Or perhaps, merely demonstrating an excess of symptomatic behaviors? This is a crucial question because an individual or society's definition of mental health will determine what symptoms they pay attention to, whether or not they seek help, the context within which they present their symptoms, and ultimately treatment compliance (U.S. Department of Health and Human Services 2001). In other words, mental health is a subjective concept that may influence how ethnic minority clients perceive severity of and need for professional help.

The *Diagnostic and Statistical Manual* (DSM-IV-TR) defines mental illness or mental disorder as "a clinically significant behavioral or psychological syndrome or pattern that occurs in an individual and that is associated with present distress (e.g., a painful symptom) or disability (i.e., impairment in one or more important areas of functioning) or with a significantly increased risk of suffering death, pain, disability, or an important loss of freedom" (American Psychiatric Association 2000, xxxi). The authors of the DSM further emphasize the importance of making a distinction between conditions that are expected or acceptable within a given culture or those that represent a conflict between an individual's and society's values or norms such that it denotes a "manifestation of a behavioral, psychological, or biological dysfunction" (xxxi). Although the DSM-IV-TR definition is not as comprehensive as may be desired, the importance of an individual's culture in assessment, diagnosis, and treatment is highlighted quite well.

The importance of culture in conceptualizing, assessment, and developing treatment plans for mental health has been emphasized by both the American Psychological Association (2003) and the American Psychiatric Association (2000) in the past two decades. For example, as briefly discussed earlier, an area of improvement in the current version of the *Diagnostic and Statistical Manual* (DSM-IV-TR) is the inclusion of culture-bound syndromes and the Cultural Formulation in Appendix I. Thorough assessment of ethnic minority populations call for familiarity with common culture-bound syndromes such as *amok* (among Puerto Ricans and Navajos), *Ataque de nervios* among Latinos, *boufée delirante* among west African and Haitian immigrants, Ghost sickness among Native American Indians, and Rootwork or *mal puesto* among African Americans and European Americans in the Southern United States, as well as some Latino groups (American Psychiatric Association 2000). It is common for health professionals to see culture-bound syndromes as a category that is only applicable to individuals from different nations or recent immigrants. However, caution needs to be taken because the values, beliefs, concepts, and ideas may have been passed on to younger generations even if they were born and raised in the United States.

Castillo (1997) identified that culture influences mental health based on (1) the individual's own personal experience of the illness and associated symptoms; (2) how the individual expresses symptoms within the context of his/her cultural norms; (3) how the symptoms expressed are interpreted and diagnosed; and (4) the treatment outcome. In general there tends to be a stigma associated with mental illness among ethnic minority groups, which discourages help seeking behaviors (Menke and Flynn 2009). These cultural influences have also been recognized in the DSM-IV-TR, Cultural Formulation section, in an understanding that the individual's self-perception and ethnic identity is crucial to the process of assessment, diagnosis, treatment planning, and compliance. Specifically, clinicians are strongly encouraged to consider (1) cultural identity of the individual, such as ethnic/cultural reference group and level acculturation; (2) cultural explanations of the individual's illness, including common symptoms or expressions of distress and severity of illness as well as beliefs about the cause of illness; (3) cultural factors related to psychosocial environment and levels of functioning such as role of religion, the extended family and other forms of social support or resources; and (4) cultural elements of the relationship between the individual and the clinician, including differences in social status, communication problems related to differences in spoken and expressed language, as well as lack of equivalence or difference in the meaning of behaviors and concepts discussed (American Psychiatric Association 2000, 897–898).

As has been noted in other chapters in this volume, failure to seriously consider the cultural perspective of patients may have serious implications, for assessment, diagnosis, and treatment planning. For instance, ethnic variations in diagnosis of affective and psychotic disorders: with whites and Asians being more likely to be diagnosed with affective disorders and African Americans being diagnosed more with schizophrenia may be partly due to a lack of cultural acuity on the part of the clinician or miscommunication due to lack of equivalence in meanings and expressions of distress from the perspectives of the clinician and the patient (Foulks 2004).

Selecting a Mental Health Assessment Instrument

In general the purpose of a mental health measure is to separate normal from abnormal functioning, and to assist in determining the extent that mental health care is needed. Green (2009) summarized that "Proper test selection is key, keeping in mind the following:

1. Purpose of the measure;
2. Population for which the measure was design and normed;

3. Recentness of norming the measure;
4. Test construction and/or translation that involves members of the culture of interest;
5. Appropriate validation that is culturally inclusive."

An important consideration in selecting assessment instruments for evaluating ethnic minorities (or any group) is the psychometric values. These include reliability, validity, standardization, and norming.

The major question in test selection ought to be, who was the test normed for? It is unethical to blindly administer a test that was never normed for a group and expect accurate results. For instance, if a health practitioner decides to use the Beck Depression Inventory-II or BDI-II (Beck, Brown, and Steer 1996) to measure depression levels, it is important to note that the inventory was originally normed on a sample that was predominantly white or Caucasian (approximately 95 percent) and only included two ethnic minority groups (African Americans and Asian Americans), together representing about 5 percent of the sample. Researchers continue to work on generalizability to other cultural groups with positive results.

Reliability is basically looking at consistency in responses: typically standardized assessment instruments should report data indicating test-retest, split-half or coefficient alpha value. Still using the BDI-II as an example, the authors reported a coefficient alpha of .92 for an outpatient sample and a one-week test-retest reliability of .93 for another outpatient sample (Beck et al. 1996). However, given that ethnic minorities comprised only 5 percent of the norming sample, it is crucial to consider studies that have focused on those specific samples with reports of acceptable reliability (Joe et al. 2008, Ames, Gatewood-Colwell, and Kaczmarek 1989, Contreras et al. 2004).

Validity is a measure of the degree to which the instrument assesses the psychological construct (or psychological condition) of interest. In working with members of ethnic minority groups, validity is extremely crucial because whatever instrument or means of assessment we select must capture culturally unique symptoms that may not be relevant to mainstream America. For instance, if an instrument uses DSM-IV-TR as the standard for symptom measurement, it may be necessary to ensure that you apply the cultural formulation presented in Appendix I in interpreting and formulating treatment (American Psychiatric Association 2000). Furthermore, to increase accuracy and reduce possible measurement bias or errors, standardization is important. In other words, the selected assessment instrument has to be administered as per instructions—the same way to all respondents. Any alterations in standardization may influence the validity of the instrument and ultimately the accuracy of responses.

Aside from the psychometric qualities discussed earlier in this section, issues of culture and test fairness ought to be considered as well. Generally it has been argued that variations in familiarity of test items may exist for different ethnic groups. Several factors need to be taken into account. First is cultural relevance, which refers to how easy it is to understand test items. Second is cultural equivalence, which pertains to the extent to which items on the assessment instrument measure the same concept among different ethnic groups, in spite of variations in cultural experiences. It has been argued that cross-cultural comparisons and applications are only accurate if the meaning of items on the assessment instrument is more or less similar across the respective ethnic groups (Norenzayan and Heine 2005). Last is generalizability of assessment results to the individual's life and their ability to predict psychological well-being in the future. For instance the Center for Epidemiologic Studies–Depression scale (CES-D) has been used quite extensively in research of Latino samples in the United States and has been found to predict depression levels associated with acculturative stress (Torres 2010). In general, bias associated with cultural relevance, cultural equivalence, and generalizability could be minimized by employing existing instruments that have been documented to possess good reliability and validity for diverse ethnic populations. It is also important to use an additional mode of assessment where possible (e.g., follow up questionnaire with a brief face-to-face interview as a way of confirming items endorsed, and also for further elaboration where necessary). Finally, regardless of assessment instrument selected, it is important to consider the sociopolitical setting and document the following factors, as per recommendation of the American Psychological Association guidelines (American Psychological Association 1990):

a. number of generations in the country
b. number of years in the country
c. fluency in English
d. extent of family support (or disintegration of family)
e. community resources
f. level of education
g. change in social status as a result of coming to this country (for immigrant or refugee)
h. intimate relationship with people of different backgrounds
i. level of stress related to acculturation

Important Factors in Assessment of Mental Health Status

In this section, we discuss important cultural factors that may influence individual responses even after selecting an appropriate assessment instrument, and ultimately impact interpretation and application of scores on the selected tool. Six factors are considered: the individual's explanatory style, level of acculturation, tendency towards individualism or collectivism, language or linguistic barriers, cultural equivalence, and past experiences of prejudice and perceptions about the healthcare system.

(I) Individual's Explanatory Model of Illness

According to Kleinmann (1988) an individual's explanatory style or their cultural interpretation of mental illness influences how they perceive symptoms and whether or not they acknowledge the condition. For instance, whereas a European American individual may focus on genetic predisposition or psychological trauma in explaining depression, an African American from the southern United States or one with a direct Caribbean ancestry may explain their depression as a result of witchcraft, and a Native American Indian may attribute the condition to a spirit or taboo. These examples ought to be taken with great caution, so as not to generalize blindly to all individuals belonging to the various ethnic groups because several other sociodemographic factors (e.g., gender, socioeconomic status, religiosity or spirituality, level of education, etc.) interact with ethnic values and beliefs to influence one's explanatory style.

Foulks (2004) suggests that a patient's explanatory model could be evaluated by asking six simple questions:

1. What has happened?
2. Why?
3. Why now?
4. What will happen if nothing is done?
5. What effect will the experience have on others?
6. What can be done about it?

Again, in asking these questions, it is crucial to be wary about cultural biases that tend to impact how the health practitioner receives or records, interprets, and utilizes information in working with the ethnic minority individual.

The American Psychological Association (2003b) has summarized information pertaining to general world view of ethnic minority groups. According to APA guidelines, African American clients value interconnectedness of all things, group welfare, extended kinship networks, and tend to prefer a treatment approach that includes important support systems such as church and extended family members. Native American Indian/Alaskians tend to possess spiritual/holistic values, view illness as a result of disharmony, value cooperation, and prefer a value-free, collaborative approach that includes their traditions. Asian Americans (depending on their country of origin) may value a hierarchical family structure, harmony, a sense of allegiance, dependence on each other, and may prefer a direct, structured approach with focus on specific goals. Last, Hispanic/Latin Americans have been reported to value family welfare, sharing, a sense of connection, religious attributions, and prefer an active and direct approach that emphasizes the affective, cognitive, and biological modalities. It is worth mentioning that the APA guidelines emphasize the tendency for African Americans to demonstrate healthy paranoia, Asian Americans to restrain from expressing strong emotions, and Latino Americans to report more somatic symptoms.

As indicated by the American Psychological Association in their first guideline, "Psychologists are encouraged to recognize that, as cultural beings, they may hold attitudes and beliefs that can detrimentally influence their perceptions of and interactions with individuals who are ethnically and racially different from themselves" (American Psychological Association 2003a, 382). Health practitioners are strongly encouraged to be open to the reality that beyond explicit biases, implicit biases have an even stronger impact on their perceptions and interpretations of behaviors presented by ethnic minorities. For instance in a study Peris, Teachman, and Nosek (2008), they found that explicit biases predicted negative patient prognoses while implicit biases predicted over-diagnoses.

Furthermore, research on interpersonal expectancy effects have informed us has shown that the way we perceive an individual influences how we behave towards them and ultimately predicts how he or she will behave towards us (Rosenthal 2002). So our expectations are likely to influence the results we obtain from an individual who is culturally different from us. Similarly, the anxiety associated with an individual's belief or concerns about others thinking about them in stereotypical ways (i.e., stereotype threat) could influence their behavior. Henry, von Hippel, and Shapiro (2010) reported that people diagnosed with schizophrenia performed poorly in a social environment in which they felt stereotyped as being mentally ill. Other studies have reported negative impact of stereotype threat on mental health status of ethnic minorities (see Burgess et al. 2010). All in all, it is vital to consider the possibility of ethnic minority clients either underreporting or over-reporting symptoms based on their beliefs, values, personal experiences, and expectations.

(II) Acculturation

As mentioned earlier in this chapter, specific cultural issues in mental health assessment significantly influence individual responses. In addition to background history of discrimination, racism, and issues of mistrust, other issues such as acculturation, individualism/collectivism, and spirituality or religion are crucial points of assessment in any mental health system (see also chapter 2 in volume 1 of this series). In other words, an individual's country of origin, how long they have lived in the United States and the extent to which they identify with and interact routinely with members of their ethnic group are crucial assessment factors for any comprehensive mental health evaluation. Acculturation has been defined as a transition in which a person gradually accommodates to and eventually takes on some of the values and beliefs of the dominant culture (see also chapter 4, volume 1). Berry described acculturation as a process of "culture shedding and culture learning," that involves intentionally or unintentionally losing selected cultural values or behaviors with the passage of time, while adopting new values and behaviors from the new group (Berry 1992, 2001). This is particularly important to ethnic groups in the United States, many of who continue to maintain close interaction with relatives in their country of origin.

In earlier publications, Berry described four different forms of acculturation based on the extent to which an individual has preference for his or her own culture and the extent to which he or she prefers the values and norms of the new culture. They are integration, assimilation, separation, and marginalization (Berry 1970). Integration is when the individual (or immigrant) is willing to adopt behaviors and adapt to the host culture while also maintaining his or her own cultural norms and values—some form of a balance between the two. This is different from separation, in which the individual focuses almost exclusively on adopting the cultural norms of the host group (or country) and basically disregards his or her own cultural heritage. Assimilation is more or less the opposite of separation. With assimilation, the person puts most of his or her efforts toward maintaining their own cultural heritage, and very little effort toward adopting the norms of the host group. Last, marginalization refers to an individual who neither adopts their own cultural heritage, nor that of the host or dominant group. Marginalization is the least preferred type of acculturation and has been associated with many adjustment and mental health challenges.

The applicability of Berry's initial conceptualization of acculturation has been analyzed by some authors in recent times. For instance, in their application of acculturation to Native Americans, Garrett and Pichette (2000) outlined five levels:

1. Traditional—speaks native language, sticks to traditional beliefs and values, and practices traditional customs;
2. Marginal—speaks both native and English language, does not necessarily abide by native cultural values, but is not identified with mainstream American values or norms;
3. Bicultural—identifies with values and norms, and practices customs of natives as well as mainstream Americans;
4. Assimilated—identifies mostly with values, norms and customs of mainstream America; and
5. Pantraditional—after reaching level of assimilation, chooses to go back to the traditional native values, beliefs, and customs.

Thus, when working with a Native American, it is beneficial to have a rough idea of his or her level of acculturation as a tool in treatment planning. It is worth mentioning that Berry's model of acculturation may not equally apply to all ethnic and migrant groups and therefore might need some adjustments or modifications (Chirkov 2009). For instance, an ethnic minority individual who migrates to the United States and lives in a neighborhood predominated by people of his country of origin may have a different experience with the acculturation process, especially if his or her native language (e.g., Spanish or Chinese) is spoken more often in that neighborhood (Portes and Rumbaut 2001). Furthermore, acculturation may not be an issue for second generation immigrants, most of whom are born in the receiving country and therefore adopt its values, customs, and norms while growing up.

Acculturation is an important factor in the assessment of an ethnic minority individual's mental health status because levels of acculturation have been associated with physical and mental health (for review, see Suinn 2010, Schwartz et al. 2010). It has been associated with health behaviors in general, including nutrition, smoking, alcohol use, and exercise behavior. In general, low acculturation levels have been associated with high levels of psychological distress among Asian Americans (Wang and Mallinckrodt 2006), Latino Americans (Torres 2010), and African Americans (Koneru and Weisman de Mamani 2006). Other studies have demonstrated a negative relationship between acculturation levels and depression among Asian Americans (Wong, Tran, and Lai 2009), Mexican American (Gonzalez, Haan, and Hinton 2001). Similarly, studies have reported an inverse relationship between low acculturation and suicidal behavior among Asian Americans (especially within the context of high parent-child conflict—Groves, Stanley, and

Sher 2007). In general, integration or bicultural acculturation has been associated with psychological wellbeing, high self-esteem, and lower levels of depression (Coatesworth et al. 2005, Chen, Benet-Martinez, and Bond 2008, David, Okazaki, and Saw 2009).

Over the years many instruments have been developed to assess acculturation (see Suinn 2010). Some of the scales are specific for an ethnic group (Kim and Hong 2004, Suinn et al.1987, Suinn 2010). Yet others are more generic and suited for any cultural group (e.g., Wong-Riegner and Quintana 1987, Ryder, Alden, and Paulhus 2000).

(III) Individualism/Collectivism

Another cultural construct that is known to influence perceptions and ultimately health-seeking behaviors of ethnic minorities is individualism/collectivism (see also Chapter 1, volume 1 of this series). Hofstede (1983) originally presented individualism and collectivism as two opposing views, with individualism referring to a general affinity towards independence, self-reliance, and competitiveness and collectivism referring to a preference for the group, a need to fit into the group, and increased concern for harmony within the group. In general, Hofstede linked these concepts to national cultures, so that westerners (such as Canadians or Americans) were typically perceived as individualistic in their views, whereas non westerners (such as Indians and Mexicans) were perceived as collectivistic. Past studies have described African American and other ethnic minority groups as more collective (Triandis 2001a). However, a review of studies actually demonstrate that we tend to portray either individualism or collectivism, depending on the situation, so that an Asian American who has lived in the United States for decades may lean more towards individualism through acculturation.

Although Hofstede's initial conceptualization of individualism and collectivism portrayed people from different western and nonwestern nations, we have now come to understand that it is erroneous to make generalized statements about nations or people from a particular region without making provision for differences within the group. Triandis (2001b) explained that individualism/collectivism could be either vertical or horizontal, depending on whether the individual or group of people is more concerned with equality or likeness (horizontal) or whether they are concerned with hierarchy or difference (vertical). Thus, he identified two levels each of individualism and collectivism, namely, horizontal individualism-HI, vertical individualism-VI, horizontal collectivism-HC, and vertical collectivism-VC (Triandis and Gelfand 1998). HI pertains to a desire to be distinct, but not necessarily better than one's group and VI applies to a desire to be distinct and better than the group (connoting competitiveness). On the other hand, HC refers to an individual who emphasizes interdependence or the willingness to share common goals with others in the group, while VC describes an individual who places his or her group's goals over his or her personal goals. Collectivism and individualism have both been associated with poor mental health, especially when an individual's personality style is inconsistent with his or her cultural society's values (Caldwell-Harris and Ayçiçegi 2006).

Cultural differences and the tendency towards individualism or collectivism can affect an individual's explanation of his or her mental illness and influence his or her typical responses on assessment tools, as well as preference for treatment. Chen, Lee, and Stevenson (1995) reported a moderacy response style among collectivist Asian respondents, where they are more likely to respond using midpoint choices on a Likert scale, while people from individualistic cultures are more likely to respond using extreme choices. Furthermore, when using Likert scale questions, health practitioners need to cautiously evaluate responses for a possible reference-group effect. This occurs because members from different ethnic groups tend to use a different reference point in making judgments on self-report inventories (Peng, Nisbett, and Wong 1997, Heine et al. 2002). In other words, African Americans tend to compare themselves to other African Americans, while Latinos tend to compare themselves to other Latinos. Cultural factors associated with the moderacy effect and reference-group effect may result in underreporting of psychopathology among some ethnic groups.

(IV) Language/linguistic Barriers and Non-Verbal Cues

Language is a major communication tool in any system and certainly plays an important role in an individual's attitudes about mental illness and help-seeking behaviors. Specifically, proficiency in English language has been found to influence help-seeking behaviors among some ethnic minority groups (Chu, Hsieh, and Tokars 2011, Le Meyer et al. 2009). Issues pertaining to language difficulties may be more pronounced for recent Asian American and Hispanic American immigrants. Data from the U.S. Census Bureau suggests that quite a significant proportion of ethnic minorities either speak a second language or have a primary language other than English. For instance, the 2009 American Community Survey found that an estimated 35 million residents five and older spoke Spanish at home, and one half of this number did not speak English very well

(U.S Census Bureau 2011a). This number implies that approximately 75 percent or more of Hispanics spoke Spanish at home. Similarly, 2.6 million people five years and older spoke Chinese at home, and an additional one-plus million spoke either Tagalog, Vietnamese, or Korean language at home (U.S. Census Bureau 2011b). Furthermore, 28 percent of Native Americans five years and older spoke another language at home: This number is slightly greater than the overall percent of 21 percent for the entire United States (U.S. Census Bureau 2011c).

The preponderance of the data from the U.S. Census Bureau point to the importance of providing assessment instruments in alternate major languages such as Spanish and Chinese. Although it is arguable that immigrants to the United States should make every effort to speak and if possible write English, health professionals do not have the luxury of waiting for individuals to fulfill that English requirement before working with them. It is therefore advisable to be ready in any way possible by using existing assessment instruments that have been translated into other languages. Instruments include Spanish versions of the Beck Depression Inventory (Bonilla et al. 2003), Center for Epidemiologic Studies Depression Scale—CES-D (Reuland et al. 2009), Wechsler Intelligence Scale for Children-IV—Spanish version (Wechsler 2004), and Primary Care Evaluation of Mental Disorders—PRIME-MD-9 (Reuland et al. 2009). Similarly commonly used assessment and screening instruments have been translated to traditional Chinese versions. These include Chinese versions of the Beck Depression Inventory (Yeung et al. 2002, Wang, et al, 2011), Center for Epidemiologic Studies Depression Scale—CES-D (Li and Hsiao-Rei Hicks 2010), Beck Anxiety Inventory (Cheng et al. 2002), and Primary Care Evaluation of Mental Disorders—PRIME-MD-9 (Lubetkin, Jia, and Gold 2003).

There also exist non-verbal, self-rated, assessment instruments which limit the need for proficiency in English language. One example is the Visual Analogue Scale (VAS), which consists of a 100mm line with two well-defined end points, such as *No Pain* and *Extreme Pain* (Wewers and Lowe 1990). The respondent is asked to mark a point on the line that best describes the intensity of his or her symptom. Thus the length from the lower end point (e.g., No Pain) to the respondent's mark represents the intensity of the symptom being measured. Although using the VAS could be time consuming, it is a great way to get around the complexity and bias associated with lack of language proficiency among some ethnic minorities. The VAS has been used in assessment of depression among cognitively impaired patients (Kertzman et al. 2004), anxiety in preoperative patients (Kindler et al. 2000), and pain in patients undergoing spinal procedures (Fish et al. 2010).

Furthermore, the VAS has also been found to correlate significantly with existing measures of anxiety (Williams, Morlock, and Feltner 2010), depression (McCoy et al. 2005), and pain (Fish et al. 2010). Alternatively, some non-verbal assessment tools employ pictures of different facial expressions depicting severity in measuring the patient's feelings and symptoms (Warden, Hurley, and Volicer 2003).

In keeping with ensuring bilingual patients, and other patients who lack proficiency in English language, have an opportunity to be assessed accurately and treated efficaciously, it is vital that health practitioners create a welcoming atmosphere. For instance, having signs up in English, Spanish, and a major Chinese language in the waiting room, could connote a sense of warmth, trust, and acceptance to bilingual or multilingual ethnic minorities. It is a common practice to see written instructions to "please sign in" when one enters the waiting area of a healthcare facility or clinic, which assumes that all patients entering the waiting area speak and understand English language, but having that same instruction also written in another language, such as Spanish (registre por favor) or traditional Chinese (请登录) speaks volumes to people of color. Beyond a welcoming atmosphere in the waiting area, another way to increase accuracy in assessing an ethnic minority is to provide translated versions of surveys and other assessment instruments where possible, as well as to make provision for extra time to complete forms.

(V) Cultural Equivalence

Cultural equivalence refers to the extent to which concepts, assessment instruments and treatment procedures have the same meaning in different ethnic or cultural groups. The importance of communication between providers and patients has been highlighted in the literature (Perloff et al. 2006). As summarized by Street (2003) "another way the cultural context may have an impact on communication in a consultation is with respect to ethnicity-related attitudes and stereotypes possessed by clinicians and patients" (79). A crucial initial step to awareness of a lack of cultural equivalence is for clinicians to recognize and be willing to address their own ethnocentric views about mental illness. In other words, clinicians ought to seriously consider the extent to which their own views about mental health may be influenced by their individual cultural perspectives and inadvertent ignoring of the perspective of a culturally different client (Capell, Dean, and Veenstra 2008). This is even more important with modes of assessment that are predominantly based on face-to-face interviews and may require the interviewer (clinician) to make subjective judgments about severity and type of illness.

Other studies have emphasized patients' perceptions about health practitioners' cultural competence. For instance, Ahmed and Bates (2010) found a negative relationship between patients' own ethnocentric views and their perceptions of cultural competence regarding language (e.g., using translator if available) and other macro-cultural issues (e.g., knowledge about health-related religious practices) amongst their health practitioners or physicians. In other words, the more ethnocentric a patient is, the less likely he or she is to perceive their physician as one who is concerned with the patient's cultural beliefs and norms (e.g., customs, religion, and language). These results support the importance of assessing patients' level of ethnocentrism and cultural identity, as well as their perceptions of the health care practitioner's cultural competence prior to clinical formulation and development of treatment plans.

Maintaining cultural equivalence also means that clinicians ought to be trained in the selection of assessment tools so that they make an effort to include assessment tools or mechanisms derived from research conducted using emic as well as etic approaches. Simply put, research using the emic approach considers the perspective of native or ethnic groups (e.g., assessment tools validated using an ethnic sample), while research using the etic approach is typically based on information from external sources.

(VI) Past Experiences of Prejudice and Perceptions about the Healthcare System

Effectively working with and serving ethnic minorities suffering from mental health challenges requires knowledge of how factors such as immigration, acculturation, alienation, and the long history of prejudice and discrimination have influenced their level of trust in healthcare workers or the health system in general (Rodenhauser 1994). In general, attitudes and perceptions of ethnic minorities towards healthcare workers connote mistrust of health professionals and have been associated with a history of racism, oppression, prejudice, and discrimination against ethnic minority groups (Williams and Williams-Morris 2000, Whaley 2001, Rajakumar et al. 2009, David 2010). These factors are crucial in any form of assessment, as they tend to influence the extent to which a patient may feel comfortable disclosing personal information, which in turn may influence the accuracy of a clinician's diagnosis and treatment plan, as well as the patient's likelihood to comply with treatment.

Summary and Conclusions

In this chapter we have provided information unique to assessment of ethnic minorities within the context of their background histories, values, beliefs, and conceptualizations of the etiology, course and treatment of mental illness. In selecting a test, health practitioners are encouraged to consider several psychometric factors, including validity, reliability, and consider the sample included in norming the assessment instrument. It is also important to seriously take a look at cultural relevance (e.g., Does it make sense to the ethnic group in question?); cultural equivalence (e.g., Does the assessment tool evaluate the same symptoms among different ethnic groups with different cultural experiences?); generalizability (i.e., whether results are applicable to situations unique to ethnic minorities and able to predict future mental health or psychological well-being); and systematic errors (e.g., Is the measure applicable to ethnic minorities or does it systematically show them as possessing a specific quality?).

Furthermore, when working with members of ethnic minority groups, health practitioners ought to be aware of their own personal biases. As noted by the American Psychological Association, "psychologists are encouraged to recognize that, as cultural beings, they may hold attitudes and beliefs that can detrimentally influence their perceptions of and interactions with individuals who are ethnically and racially different from themselves" (American Psychological Association 2003, 382). Awareness of one's own biases means recognizing and understanding that such biases may influence our assessment, diagnosis, and treatment of minority patients, which could be fatal to their well-being. In other words, healthcare practitioners ought to be "aware of their own attitudes and values," and make every effort to change the "automatically favorable perceptions of the in-group," and the "automatically . . . negative perceptions of the out-group" (American Psychological Association 2003, 384).

Finally, actions speak louder than words . . . sensitivity to the norms, values, beliefs and expectations of ethnic minority patients should connote reducing the impact of language barriers, incorporating the impact of cultural constructs, such as acculturation, individualism and collectivism, cultural equivalence, and unique experiences of racism, prejudice, and discrimination (particularly from the healthcare system). Also, imperative is inclusion of alternate forms of treatment that are more common to ethnic minorities (e.g., herbal treatments, curanderos, medicine men, clergy, pastors, etc.).

Last, when the opportunity arises for hiring, it is essential to recruit health practitioners and other staff members who are professionally qualified, possibly proficient in a second language, have some knowledge, training, and possibly experience with people of color. Training needs to focus on cultural competence as well as patient-centered care (Ahmed and Bates 2010). Cultural competence as defined by Ahmed and Bates refers to "a process that acknowledges health care providers' and receivers' perspectives, and promotes knowledge and awareness of individual and cross-cultural differences in order to facilitate adaptation" (112). Patient-centered care focuses on "compassion, empathy, and responsiveness to the needs, values, and expressed preferences of the individual patient" (Betancourt 2006, 9), Although the two concepts have been viewed separately, comprehensive training for effective and accurate assessment of patients calls for a much needed "balance [in] . . . treatment of patients as individuals and [also] as members of a group" (Ahmed and Bates 2010, 121).

Acknowledgment

Portions of this chapter are reprinted from Eshun, S. and Gurung, R. A. R. (2009). "Introduction to Culture and Psychopathology," Chapter 1, in *Culture and Mental Health: Sociocultural Influences Theory and Practice,* edited by S. Eshun and R. A. R. Gurung. Boston, MA: Wiley-Blackwell.

References

Ahmed, R. and B. R. Bates. 2010. "Assessing the Relationship between Patients' Ethnocentric Views and Patients' Perceptions of Physicians' Cultural Competence in Health Care Interactions." *Intercultural Communication Studies XIX*(2): 111–127.

American Psychiatric Association. 2000. *Diagnostic and Statistical Manual of Mental Disorders* (4th ed., text revision). Washington, DC: Author.

American Psychological Association. 1990. *Guidelines for Providers of Psychological Services to Ethnic, Linguistic, and Culturally Diverse Populations.* http://www.apa.org/pi/oema/resources/policy/provider-guidelines.aspx

American Psychological Association. 2003a. "Guidelines on Multicultural Education, Training, Research, Practice, and Organizational Change for Psychologists." *American Psychologist 58*: 377–402.

American Psychological Association. 2003b. *Psychological Treatment of Ethnic Minority Populations.* http://www.apa.org/pi/oema/resources/brochures/treatment-minority.pdf

Ames, M. H., G. Gatewood-Colwell, and M. Kaczmarek. 1989. "Reliability and Validity of the Beck Depression Inventory for White and Mexican American Gerontic Population." *Psychological Reports 65*: 1163–1165.

Ayalon, L. and M. A. Young. 2005. "Racial Group Differences in Help-Seeking Behaviors. *Journal of Social Psychology 145*: 391–403.

Beck, A. T., G. Brown, and R. A. Steer. 1996. *Beck Depression Inventory II Manual.* San Antonio, TX: The Psychological Corporation.

Berry, J. W. 1970. "Marginality, Stress and Identification in an Acculturating Aboriginal Community." *Journal of Cross-Cultural Psychology* 1: 239–252.

Berry, J. W. 1992. "Acculturation and Adaptation in a New Society." *International Migration 30:* 69–85.

Berry, J. W. 2001. "A Psychology of Immigration." *Journal of Social Issues* 7(3): 615–631.

Betancourt, J. R. 2006. *Improving Quality and Achieving Equity: the Role of Cultural Competence in Reducing Racial and Ethnic Disparities in Health Care.* New York: The Commonwealth Fund. Retrieved February 16, 2013, from http://www .commonwealthfund.org/usr_doc/Betancourt_improvingqualityachievingequity _961.pdf

Bonilla, J., G. Bernal, A. Santos, and D. Santos. 2004. "A Revised Spanish Version of the Beck Depression Inventory: Psychometric Properties with a Puerto Rican Sample of College Students." *Journal of Clinical Psychology* 60(1): 119–130.

Burgess, D. J., J. Warren, S. Phelan, J. Dovidio, and M. van Ryn. 2010. "Stereotype Threat and Health Disparities: What Medical Educators and Future Physicians Need to Know." *Journal of General Internal Medicine* 25(2): 169–177. doi:10.1007/s11606-009-1221-4

Caldwell-Harris, C. L. and A. Ayçiçegi. 2006. "When Personality and Culture Clash: The Psychological Distress of Allocentrics in an Individualist Culture and Idiocentrics in a Collectivist Culture." *Transcultural Psychiatry* 43(3): 331–361, doi: 10.1177/1363461506066982

Capell, J., E. Dean, and G. Veenstra. 2008. "The Relationship between Cultural Competence and Ethnocentrism of Health Care Professionals." *Journal of Transcultural Nursing* 19(2): 121–125.

Castillo, R. J. 1997. *Culture and Mental Illness.* Pacific Grove, CA: ITP.

Chen, C., S. Lee, and H. W. Stevenson, H. W. 1995. "Response Style and Cross Cultural Comparison among East Asians and North American Students." *Psychological Science* 6: 170–175.

Chen, S. X., V. Benet-Martinez, and M. H. Bond. 2008. "Bicultural Identity, Bilingualism, and Psychological Adjustment in Multicultural Societies: Immigration-Based and Globalization-Based Acculturation." *Journal of Personality* 76: 803–838. Doi:10.1111/j.1467-6494.2008.00505.x

Cheng, S. K. W., C. S. Wong, K. C. Wong, G. H. C. Chong, M. T. P. Wong, and S. S. Y. Chang. 2002. "A Study of Psychometric Properties, Normative Scores, and Factor Structure of the Beck Anxiety Inventory—the Chinese Version." *Chinese Journal of Clinical Psychology* 10: 4–6.

Chirkov, V. 2009. "Summary of the Criticism and of the Potential Ways to Improve Acculturation Psychology." *International Journal of Intercultural Relations* 33: 177–180.

Chu, J. P., K.Y. Hsieh, and D. A. Tokars. 2011. "Halo-Seeking Tendencies in Asian Americans with Suicidal Ideation and Attempts." *Asian American Journal of Psychology* 2(1): 25–38.

Coatsworth, J. D., M. Maldonado-Molina, H. Pantin, and J. Szapocznik. 2005. "A Person-Centered and Ecological Investigation of Acculturation Strategies in Hispanic Immigrant Youth." *Journal of Community Psychology* 33: 157–174. Doi:10.1002/jcop.20046.

Contreras, S., S. Fernandez, V. L. Malcarne, R. E. Ingram, and V. R. Vaccarino. 2004. "Reliability and Validity of Beck Depression and Anxiety Inventories in Caucasian American and Latinos." *Hispanic Journal of Behavioral Sciences* 26(4): 446–462.

Cross, T. L. 2003. "Culture as a Resource for Mental Health." *Cultural Diversity and Ethnic Minority Psychology* 9(4): 354–359.

David, E. J. R. 2010. "Cultural Mistrust and Mental Health Help-Seeking Attitudes among Filipino Americans." *Asian American Journal of Psychology* 1 (1): 57–66.

David, E. J. R., S. Okazaki, and A. Saw. 2009. "Bicultural Self-Efficacy among College Students: Initial Scale Development and Mental Health Correlates." *Journal of Counseling Psychology* 56: 211–226. doi:10.1037/a0015419.

Eshun, S. and R. A. R. Gurung. 2009. "Introduction to Culture and Psychopathology." In *Culture and Mental Health: Sociocultural Influences, Theory and Practice*, edited by S. Eshun and R. A. R. Gurung. Boston, MA: Wiley-Blackwell.

Fish, D. E., P. C. Lee, A. Parti, and Q. Pham. 2010. "Evaluating Correlation of Two Pain Scales in Spinal Procedures." *Federal Practitioner,* 27(5): 24–28.

Foulks, E. F. 2004. "Cultural Variables in Psychiatry." *Psychiatric Times* 24(4): 28–30.

Garrett, M.T. and E. F. Pichette. 2000. "Red as an Apple: Native American Acculturation and Counseling with or without Reservation." *Journal of Counseling and Development* 78: 3–13.

Gonzalez, H. M., N. M. Haan, and L. Hinton. 2001. "Acculturation and the Prevalence of Depression in Older Mexican Americans: Baseline Results of the Sacramento Area Latino Study on Aging." *Journal of American Geriatrics Society* 49 (7): 948–953.

Green, B.A. 2009. "Culture and Mental Health Assessment." In *Culture and Mental Health: Sociocultural Influences, Theory and Practice*, edited by S. Eshun and R. A. R. Gurung. Boston, MA: Wiley-Blackwell.

Groves, S., B. Stanley, and L. Sher. 2007. "Ethnicity and the Relationship between Adolescent Alcohol Use and Suicidal Behavior." *International Journal of Adolescent Medicine and Health* 19: 19–25.

Guarnaccia, P., I. Pincay, M. Alegria, P. Shrout, R. Lewis-Fernandez, and G. Canino. 2007. "Assessing Diversity Among Latinos: Results from the NLAAS." *Hispanic Journal of Behavioral Sciences* 29(4): 510–534.

Heine, S. J., D. R. Lehman, K. Peng, and J. Greenholtz. 2002. "What's Wrong with Cross-Cultural Comparisons of Subjective Likert Scales?: The Reference Group Effect." *Journal of Personality and Social Psychology* 82: 903–918.

Henry, J. D., C. von Hippel, and L. Shapiro. 2010. "Stereotype Threat Contributes to Social Difficulties in People with Schizophrenia." *British Journal of Clinical Psychology* 49: 31–41.

Hofstede, G. 1983. "National Cultures Revisited." *Behavioral Research, 18*: 285-305.

Hwang, W. C., H. F. Myers, J. Abe-Kim, and J. Y. Ting. 2008. "A Conceptual Paradigm for Understanding Culture's Impact on Mental Health: The Cultural Influences on Mental Health (CIMH) Model." *Clinical Psychology Review 28*(2): 211–227.

Joe, S., M. E. Woolley, G. K. Brown, M. Ghahramanlou-Holloway, A. T. Beck. 2008. "Psychometric Properties of the Beck Depression Inventory-II in Low Income African American Suicide Attempters." *Journal of Personality Assessment 90*(5): 521–523.

Kertzman, S., Z. Aladjem, R. Milo, Z. Ben-Nahum, M. Birger, H. Grinspan, A. Weizman, and M. Kotler. 2004. "The Utility of the Visual Analogue Scale for the Assessment of Depressive Mood in Cognitively Impaired Patients." *International Journal of Geriatric Psychiatry 19*(8): 789–96.

Kleinmann, A. 1988. "Do Psychiatric Disorders Differ in Different Cultures?" In *Understanding and Applying Medical Anthropology,* edited by P. Brown, 185–196. CA: Mayfield Publishing Company.

Kim, B. and S. Hong. 2004. "A Psychometric Revision of the Asian Values Scale Using the Rasch Model." *Measurement and Evaluation in Counseling and Development 37*: 15–27.

Kindler, C. H., C. Harms, F. Amsler, T. Ihde-Scholl, and D. Scheidegger. 2000. "The Visual Analog Scale Allows Effective Measurement of Preoperative Anxiety and Detection of Patients' Anesthetic Concerns." *Anesthesia and Analgesia 90*: 706–712.

Kirmayer, L. J. and R. Santhanam. 2001. "The Anthropology of Hysteria." In *Contemporary Approaches to the Study of Hysteria: Clinical and Theoretical Perspectives,* edited by P. W. Halligan, C. Bass, and J. C. Marshall, 251–270. Oxford: Oxford University Press.

Koneru, V. K. and A. G. Weisman de Mamani. 2006. "Acculturation, Ethnicity, and Symptoms of Schizophrenia." *Interamerican Journal of Psychology 40*(3): 355–362.

Le Meyer, O., N. Zane, Y. Cho, and D. T. Takeuchi. 2009. "Use of Specialty Mental Health Services by Asian Americans with Psychiatric Disorders." *Journal of Consulting and Clinical Psychology 77*: 1000–1005. Doi:10.1023/A:1013177014788.

Li, Z. and M. Hsiao-Rei Hicks. 2010. "The CES-D in Chinese American Women: Construct Validity, Diagnostic Validity for Major Depression, and Cultural Response Bias." *Psychiatry Research 175*(3): 227–232.

Lubetkin, E. I., H. Jia, and M. R. Gold. 2003. "Depression, Anxiety, and Associated Health Status in Low-Income Chinese Patients." *American Journal of Preventive Medicine 24*(4): 354–360. DOI: 10.1016/S0749-3797(03)00017-5)

Magán, I., J. Sanz, and M. P. Garcia-Vera. 2008. "Psychometric Properties of a Spanish Version of the Beck Anxiety Inventory (BAI) in General Population." *Spanish Journal of Psychology 11*(2): 626–640.

McCoy, S. J., J. M. Beal, M. E. Payton, A. L. Stewart, A. M. DeMers, and G. H. Watson. 2005. "Correlations of the Visual Analog Scales with Edinburgh Postnatal Depression Scale." *Journal of Affective Disorders 86*(2–3): 295–297. PMID: 15935250

Menke, R. and H. Flynn. 2009. "Relationships between Stigma, Depression, and Treatment in White and African American Primary Care Patients." *The Journal of Nervous and Mental Disease* 197(6): 407–411.

Mills, T. L. and C. A. Edwards. 2002. "A Critical Review of Research on the Mental Health Status of Older African Africans." *Aging and Society* 22: 273–304.

Norenzayan, A. and S. J. Heine. 2005. "Psychological Universals: What Are They and How Can We Know?" *Psychological Bulletin* 131(5): 763–784.

Peng, K., R. E. Nisbett, and N. Wong. 1997. "Validity Problems of Cross-Cultural Value Comparison and Possible Solutions." *Psychological Methods* 2(4): 329–41.

Perloff, R. M., B. Bonder, E. B. Ray, and L. A. Siminoff. 2006. "Doctor-Patient Communication, Cultural Competence, and Minority Health: Theoretical and Empirical Perspectives." *American Behavioral Scientist* 49(6): 835–852.

Perris, T. S., B. A. Teachman, and B. A. Nosek. 2008. "Implicit and Explicit Stigma of Mental Illness: Links to Clinical Care." *Journal of Nervous and Mental Disorders* 196(10): 752–760.

Portes, A., and R. G. Rumbaut. 2001. *Legacies: The Story of the Immigrant Second Generation.* Berkeley: University of California Press.

Rajakumar, K., S. B. Thomas, D. Musa, D. Almario, and M. A. Garza. 2009. "Racial Differences in Parents' Distrust of Medicine and Research." *Archives of Pediatric and Adolescent Medicine* 163: 108–114.

Reuland, D. S., A. Cherrington, G. S. Watkins, D. W. Bradford, R. A. Blanco, and B. N. Gaynes. 2009. "Diagnostic Accuracy of Spanish Language Depression-Screening Instruments." *Annals of Family Medicine* 7(5): 455–462. doi: 10.1370/afm.981PMCID: PMC2746515

Rodenhauser, P. 1994. "Cultural Barriers to Mental Health Care Delivery in Alaska." *Journal of Mental Health Administration* 21(1): 60–70.

Rosenthal, R. 2002. "Experimenter and Clinician Effects in Scientific Inquiry and clinical Practice." *Prevention and Treatment* 5(1). doi:10.1037/1522 -3736.5.1.538c

Russell, G. 2004. *American Indian Facts of Life: A Profile of Today's Tribes and Reservations.* Phoenix: Native Data Network.

Ryder, A. L. Alden, and D. Paulhus. 2000. "Is Acculturation Unidimensional or Bidimensional?" *Journal of Personality and Social Psychology* 79: 49–65.

Schwartz, S. J., B. L. Zamboanga, R. S. Weisskirch, and S. C. Wang. 2010. "The Relationships of Personal and Cultural Identity to Adaptive and Maladaptive Psychosocial Functioning in emerging adults." *Journal of Social Psychology* 150(1): 1–33.

Seccombe, K. 2007. *Families in Poverty.* New York: Allyn and Bacon.

Street, R. L. Jr. 2003. *Communicating in Medical Encounters: An Ecological Perspective in Health Communication.* London: Lawrence Erlbaum.

Suinn, R. 2010. "Reviewing Acculturation and Asian Americans: How Acculturation Affects Health, Adjustment, School Achievement, and Counseling." *Asian American Journal of Psychology* 1(1): 5–17.

Suinn, R., K. Rickard-Figueroa, S. Lew, and P. Vigil. 1987. "The Suinn-Lew Asian Self-Identity Acculturation Scale: An Initial Report." *Educational and Psychological Measurement* 47: 402–407.

Torres, L. 2010. "Predicting Levels of Latino Depression: Acculturation, Acculturative Stress and coping." *Cultural Diversity and Ethnic Minority Psychology* 16(2). doi: 10.1037/a0017357

Triandis, H. C. 2001a. "Individualism and Collectivism: Past, Present, and Future." In *Handbook of Culture and Psychology*, edited by D. Matsumoto, 35–50. New York: Oxford University Press.

Triandis, H. C. 2001b. "Individualism-Collectivism and Personality." *Journal of Personality* 69: 907–924.

Triandis, H. C. and M. J. Gelfand. 1998. "Converging Measurements of the Horizontal and Vertical Individualism and Collectivism." *Journal of Personality and Social Personality* 74: 118–128.

Urban Indian Health Institute. 2009. *Urban Native American and Alaska Native Youth: An analysis of Select National Data Sources*. Seattle: Seattle Indian Health Board.

U.S. Census Bureau. 2002. "The Asian population: 2000." Census 2000 Brief. http://www.cdc.gove/omhd/populations/AsianAm.htm/

U.S. Census Bureau. 2009a. "American Fact Finder: United States DP-1." http://factfinder2.census.gov

U.S. Census Bureau. 2009b. "Profile America: Facts for Features. Population Estimates." http://www.census.gov/popest/national/asrh/NC-EST2009-srh.html

U.S. Census Bureau. 2010a. "American Fact Finder: United States." http://www.census.gov/prod/cen2010/briefs/c2010br-04.pdf

U.S. Census Bureau. 2010b. "2010 Census Brief—Overview of Race and Hispanic Origin." http://www.census.gov/prod/cen2010/briefs/c2010br-02.pdf

U.S. Census Bureau. 2010c. "2010 Census Brief: Overview of Race and Hispanic Origin." http://www.census.gov/prod/cen2010/briefs/c2010br-02.pdf

U.S. Census Bureau. 2011a. "2009 American Community Survey: Table B16001." http://www.census.gov/acs/www/

U. S. Census Bureau. 2011b. "2009 American Community Survey." http://factfinder.census.gov

U. S. Census Bureau. 2011c. "2010 American Community Survey for the American Indian and Alaska Native Alone Population." http://factfinder2.census.gov

U.S. Department of Health and Human Services. 2001. "Mental Health: Culture, Race, and Ethnicity—A Supplement to Mental Health: A Report of the Surgeon General." Rockville, MD: U.S. Department of Health and Human Services, Public Health Office, Office of the Surgeon General.

Wang, C. and B. Mallinckrodt. 2006. "Acculturation Attachment, and Psychological Adjustment of Chinese/Taiwanese International Students." *Journal of Counseling Psychology* 53: 422–433.

Wang Z., C. Yuan, J. Huang, Z. Li, J. Chen, et al. 2011. "Reliability and Validity of the Chinese Version of Beck Depression Inventory-II among Depression Patients." *Chinese Mental Health Journal* 25: 476–480.

Warden, V., A. C. Hurley, and L. Volicer. 2003. "Development and Psychometric Evaluation of the Pain Assessment in Advanced Dementia (PAINAD) Scale." *Journal of the American Medical Directors Association* 4: 9–15.

Wechsler, D. 2004. "Wechsler Intelligence Scale for Children—Fourth Edition, Spanish (WISC-IV—Spanish)." http://www.pearsonassessments.com/HAIWEB/Cultures/en-us/Productdetail.htm?Pid=015-8978-846

Whaley, A. 2001. "Cultural Mistrust: An Important Psychological Construct for Diagnosis and Treatment of African Americans." *Professional Psychology: Research and Practice* 32(6): 555–562.

Wewers, M.E. and N. K. Lowe. 1990. "A Critical Review of Visual Analogue Scales in the Measurement of Clinical Phenomena." *Research in Nursing and Health* 13: 227–236.

Williams, D. R., and R. Williams-Morris. 2000. "Racism and Mental Health: The African American Experience." *Ethnicity & Health,* 5: 243–268. doi:10.1080/713667453

Williams, V. S. L., R. J. Morlock, and D. Feltner. 2010. "Psychometric Evaluation of a Visual Analog Scale for the Assessment of Anxiety." *Health and Quality of Life Outcomes* 8: 57. doi: 10.1186/1477-7525-8-57

Wong, Y. K. Tran, and A. Lai. 2009. "Association among Asian Americans' Enculturation, Emotional Experiences, and Depressive Symptoms." *Journal of Multicultural Counseling and Development* 37: 105–116.

Wong-Riegner, D. and D. Quintana. 1987. "Comparative Acculturation of Southeast Asian and Hispanic Immigrants and Sojourners." *Journal of Cross-Cultural Psychology* 18: 345–362.

Yeung, A., S. Howarth, R. Chan, S. Sonawalla, A. A. Nierenberg, and M. Fava. 2002. "Use of the Chinese Version of the Beck Depression Inventory for Screening Depression in Primary Care." *Journal of Nervous and Mental Disorders* 190(2): 94–99.

CHAPTER THREE

The Mental Health of Latina/os: A Cultural Focus

Rocío Rosales Meza
and Leticia Arellano-Morales

Responding to the mental health needs of the Latina/o community is critical to our health as a nation. Latina/os are the largest and fastest growing racial/ethnic minority within the United States, and their growth is expected to continue. Despite this tremendous growth, mental health disparities pose several challenges to the Latina/o community and the field of mental health. Latina/os in the United States are at high risk for anxiety, depression, and substance abuse. They have less access to mental health care, receive lower quality care, receive services that poorly match their needs, and are thus more likely to drop out after the first treatment session (National Alliance for Hispanic Health 2001, U.S. Department of Health and Human Services [USDHHS], 2001). In addition, they demonstrate more persistent mental illnesses, are more likely to somaticize distress, and have lower medication adherence (Alegria and Woo 2009, Marin, Escobar, and Vega 2005). Experts state these findings are largely associated with broader sociocultural factors that pose obstacles for Latina/os engaging in and receiving effective care within the U.S. mental health system.

These issues highlight the need that within the mental health field, a culturally centered understanding is needed, followed by a delivery of culturally effective services for Latina/os. Accordingly, the purpose of this chapter is to provide recent developments in Latina/o mental health research and practice, with a focus on cultural issues. First we provide a discussion of the cultural influences and processes that may impact Latina/o clients. Next we address mental health and illness beliefs, along with coping styles and cultural strengths. We then provide a mental health profile of the Latina/o population. Finally, we discuss barriers to mental health and treatment, and research regarding effective practices. It is important to note that Latina/os are a highly heterogeneous group and large variations exist depending on country of origin, age, generation, acculturation status, language, social class, documented status, education, religion, gender, and sexual orientation (for more detail see Arellano-Morales and Rosales Meza chapter in volume 1).

Understanding Latina/o Culture

A description of Latina/o culture is necessary to understand the experiences and lives of Latina/o clients. Culture influences one's behavior, thoughts, feelings. Culture and may also dictate the meaning of mental health, expression and experiences of symptoms, and coping. By deepening the understanding of Latina/o culture, mental health providers can strengthen the delivery and quality of services. Following is a discussion of cultural values and norms.

Cultural Values and Beliefs

Cultural values are conceptualized as conscious or unconscious culturally significant assumptions upon which a group centers its thinking, feelings, and behaviors. Cultural values also relate to "cultural nuances or unwritten rules" that may direct social interactions (National Alliance for Hispanic Health 2001). Although Latino subgroups are heterogeneous, research demonstrates that adherence to these values remain. A brief overview of Latina/o cultural values is provided.

Familismo refers to the deep affection, respect, and connectedness among family members that permeates Latina/o culture (Falicov 1998). The cultural value and practice of *familismo* stems from a collectivist worldview that includes a willingness to sacrifice the self for the welfare of the family, and an allocentric worldview where individuals understand their selves through others, emphasize relationships, and focus on group goals. *Familismo* reflects solidarity, family pride, loyalty, reciprocity, mutual empathy, and a sense of belonging to one's family. Irrespective of generation and acculturation, Latina/os place special emphasis, sentiment, closeness, and value upon the family when compared to Whites and the U.S.

population in general (Santiago-Rivera, Arredondo, and Gallardo-Cooper 2002).

Among Latina/os, the family has been described as the basic social unit and the single most important institution. In general, Latina/os have a strong family orientation and value close relationships with family, including immediate and extended family members. A unique embodiment of *familismo* involves the extension of the family system: one between *padrinos* (godparents) and *ahijados* (godchildren), and the other between the parents and the godparents, who become *compadres* and *comadres* (coparents). In Latina/o culture, to be chosen as a *padrino* or *madrina* (godparent) is a great honor and associated with significant status within the family (for more detail see Falicov 1998, Santiago-Rivera et al. 2002).

Latina/o families tend to value interdependence over independence, cohesiveness and cooperation over competition, and harmony over confrontation. Shared decision making among the family may be common and family members may be considered, and consulted, when making decisions due to the cohesiveness and interdependence of family members (Santiago-Rivera et al. 2002). *Familismo* also entails respect, deference, and obedience to parents, elders, and revered relatives throughout the life cycle. Moreover, Latina/os place a high value upon children, parents, family unity, and family honor.

This collectivist orientation provides Latina/os with a great deal of support, as it manifests itself within a shared responsibility to care for children, companionship, financial and emotional support, mutual support and reciprocity, consultation, and problem solving. For Latina/os, family members are often the main source of help and provide strong support for each other during difficult periods. Families are also a great source of strength that may provide self-worth and a supportive environment, especially during times of crisis.

Familismo has lifelong implications for how Latina/os place the needs of their family above self and how they maintain the strength of the family bond. Both strengths and challenges may be experienced as adherence to *familismo* provides a great deal of support but also results in increased responsibility, and added stress and increased conflict when family members do not adhere to this cultural script (Rivera et al. 2008). Unfortunately, when viewed with a Eurocentric lens, Latina/o families and their closeness have been misunderstood and pathologized (Falicov 1998). However, when viewed through a cultural lens, close family relationships and sacrificing for the benefit of the family are normative within Latina/o culture. Thus, mental health professionals are urged to view *familismo* as a source of strength and a resource that can buffer distress.

Indeed, research indicates that family cohesion may increase life satisfaction and health and also serve as a protective factor (Hill, Bush, and Roosa 2003). Strong family ties provide a safety net, protection and/or relief from life's hardships, and security that help is always available. Clearly, family cohesion and a strong family support system serve to mitigate psychological distress. Clinicians who work with Latina/os are strongly advised to examine their biases about family structure and closeness, maintain a Latina/o cultural lens when exploring the specific meanings of closeness and attachment, and work with the family's personal construction and unique background. It is important to note that while *familismo* is a Latina/o value, family organization and structure may vary greatly. Heterogeneity exists among and within Latina/o families which may include cultural differences, acculturation differences, language differences, difference in adherence to values, and spiritual and religious differences, among others. Working with each family's unique background is critical.

Respeto refers to the high cultural value of respect and mutual deference afforded to individuals (Añez et al. 2008). *Respeto* also includes tactfulness, diplomacy, being well-mannered, respectable, and always showing respect to others. In addition, this cultural value encourages cooperative behavior, creates a boundary within which conversations should be contained to avoid conflict, and discourages confrontation due to the fear of committing *una falta de respeto* (an act of disrespect)—a great offense within Latina/o culture (Añez et al. 2008, Santiago-Rivera et al. 2002). Further, interactions occur within a hierarchical structure, and *respeto* represents sensitivity to the individual's position such that elders, parents, professionals, and authority figures are afforded deference. *Respeto* is also displayed through the use of titles, such as *Don, Doña, Señor,* and *Señora* that reinforce relational boundaries and hierarchical positions (Añez et al. 2008, Santiago-Rivera et al. 2002). Thus, *respeto* relates to being aware of a level of courtesy and decorum required within interactions with others and social situations.

While Latina/o families may be characterized as having "affectional closeness and cohesion" (Falicov 1998), boundaries between parents and children are fairly impermeable due to the value of *respeto,* which ensures that parents maintain their authority (168). A child that is *buen educado* (well-mannered and/or respectable) is highly valued among Latina/os because these children engage in appropriate and respectful behavior. Thus, children are socialized to demonstrate "proper demeanor" and respect their parents, elders, and those within positions of authority; however, adults are also expected to adhere to this code (Añez et al. 2008, Falicov 1998). As Santiago-Rivera and colleagues (2002) state "*no faltarle el respeto* (not disrespecting) is a golden rule that children and adults abide by with peers, parents, elders, and authority figures" (159). *Falta de respeto* or lack of respect is considered a personal offense among Latina/os and is a "pervasive cause" of failures within relationships, communication problems, and negative interactions (Santiago-Rivera et al. 2002). *Respeto* serves many functions, including maintaining hierarchical structure, defining boundaries within relationships, and providing directives to respond to interpersonal conflict.

Personalismo also relates to Latina/os valuing and nurturing their relationships. *Personalismo* refers to a direct interest, concern, and consideration for others, and valuing warmth rather than distance within relationships. It also refers to a preference for pleasant exchanges with others, and a belief in building nurturing, loving, intimate, and respectful relationships (Garza and Watts 2010). The intersection of the values of *familismo, respeto, and personalismo* also relate to Latina/os highly valuing privacy due to the belief that close, trustworthy relationships should be respected. *Personalismo* also reflects the belief and communication style that individuals are always more important than the task at hand. Latina/os may give someone "personalized attention which facilitates the development and maintenance of warm, genuine, and friendly exchanges" (Añez et al. 2008). Accordingly, Latina/o children are also socialized to be considerate, helpful, and use a warm approach when interacting with others.

Related to *personalismo*, Latina/os engage in *platica* (personable small talk) which eases conversation, promotes familiarity, and is a necessary prerequisite before engaging in serious conversations (Santiago-Rivera et al. 2002). This personable style of relating also encompasses Latina/os' efforts and preference for engaging in pleasant and conflict-free exchanges and interactions—behaviors that foster personal relationships. Describing others as *una persona simpatica* (a likeable person) or *buena gente* (friendly people) is used when individuals engage and display behaviors that convey value for interpersonal relationships (Añez et al. 2008). *Amabilidad* is also associated with *personalismo* as it relates to a valuing of gentility, politeness, and civility within one's demeanor, language, and communication (Falicov 1998).

Individuals who adhere to *personalismo* may avoid expressing disagreement, confrontations, communicating assertively, and direct interactions to preserve harmony within their relationships. *Personalismo* may also lead to presenting a pleasing, noncontroversial attitude, and agreeing, or at least not disagreeing, in public to preserve harmony. It also serves avoid displeasure, avoid conflict, and avoid making others uncomfortable. Thus, direct interactions and demands may not be preferred among Latina/os, as they prefer harmonious and smooth relationships. Latina/os may perceive directness as rude, insensitive to others' feelings, and as a sign of conflict and possible disrespect. Like other collectivistic cultures, Latina/os prefer indirect, implicit, and covert communication styles to preserve harmony.

Dignidad (dignity) is also related to *personalismo* and *respeto*. *Dignidad* refers to the belief that an individual, regardless of his or her position, should engage in behaviors that increase a sense of pride, thus being worthy and respected. Thus, a *falta de respeto* is perceived as a personal attack upon an individual's *dignidad* (Santiago-Rivera et al. 2002). Further, protecting an individual's *dignidad*, or sense of dignity, is considered and valued in interactions as it is a form of honor and respect.

Latina/os also maintain harmony within their relationships through the use of *indirectas*, or indirect messages, *bromas* or *choteo* (jokes and use of humor), and *dichos* (parables or proverbs) (Añez et al. 2008, Falicov 1998, Santiago-Rivera et al. 2002). Tension or discomfort associated with direct conversations is offset by *indirectas*. These are indirect messages related to the emotion of anger, and consist of criticisms that take the form of insinuations, and "diminutives used in a sarcastic way, and belittlement" (Falicov 1998, 179). The use of humor is also useful to decrease conflict and preserve harmony. *Bromas* are used as a way of making fun of situations, things, or people and may also involve exaggerations or satire to lessen tense exchanges and situations (Falicov 1998). *Indirectas* may also take the form of a *dicho*—metaphors that address themes and problems in life, and involve cultural and folk wisdom. *Dichos* are identified as a resource to acknowledge feelings, make points and convey opinions, address resistance, soften messages, and reframe perspectives or situations. The use of *indirectas* and *bromas* may avoid conflict and uncomfortable interactions, as they are covert methods of communication involving metaphorical, indirect messages, and humor. While the use of these indirect ways may decrease conflict, they may also result in outward and illusory harmony, confusion, a misunderstanding of the messages and intentions of others, concealment, and overavoidance of conflict when used excessively (Falicov 1998). Nonetheless, a balanced use of these methods is useful in acknowledging emotions while undercutting conflict.

With time, Latina/os may develop *confianza* within their interpersonal relationships which refers to a sense of trust, intimacy, and familiarity. *Confianza* implies a sense of *familismo* and informality and "ease of interpersonal comfort" that allows Latina/os to be more direct in conversations (Santiago-Rivera et al. 2002, 114). However, this intimacy and trust takes time to build, strengthens through positive interactions over time, and must be earned and maintained. Latina/os may describe their relationships in relation to this characteristic as a *persona de confianza* (trustworthy) or *de confianza* (can be trusted). Further, *una persona de confianza* may be privy to certain information, may be allowed to witness an act or personal comment, or consulted for advice. Taken together, these cultural values reflect the high importance given to relationships with family and to the qualities of positive interpersonal skills.

An intimate union and synthesis exists between spirituality, religion, and folk/cultural practices and is fundamental to Latina/o culture. These core components and interrelationships between spirituality, religion, and culture reflect Latina/os' cultural heritage as it represents a melding of their indigenous, Spanish, and African roots. Taken together, Latina/os, spirituality and religion reflects their belief in higher powers and the notion that God, destiny, fate, spirits, deities, and other higher powers, are in charge. In terms of religion and spirituality, Latina/os ultimately believe in achieving harmony with self and the higher powers (Castellanos and Gloria 2008). Unfortunately, this cultural value has been misunderstood as a fatalistic locus of control, without acknowledging the cultural context and belief in interconnectedness with all things, including the spiritual world (Santiago-Rivera et al. 2002). Interpreting this value without the context of religious views and spirituality may lead to wrong assumptions about Latina/os.

Religious and spiritual beliefs play such a significant role within the daily lives of Latina/os that they are part of their daily vernacular. These daily expressions include *solo Dios sabe* (only God knows), *en las manos de Dios* (In God's hands), *Dios sabe lo que hace* (God knows best), *es la voluntad de Dios* (it is God's will), *si Dios quiere* (if it is God's will) and *primero Dios* (God first), when speaking of their plans in the near or distant future (Falicov 1998, Santiago-Rivera et al. 2002). Within these expressions, Latina/os' belief and trust in God's will and wisdom is reflected. Latina/os summon their belief in God and higher powers as ways of coping and meaning making, particularly with life's difficulties and unfortunate life events.

In terms of religion, Latina/os are primarily Roman Catholic This religion influences the beliefs and values of many, and significantly impacts their marital, family, and community life. Catholicism consists of primarily Christian beliefs in God as a supreme being, in spiritual life after death, and in the existence of a soul. There are several important religious figures including Jesus Christ, the Virgin Mary, and other Catholic saints or *santos* who are prayed to for various specific intercessions and support. Nonetheless, the practice of the organized religion varies among Latina/os. Mexicans have been described as a devout group to whom church attendance and observance of religious holidays and rituals are vital. However, while Cubans and Puerto Ricans may partake in Catholic rituals, they may not necessarily regard church attendance as obligatory to reach God (Falicov 1998). Heterogeneity exists among subgroups, families, and communities.

Diversity also exists in the various religious ceremonies, rituals, and traditions that reflect the unique blending of Catholicism, native indigenous influences, and African elements. For instance, one of the most cherished and beloved religious figures, especially among Mexicans, is *la Virgen de Guadalupe,* patron saint of Mexico, considered "a perfect fusion of indigenous Aztec and Catholic elements" (Falicov 1998, Santiago-Rivera et al. 2002). She is the only brown-skinned virgin and is a symbol of love and hope who also "offers enormous psychological protection and unity" (Falicov 1998). In addition, among Cubans, Puerto Ricans, Dominicans and other subgroups, the practice of *santeria* exemplifies the syncretism of Catholic and African influences in which African Gods and deities, *orishas,* are worshipped in addition to Catholic figures (McNeill et al. 2008). Latina/os' unique blending of Catholic, indigenous, and African elements also incorporate magical thinking, belief in miracles, *promesas* (promises), prayers, pilgrimages, and "propitiatory rituals" to either request help or express gratitude to the higher powers (Falicov 1998, Santiago-Rivera et al. 2002).

Latina/os also place great trust, faith, and assurance in God which is reflected in the practices of *resignarse* (resignation) and *enconmendarse* (entrusting or turning over to God) (Castellanos and Gloria 2008). These practices involve giving oneself to God and resigning or releasing a concern or life difficulty, surrendering it to God, and having faith in the process, with the understanding that God knows best. These practices reflect trusting in the will and wisdom of God. Generally, Latina/os believe that life is influenced by the spiritual world and that religious beliefs provide spiritual meaning to their lives. Latina/os also believe in the importance and interconnectedness of spirituality and religion in human life and the world. These beliefs and practices are identified as important resources when encountering difficulties in life and provide healing, a sense of community, and support.

Professionals working with Latina/o clients must be knowledgeable of their specific health and illness beliefs to provide effective treatment. Researchers accept that individuals develop beliefs about illness and disease, and thus healing is facilitated by various factors including religion, spirituality, family, social roles, language, and values. Lack of cultural knowledge may create difficulties and result in inadequate care provided to Latina/o clients. Understanding Latina/os' definitions and causes of mental illness, and ways of coping are critical to their mental health care.

Nuanced differences within these beliefs may exist depending upon country of origin, adherence to spirituality and religion, and acculturation and generation level. However, most Latina/os hold beliefs, or may be socialized with beliefs, that include traditional folk illnesses and/or beliefs in spiritual or religious elements that relate to their mental health (Ortiz, Davis, and McNeill 2008). Views of mental health also stem from the historical influences of Latina/o culture originating from a combination of Spanish, indigenous, and African origins.

Mental Health and Illness Beliefs

Latina/os generally adhere to traditional cultural beliefs and practices regarding mental health and illness, which uniquely differs from White dominant cultural beliefs. Latina/os adhere to a unique view that mental health is reached through a harmony of mind, body, and spirit. Additionally, mental health is achieved through their harmonious connection with God and their relationships with others (Comas-Diaz 2006, Falicov 2009). Distress may also be caused by serious disruptions within social relations, such as family conflict and through inharmonious social interactions (Falicov 2009, Holliday 2008, Pumariega 2007). Latina/os may also view mental illness as God's will, as a test from God they must endure to demonstrate their faith, and/or caused by sinful or wrong living. In addition, they may regard mental illness as the result of a spiritual crisis (Comas-Diaz 2006, Organista 2000, Prieto, McNeill, Walls, and Gomez 2001). Thus, mental health for Latina/os is often defined by spirituality and relationships with others. Accordingly, Latina/os' views of mental illness are unique as they may be perceived as an imbalance in the mind, body, and/or spirit. Additionally, views of mental illness may include a disconnection from God, spirituality, self, family, culture, and community.

Further, some may attribute their distress to spirits, bad energy or luck, the result of a spell, hex, or supernatural event (Holliday 2008, Pumariega 2007). Some Latina/os may also incorporate spirits into their view of mental illness. For instance, spiritualism or *espiritismo* refers to the world of good and evil spirits that influence human behavior in doing good or evil. Latina/os that ascribe to these beliefs may experience spiritual and religious visions and perceive presences after the death of a loved one, hear the voice and feel the presence of God, or a ghost or spirit (Falicov 1998, Santiago-Rivera et al. 2002). Unfortunately, clinicians failing to integrate this spiritual perspective within their treatment have misdiagnosed Latina/os as having psychosis (Alegria and Woo 2009). Distress caused by any of these forms may also be experienced spiritually, emotionally, psychologically, or physically.

Views regarding mental health and illness among Latina/os involve a complex array of systems and are interpreted through their connection and harmony with God, the higher powers, and their interpersonal relationships with others. Healing takes place in the context of a larger environment that addresses mental health, physical health, spirituality, relationships, and the interconnectedness of these qualities, and also involves reconnecting with these aspects of self. Other unique views of mental health involve folk illnesses, hot/cold theories of illness, and traditional remedies and healers (for more details, see Arellano-Morales' and Rosales Meza's chapter in volume 1).

Health symptomatology also presents in the form of the mind, body, and spirit connection. Latina/os have a tendency to experience symptoms in a physical or somatic form (Alegria and Woo 2009, Willerton, Dankoski, and Martir 2008). Emotional states are not considered separate from bodily or physical reactions. Latina/os' view of mental health as an integration of mind, body, and spirit differs from Western cultures that regard the mind, body, and spirit as separate. Latina/os are likely to integrate mind-body experiences and express them somatically. For instance, Latina/os may express and experience depression and anxiety through a combination of physical and emotional complaints (Guarnaccia and Martinez 2002, National Alliance for Hispanic Health 2001). Additionally, Latina/os may be expressive of their physical and emotional pain through "rich somatic idioms" (Falicov 1998, Guarnaccia and Martinez 2002). Emotional and physiological concerns are not necessarily viewed as separate from one another, and emotional concerns are seen as capable of causing physical problems.

In addition to these interrelationships, mental health problems may not be validated within Latina/o culture (Aguilar-Gaxiola et al. 2012, Varela et al. 2007). The stigma of mental illness also exists. Some may view mental illness as a sign of weakness and lack of strength of character (Prieto et al. 2001, Varela et al. 2007). This stigma may also manifest in the form of shame, fear of being judged, and serve as a barrier to treatment. Being in therapy may be viewed as an admission of weakness, instability, or worse, being "crazy" (Vega, Rodriguez, and Ang 2010). Specifically, the label of "*loco*" (crazy or insane) and/or "*locura*" (madness) is especially troubling as it carries strong negative connotations of someone who is severely mentally ill, completely out of control, incurable, and possibly violent (Guarnaccia and Martinez 2002).

However, Latina/os make a distinction regarding folk illnesses, such as *nervios,* which are viewed with less stigma, socially understood and accepted, accepted as temporary conditions in reaction to life stressors, and viewed as curable (Falicov 1998, Varela et al. 2007). Some researchers contend that because of this stigma, physical symptoms may be viewed or taken more seriously, are perhaps a more acceptable manifestation of distress, and thus, physical symptoms or somaticizing are more of a conduit for support. This hypothesis is validated by the findings that Latina/os are more likely to present within primary health care services (Aguila-Gaxiola el al. 2012, Prieto et al. 2001, USDHHS 2001)

The expression of distress through somatic symptoms has been misunderstood and evaluated from a deficit-oriented perspective in the mental health field. In particular, the groundbreaking U.S. Surgeon General's Report on Mental Health Care (USDHHS 2001) explicitly states that the DSM-based mental health system is flawed, as it provides inadequate flexibility to account for cultural forms of distress and disorder. For example, earlier research suggested that distress expressed somatically reflected limited psychological development, a lack of insight, lack of "psychological sophistication," or an inability to express the distress within psychological terms or dimensions (Guarnaccia and Martinez 2002, USDHHS 2001). Current perspectives acknowledge that expressing distress though somatic and psychological forms are valid and reflect an individual's sociocultural context. Researchers and clinicians are beginning to acknowledge the mind/body/spirit connection and the sociocultural influences of distress for Latina/os. Additionally, they acknowledge that physical symptoms of distress may not have the same meaning as the pathology of the DSM and the medical model (National Alliance for Hispanic Health 2001, USDHHS 2001). Still, significant work is needed, as Latina/os are often misdiagnosed, mislabeled as "somaticizers," and mistreated. This inadequate care is particularly troubling as Latina/os may have higher risk for mental illness, less access to care, and encounter several barriers.

It is clear that mental health and illness for Latina/os involves "a complex interaction of physical, psychological, social, and spiritual factors" (Falicov 1998). Further, these cultural elements are interconnected and influence each other in a multitude of ways. Thus, Latina/o clients' presenting issues may contain numerous levels of interpretation depending upon the context through which their symptoms and problems are viewed (USDHHS 2001). Accordingly, researchers and clinicians call for an integration of clients' interconnected beliefs about mental health and cultural responsiveness to increase mental health access, engagement, and outcomes. Another key issue involves acknowledging cultural protective factors. To fully understand the meaning of mental health among Latina/os, we must also understand the ways they cope and the resources that serve to buffer their distress. This knowledge may allow practitioners to build upon these strengths and maximize the existing resources within the Latina/o community.

Coping Styles and Cultural Strengths: Familial and Social Support

Latina/os' high value of family and interpersonal relationships provides a great and ever present source of support. The cultural value of *familia* serves as a protective factor to mental illness, and may decrease symptomology (Ayon et al. 2010, Mendelson, Rehkopf, and Kubzansky 2008). Indeed, improvements within an individual's outlook on life and health result from treatment that incorporates the cultural value of *familismo* by focusing upon family (Garza and Watts 2010, Hill, Bush, and Roosa 2003). Latina/o families fulfill several functions that include problem solving and support during periods of crisis, mutual support and reciprocity, financial support, caretaking, consultation, emotional support, and companionship. A strong sense of *familismo* may also contribute to individual and family well-being, as family members may feel a sense of responsibility to be healthy or to become healthy to support their family.

Similarly, researchers consistently find that spirituality provides a great source of strength and coping during periods of distress. Spirituality provides the necessary elements to understand life stressors and accept problems that are often needed to move beyond difficulties and improve functioning. The mental health benefits, resources, and protective roles of family and spirituality cannot be overlooked. The cultural values of *familismo* and spirituality are critical to mental health and must be cultivated to increase wellness. Researchers suggest that interventions and programs should be grounded within the values and strengths of Latina/o culture, particularly the Latina/o family and the higher powers, to strengthen well-being and reduce or eliminate disparities. Building on these strengths is strongly suggested.

The discussion of cultural values and beliefs related to mental health and illness was provided to educate professionals in their provision of effective and quality services to Latina/os. Particularly, as data suggest that acknowledging and integrating cultural values within treatment can increase service utilization, motivation for engagement, and increase retention among Latina/o clients. A detailed explanation of Latina/o mental health research follows.

Mental Health Profile

Research findings regarding the rates of mental illness among Latina/os are mixed, with some studies reporting higher rates than Whites, others reporting lower rates than Whites, and other studies reporting similar rates to that of Whites (Alegria et al. 2008, Kessler et al. 2005). Several hypotheses have been suggested to explain these mixed findings. For instance, researchers state that the mixed findings may be attributed to within-group and between-group differences in mental illness rates and ethnocultural variability of Latina/o samples (Alegria and Woo 2009, Mendelson et al. 2008). Researchers also report methodological difficulties within these studies. These include sampling bias, untrained researchers and interviewers, diagnoses that are based upon questionnaires, use of measurements that have not been normed with Latina/os causing validity problems, and not controlling for confounding variables within analyses (Alegria and Woo 2009). Clearly, further research is needed to understand the scope of mental illness among specific Latina/o subgroups.

However, despite this knowledge, significant mental health care disparities for Latina/os continue to exist. Of great concern is the finding that these disparities in mental health care for Latina/os, and other racial/ethnic minorities, appear to be widening over time. Latina/os are at a higher risk and may suffer disproportionately from mental health disorders, particularly depression, anxiety, and substance abuse (National Alliance for Hispanic Health 2001, Rios-Ellis 2005). Latina/os may also be at increased risk for domestic violence and suicide, and may have more persistent mental health disorders (Breslau et al. 2005). Moreover, certain Latina/o subpopulations are at higher risk for mental illness and warrant immediate and further attention. These include Latinas, the elderly and their caregivers, children and youth, undocumented immigrants, the poor, lesbian, gay, and bisexual Latina/os, and Latina/o college students. Other vulnerable subgroups identified within the literature include Latina/o children, Latina/o military veterans, incarcerated Latina/os, and Latina/o professionals. These risks are heightened by the realities that mental health services provided to Latina/os are of poorer quality, and that the mental health needs among the Latina/o community are unmet and accelerating (National Alliance for Hispanic Health 2001, USDHHS 2001). These mental health disparities may increase the burden of disability from mental health problems and contribute to decreased health and resiliency.

A deeper investigation of the literature reveals key within-group differences in regards to the mental health of the Latina/o population. Interestingly, research indicates that higher rates of mental illness are found among U.S.-born Latina/os than recent Latina/o immigrants (Alegria et al. 2007,

Ortega et al. 2000). This phenomenon is regarded as the "immigrant or Latina/o paradox." Similarly, the "acculturation hypothesis" suggests that Latina/os who immigrated and are long-term residents of the U.S. experience a decline in mental health (Cook et al. 2009, Vega et al. 2004). These findings indicate that increased residence within the United States is associated with mental health problems for Latina/os.

However, researchers have yet to agree about which features of the U.S. culture or exposure are related to mental health. Findings related to the immigrant paradox have perplexed the field, as it was hypothesized that immigrants experienced additional stressors related to their disadvantaged socioeconomic status and adjustment to a new country. However, other researchers hypothesize that U.S.-born Latina/os may have a weaker affiliation with Latino values including family cohesiveness and spirituality which serve as protective factors against mental illness (Cook et al. 2009, Finch and Vega 2003). Additional hypotheses to explain these findings include increased intergenerational conflict among the family as contact with the U.S. culture increases, which may result in increased loneliness and isolation, decreased support, and a sense of belongingness that may limit Latina/os' protection against mental illness (Alegria and Woo 2009, Alegria et al. 2007, Cook et al. 2009).

Moreover, researchers hypothesize that declining levels of mental health among U.S.-born Latina/os and longtime residents are related to their higher expectations for quality of life because of citizen status and acquisition of skills. In addition, pressures to assimilate and acculturate, perceived inferior social status to that of the dominant culture, and exposure to racial/ethnic discrimination, U.S.-born Latina/os' mental health declines over time (Alegria and Woo 2009). Discrimination and unfulfilled expectations for quality of life may result in decreased levels of mental health. Continued research is needed as it is troubling that these findings suggest that exposure to U.S. culture may be detrimental to the mental health of Latina/os.

Researchers also report variability within rates of mental illness when the Latina/o population is separated into subgroups (Alegria and Woo 2009). Data suggest that Puerto Ricans have higher rates of psychiatric disorders (Alegria et al. 2008). Other data suggest that this may be found among Puerto Ricans who reside on the mainland but not on the island (USDHHS 2001). This supports the immigrant paradox hypothesis; however, researchers argue that higher rates of mental illness among Puerto Ricans may be related to a century of U.S. influence (Alegria and Woo 2009, Guarnaccia et al. 2005). The immigrant paradox appears to be consistent among Mexicans in relation to depressive, anxiety, and substance-abuse disorders

(Alegria et al. 2008). One finding that contradicts the immigrant paradox is research that finds that Cuban Americans South Florida report improvement in mental health when compared to Cuban immigrants and U.S.-born Latina/os (Turner and Gil 2002). Researchers hypothesize that this is due to the strong socioeconomic and political base that this community has developed (Rios-Ellis 2005).

These findings point to two different narratives related to Latina/o mental health. The first relates to an improved socioeconomic profile compared to individuals from their country of origin, while the second narrative relates to a perceived inferior social status relative to the White dominant culture (Alegria and Woo 2009). The social stressors Latina/os experience related to discrimination and perceived inferior status, even with education and employment, may lead to increased risk and lower mental health rates. Nonetheless, researchers also identify protective factors for Latina/os, such as family cohesion and support, strong cultural values, and religion and spirituality, which may be fostered to provide resiliency.

This profile highlights the reality that Latina/os differ from the mainstream population in important ways that impact their experience in the United States and with their mental health. Accordingly, providing mental health services to Latina/os must address the permeating influence of culture, regardless of contextual and individual differences, and the social inequities which they face. An understanding of the sociocultural and systemic factors that may infringe upon the mental health of Latina/os is critical, particularly as the inequities and disparities within mental health are largely related to social and economic factors that restrict access to quality care. Failure to address these underlying social and economic inequalities will result in failed or compromised approaches, as they fail to acknowledge the larger systems that serve to oppress Latina/os. Thus, a discussion of these barriers follows.

Barriers to Mental Health and Care

Latina/os demonstrate low utilization rates and encounter significant mental health barriers. Moreover, mental health disparities are complicated by premature termination and substandard mental health care. While these barriers differ among Latina/os, an ecological perspective is helpful in understanding the influence of individual, cultural, organizational, and societal factors. Further, discrimination is separately discussed, as it is experienced across these levels and research consistently identifies discrimination as a barrier to mental health.

Individual Barriers

Poverty and low socioeconomic status are significantly identified with low rates of utilization of mental health services rates among Latina/os (Bledsoe 2008, USDHHS 2001). However, research also suggests that individual characteristics, such as age, gender, educational level, and immigration status contribute to mental health barriers (Dupree et al. 2010). There is differential availability of mental health services among various age groups, with insufficient services for young and elderly Latina/os who often present with multiple needs and problems. For instance, Latina/o children experience a higher rate of unmet needs and utilization of mental health services than their White counterparts (Lopez, Bergren, and Painter 2008). Similarly, while the elderly comprise a smaller proportion of Latina/os, they also present with significant unmet needs for mental health services, as well as problems that may compete with their mental health concerns, such as poverty and health problems (Barrio et al. 2008, Dupree et al. 2010).

Gender is also a barrier, as Latino men are less likely to seek mental health treatment due to cultural notions that it is emasculating for them (Bledsoe 2008). Thus, it is not surprising that Latino men may prefer to remain self-reliant rather than enter therapy when experiencing psychological difficulties. Educational level is also associated with knowledge of available resources, income, degree of acculturation, and English proficiency (Bledsoe 2008). An understanding of mental health treatment is associated with higher levels of educational attainment and this understanding is also associated with the utilization of services. Latina/os are often distrustful of the mental health system, due to the legacy of racism within medical and mental health institutions (Falicov 1998). Anti-immigrant sentiment and fear of deportation also prevent Latina/os from seeking mental health care (Cabassa 2007, Vega and Lopez 2001).

Cultural Barriers

Level of English proficiency is regarded as a barrier, as most mental health services are provided in English. This is due to the limited number of Spanish-speaking mental health providers (Bledsoe 2008, USDHHS 2001). Unfortunately, Latina/os with limited English proficiency are less likely to receive mental health treatment and while in treatment face the risk of misdiagnosis and inappropriate treatment, as well as dissatisfaction, and premature termination. Latina/os in need of psychological care may prefer other types of resources rather than seeking mental health providers. These resources may include alternative healers or other sources of help such as natural remedies, religion, and consultations with friends or family.

These preferences are also related to cultural beliefs regarding mental illness and treatment. Latina/os may view their physical and psychological concerns as inseparable, as well as view emotional problems as a sign of weakness, a lack of strength or character, or the result of a supernatural phenomenon. Thus, working with a mental health provider is regarded as an admission of weakness or instability, as only the insane require mental health services. These perspectives are also associated with the stigma of mental illness. Latina/os are more likely to seek a physician for their psychological difficulties to avoid the stigma of seeing a mental health provider.

Organizational Barriers

Organizational factors such as geographic location, cost, scheduling of services, and availability of Spanish-speaking or bilingual providers also create mental health barriers (Barrio et al. 2008). Geographic location is a salient barrier particularly among Latina/os with limited transportation and funds. Mental health facilities that require significant travel are burdensome, as well as costly. Cost is a significant barrier to access, as a large number of Latina/os lack sufficient health insurance coverage or financial resources to afford mental health care (USDHHS 2001). Latina/os employed within low-wage positions do not have the ability to take time off from their place of employment to attend a therapy session, as doing so may entail financial hardship. Similarly, insurance co-payments or deductibles are often unaffordable. Limited evening or weekend appointments also pose challenges for Latina/os with inflexible work schedules or family responsibilities.

Limited availability of bilingual and bicultural services is also a significant barrier, particularly among monolingual Spanish-speaking Latina/os or individuals who prefer to work with a Spanish-speaking provider (Vega and Lopez 2001). Even highly acculturated, middle-class Latina/os may prefer to work with a bilingual/bicultural mental health provider who is familiar with their cultural background and unique worldviews (Bledsoe 2008). Unfortunately, experiences of racism within clinical settings and ineffective mainstream mental health approaches contribute to client dissatisfaction and premature termination among Latina/os (Sue et al. 2007). The lack of culturally sensitive assessments and treatment approaches also play a vital role in Latina/os' skepticism regarding the efficacy of mainstream mental health approaches and further contribute to disparities.

Discrimination

Most research documenting the adverse consequences of discrimination against Latina/os has focused upon Latina/os of Mexican-origin; less is known about the discriminatory experiences of other subgroups (for a review see Araújo Dawson 2009, Araújo and Borrell 2006). This literature supports the association between discrimination and poor mental health among Latina/os such as psychological distress, decreased psychological well-being, and depression (Flores et al. 2008, Zhang et al. 2012). Discrimination against Latina/os results in significant deterioration in mental health, education, and employment (Lee and Ahn 2012). Mental health indicators have the strongest associations with discrimination, such as depression, anxiety, psychological distress, job dissatisfaction, and unhealthy behaviors. Discrimination is also associated with health outcomes, such as health symptoms, somatization, and cardiovascular responses (Alamilla et al. 2010, Salomon and Jagusztyn 2008).

Language is also associated with discrimination among Latina/os. Discrimination based upon use of Spanish, accent, and limited English proficiency is experienced (Goodkind et al. 2008, Smith and Mannon 2010). Even middle-class Latina/os are ignored or silenced because of their accent (Cobas and Feagin 2008). Latina/os may also experience discrimination based upon their facial features and phenotype such as darker skin (Pew Hispanic Center 2004, Ramos et al. 2003). Black Latina/os are likely to be racialized due to their darker complexions and experience internalized racism (Araújo Dawson and Panchanadeswaran 2010).

Although researchers have documented how Latina/os experience various forms of racism within the United States from Whites, empirical research regarding within-group discrimination is sparse. Nonetheless, this research suggests that language and nativity are associated with within group discrimination (Córdova and Cervantes 2010). Rosenbloom and Way (2004) found that Puerto Rican and Dominican adolescents discriminated against one another and that foreign-born Latina/os experienced discrimination from their U.S.-born counterparts due to immigration, assimilation, and language. Additional research supports the finding that foreign-born Latina/os may also experience discrimination from their U.S.-born counterparts due to their English proficiency, citizenship, and generational status (Córdova and Cervantes 2010). To address the aforementioned cultural contexts, the following practices have been suggested.

Research on Effective Treatments and Practice

The unmet mental health needs of Latina/os are well-documented within the literature. It is also well-documented that the mental health field has failed to provide culturally responsive services. Specifically, research demonstrates that few Latina/os have access or are able to access mental health services. Further, Latina/os in the mental health system experience poorer quality services, poor treatment outcomes, lack of engagement, poor client-provider interactions, discrimination, high dropout rates, and also feel misunderstood (Aguilar-Gaxiola et al. 2012, Falicov 2009). These findings make sense when considering that mental health services often mirror the oppression that Latina/os experience within American society. For instance, given that existing mental health services and treatments were developed for White clients, and that the core components of illness, health, and therapeutic change were based upon the norms and values of the White dominant culture, it seems logical to question whether these therapies and therapeutic constructs fit the realities of Laina/os' lives (Falicov 2009).

Unfortunately, even therapeutic encounters for Latina/os may add to their oppression as often "therapists may unwittingly cause stress by encouraging rapid acculturation to new ways of thinking or behaving" to reflect and/or benefit the White dominant culture (Falicov 2009, 293). However, modifying existing treatments and/or creating new forms of therapy that are culturally and contextually relevant to Latina/os provides promise in rectifying mental health disparities (Falicov 2009). Findings indicate that these types of treatments may increase access, utilization, and effectiveness for Latina/o clients (Garza and Watts 2010, Griner and Smith 2006, Miranda et al. 2003). Treatments specifically developed for Latina/os hold the most promise, as they reflect and respond to their culture-specific views of mental health and illness (Bernal and Jimenez-Caffey 2009, Griner and Smith 2006). There are various examples of effective practices and treatments that are provided to Latina/os; those discussed will include culturally competent and best practices, cultural adaptations of existing therapies, and culture-specific treatments.

Cultural Competence

Directives for working with Latina/o clients include providing bilingual and bicultural staff, materials, and clinicians, providing knowledge related to the culture and histories of Latina/o groups, and integrating cultural values and family preferences into the treatment of Latina/o clients and their families. These suggestions also include integrating the value of *res-peto* by respecting the hierarchical structure of families and using titles such as *Señor* and *Señora* when referring to clients, *personalismo* by demonstrating genuine interest in the Latina/o client rather than procedures, the cultural value of religion and spirituality by accounting for spiritual beliefs in treatment, and *familismo* by involving family members within the therapeutic process, accounting for the influence of the client's change upon the family, and accounting for family goals (Añez et al. 2008, Calzada, Fernandez, and Cortes 2010, Gonzalez-Prendes, Hindo, and Pardo 2011). Acknowledging and integrating Latina/o cultural values and cultural family preferences into treatment can increase service utilization, engagement and collaboration, and retention of Latina/o clients and result in positive outcomes. Further, maintaining a flexible time frame along with a personalized approach in treatment is suggested. In terms of the methods and process of therapy, providers should remain present oriented, focus upon problem solving, and provide suggestions for immediate symptom relief (Falicov 1998, Organista 2000). Attending to culture-specific beliefs about mental health and illness is critical (Cardemil and Sarmiento 2009). Using a social justice perspective is also recommended, given that many of the stressors that Latina/os experience are related to social inequities.

Cultural Adaptations

Another way researchers and clinicians have accounted for culture in the mental health field relates to modifying aspects of a psychological construct, program, therapeutic approach, and/or adapting existing empirically supported treatments to make them more culturally appropriate (Castro, Barrera, and Martinez 2004, Falicov 2009). Researchers are beginning to distinguish between the types of cultural adaptations that exist. Cardemil and Sarmiento (2009) distinguish between superficial or surface and deep or core modifications. Superficial modifications may include changing the location of the treatment program to meet the needs of the population or changing the ethnicity of characters in an intervention to reflect clients. Core modifications may include modifying content to integrate cultural values into program delivery through using relevant cultural expressions, interaction styles, and innovative techniques that reflect the lives of Latina/os. Examples of this approach include the study of parenting styles in cultural context (Domenech-Rodriguez 2011) which incorporates the highly valued cultural value of *respeto* into Latina/o parenting programs. Additional examples include the variability of emotional expression in Latina/o families

(Lopez 2009), and adapting Cognitive Behavioral Therapy (CBT) to Latina/o culture (Gonzalez-Prendes, Hindo, and Pardo 2011, Miranda et al. 2003, Organista 2006).

CBT is identified as a useful intervention for Latina/o clients, as it appears to be congruent with their treatment goals, including immediate symptom relief, services that are time-limited, directive intervention such as guidance, and a problem-solving approach (Organista 2000). Further, CBT may provide psychoeducation to clients to help "demystify" therapy and may alleviate stigma (Organista and Munoz 1996, 259). While CBT may be a useful treatment, researchers emphasize tailoring the content, goals, and methods to include Latina/o culture, as this impacts the cognitive and behavioral process, facilitates cognitive restructuring, and may result in improved access and outcomes (Organista 2000). Some of the cultural adaptations to CBT have involved the use of *dichos* to help clients understand the importance of active and behavioral coping strategies (Interian and Diaz-Martinez 2007, Organista 2000). In particular, the culturally relevant *dichos* or proverbs *"Ayudate, que Dios te ayudara"*(God helps those who help themselves) or *"Dios dijo, ayudate que yo te ayudara"* (God said, help yourself and I will help you) incorporate Latina/o spiritual beliefs and address the cultural value of accepting God's will, while also addressing the importance of shifting into a more active direction (Organista 2000). Additionally, the *dicho "Poner de su parte"* (Doing your/their part) is used when framing the purpose of implementing behavioral techniques within therapy. The use of this proverb with Latina/o clients allows them to recognize that this aspect of therapy provides an opportunity to *poner de su parte* to improve their mental health and functioning (Interian and Diaz-Martinez 2007).

Strengths of cultural adaptations include the significant modifications that integrate culture into constructs, typologies, and techniques to make treatment more relevant for clients and increase engagement (Cardemil and Sarmiento 2009). These modifications may result in decreased dropout rates, increased access and utilization of services, and may even help to reduce disparities within treatment. Research reports that cultural adaptations have produced effective outcomes for Latina/os within the treatment of depression (Cardemil and Sarmiento 2009). Moreover, Falicov (2009) states that these types of therapies may present a middle ground for the treatment of Latina/o and other ethnic minority clients. Further, whether these modifications compromise the evidence-based research of the original treatments is yet to be determined (Falicov 2009). There is some concern that in adding new components for cultural relevance the treatment is not equivalent, or is more complex, and thus the research and measuring outcomes may be compromised (Castro, Barrera, and Martinez 2004). However, studies have not compared whether these cultural adaptations for Latina/os are more effective than those same treatments that are not adapted for Latina/o clients (Cardemil and Sarmiento 2009, Falicov 2009). Nonetheless, there are several advantages to these types of treatment and positive outcomes have been seen with Latina/o clients.

Culture Specific Treatments

Additional forms of integrating culture involve therapies known as either culture specific therapies or culturally centered therapies (Cardemil and Sarmiento 2009, Falicov 2009). These therapies are based upon the assumption that cultures have their own healing approaches and that traditional forms of psychotherapy are inappropriate as they impose and are rooted within White middle-class values (Cardemil and Sarmiento 2009, Falicov 2009). These types of therapies also argue that it would be "theoretically incongruent to provide a traditional form of psychotherapy for culturally specific expressions of distress" (Cardemil and Sarmiento 2009, 337). Examples of culture specific therapies include *cuento* therapy (Constantino, Malgady, and Rogler 1986), a groundbreaking therapy inspiring similar types of therapies. *Cuento* therapy was developed for at-risk Puerto Rican adolescents experiencing anxiety, low self-esteem, and behavioral difficulties. Adolescents participated in group therapy that used cultural folktales based upon Puerto Rican culture to serve as role models that overcame difficult circumstances. The group served to provide support in a culturally relevant manner, and also increased the participant's connection with their parents and culture (Constantino, Malgady, and Rogler 1986). Similarly, a *Dichos* therapy group was developed for hospitalized Spanish-speaking psychiatric patients who also benefitted from a multimodal treatment approach. Discussion and use of *dichos* formed a central focus of the therapy group. Outcomes of the group included positive attitudes toward therapy and increased functioning (Aviera 1996). Further, ethnopolitical psychology argues that healing arises from critical consciousness and sociopolitical action. This therapy acknowledges the context of oppression among people of color, validates their identity and experience, and emphasizes the importance of working together for liberation from oppression (Comas-Diaz 2006). Finally, it is also important to acknowledge the culture-specific therapies that focus upon spirituality, religion, the higher powers, and indigenous practices and rituals as healing.

Strengths of culturally centered therapies consist of their focus upon wellness, and their ability to validate and address psychosocial and sociocultural stressors within the lives of Latina/os. Cardemil and Sarmiento (2009) also identify the congruence between conceptualization of the problem and treatment approach as a strength. These therapies offer much promise because they are grounded within Latina/o culture and thus may provide culture-specific healing that may not be achieved through other types of treatments. Still, it is important to recognize that the specificity may limit the generalizability of these treatments.

Each of these treatment models provides the potential to decrease disparities as they address various types of distress. Given the heterogeneity of the Latina/o population, the ways in which they integrate culture into mental health care also offers various approaches to meet the needs of the Latina/o community.

Conclusion

Mental health disparities among Latina/os are well documented and continue to persist despite continued research. It is clear that reducing these disparities must involve partnerships and an integrated approach with several systems, such as primary health care systems and local Latina/o communities. Further, a multilayered and culturally sensitive approach is necessary given that Latina/os endorse beliefs about mental health and illness that are holistic and stressors that are comprehensive and systemic. It is hoped that the information provided within this chapter contributes to the wellness of the Latina/o community and serves to reduce disparities in the mental health field.

References

Aguilar-Gaxiola, S., G. Loera, L. Mendez, M. Sala, Concilio, and J. Nakamoto. 2012. "Community Defined Solutions for Latino Mental Health Disparities: California Reducing Disparities Project, Latino Strategic Planning Workgroup Population Report." Sacramento, CA: UC Davis.

Alamilla, S. G., B. S. K. Kim, and N. A. Lam. 2010. "Acculturation, Enculturation, Perceived Racism, Minority Status Stressors, and Psychological Symptomatology among Latino/as." *Hispanic Journal of Behavioral Sciences* 32: 55–76.

Alegria, M., G. Canino, R. Rios, M. Vera, J. Calderon, D. Rusch, et al. 2002. "Inequalities in the Use of Specialty Mental Health Services among Latino, African Americans, and Non-Latino Whites." *Psychiatric Services* 53: 1547–1555.

Alegria, M., P. Chatterji, K. Wells, Z. Cao, C. N. Chen, D. Takeuchi, et al. 2008. "Disparity in Depression Treatment among Racial and Ethnic Minority Populations in the United States." *Psychiatric Services* 59(11): 1264–72.

Alegria, M., N. Mulvaney-Day, M. Torres, A. Polo, Z. Cao, and G. Canino. 2007. "Prevalence of Psychiatric Disorders across Latino Subgroups in the United States." *American Journal of Public Health* 97(1): 68–75.

Alegria, M. and M. Woo. 2009. "Conceptual Issues in Latino Mental Health." In *Handbook of U.S. Latino Psychology Developmental and Community-Based Perspectives,* edited by F.A. Villareal, G. Carlo, J. M Grau, M. Azmitia, N. J. Cabrera, and T. J. Chahin, 15–30. Thousand Oaks, CA: Sage.

Añez, L. M., M. A. Silva, M. J. Paris, and L. E. Bedregal. 2008. "Engaging Latinos through the Integration of Cultural Values and Motivational Interviewing Principles." *Professional Psychology: Research and Practice* 39(2): 153–159.

Araújo, B. Y. and L. N. Borrell. 2006. "Understanding the Link Between Discrimination, Mental Health Outcomes, and Life Chances among Latinos." *Hispanic Journal of Behavioral Sciences* 28: 245–266.

Araújo Dawson, B. 2009. "Discrimination, Stress, and Acculturation among Dominican Immigrant Women." *Hispanic Journal of Behavioral Sciences* 31: 96–111.

Araújo Dawson, B. and S. Panchanadeswaran. 2010. "Discrimination and Acculturative Stress among First-Generation Dominicans." *Hispanic Journal of Behavioral Sciences* 32: 216–231.

Aviera, A. 1996. "'Dichos' Therapy Group: A Therapeutic Use of Spanish Language Proverbs with Hospitalized Spanish-Speaking Psychiatric Patients." *Cultural Diversity and Mental Health* 2: 73–87.

Ayon, C., F. F. Marsiglia, and M. Bermudez-Parsai. 2010. "Latino Family Mental Health: Exploring the Role of Discrimination and Familismo." *Journal of Community Psychology* 38(6): 742–756.

Barrio, C., L. A. Palinkas, A. Yamada, D. Fuentes, V. Criado, P. Garcia, et al. 2008. "Unmet Needs for Mental Health Services for Latino Older Adults: Perspectives from Consumers, Family Members, and Service Providers." *Community Mental Health Journal* 44: 57–74.

Bernal, G., M. I. Jimenez-Chafey, and M. M. Domenech-Rodriguez. 2009. "Cultural Adaptation of Treatments: A Resource for Considering Culture in Evidence-based Practice." *Professional Psychology: Research and Practice,* 40(4): 361–368.

Bledsoe, S. E. 2008. "Barriers and Promoters of Mental Health Services Utilization in a Latino Context: A Literature Review and Recommendations from an Ecosystems Perspective." *Journal of Human Behavior in the Social Environment* 18: 151–183.

Breslau, J., K. S. Kendler, M. Su, S. Aguilar-Gaxiola, and R. C. Kessler. 2005. "Lifetime Risk and Persistence of Psychiatric Disorders across Ethnic Groups in the United States." *Psychological Medicine* 35: 317–327.

Cabassa, L. J. 2007. "Latino Immigrant Men's Perceptions of Depression and Attitudes toward Help-Seeking." *Hispanic Journal of Behavioral Sciences* 26: 492–509.

Caldwell, A., A. Couture, and H. Nowotny. 2008. *Closing the Mental Health Gap: Eliminating Disparities in Treatment for Latinos.* SAMHSA. U.S. Department of Health and Human Services.

Calzada, E. J., Y. Fernandez, and D. E. Cortes. 2010. "Incorporating the Cultural Value of *Respeto* into a Framework of Latino Parents." *Cultural Diversity and Ethnic Minority Psychology* 16(1): 77–86.

Cardemil, E. V. and I. A. Sarmiento. 2009. "Clinical Approaches to Working with Latino Adults." In *Handbook of U.S. Latino Psychology Developmental and Community-Based Perspectives,* edited by F. A. Villareal, G. Carlo, J. M Grau, M. Azmitia, N. J. Cabrera, and T. J. Chahin, 329–345. Thousand Oaks, CA: Sage.

Castellanos, J. and A. M. Gloria. 2008. "Rese un Ave Maria y Encendi una Velita: The Use of Spirituality and Religion as a Means of Coping with Educational Experiences for Latina/o College Students." In *Latina/o Healing Practices. Mestizo and Indigenous perspectives,* edited by B. W. McNeill and J. M. Cervantes, 175–193. New York, NY: Routledge.

Castro, F. G., M. Barrera, and C. R. Martinez. 2004. "The Cultural Adaptation of Prevention Interventions: Resolving Tensions between Fidelity and Fit." *Prevention Science* 5: 41–45.

Cobas, J. A., and J. R. Feagin. 2008. "Language Oppression and Resistance: The Case of Middle Class Latinos in the United States." *Ethnic and Racial Studies* 31: 390–410.

Comas-Diaz, L. 2006. "Latino Healing: The Integration of Ethnic Psychology into Psychotherapy." *Psychotherapy: Theory, Research, Practice, Training* 43(4): 436–453.

Constantino, G., R. G. Malgady, and L. H. Rogler. 1986. "Cuento Therapy: A Culturally Sensitive Modality for Puerto Rican Children." *Journal of Consulting and Clinical Psychology* 54: 639–645.

Cook, B., M. Alegria, J. Y. Lin, and J. Guo. 2009. "Pathways and Correlates Connecting Latinos' Mental Health with Exposure to the United States." *American Journal of Public Health* 99(12): 2247–2254.

Córdova, D., and R. C. Cervantes, R. 2010. "Intergroup and Within-Group Perceived Discrimination among U.S. Born and Foreign Born Latino Youth." *Hispanic Journal of Behavioral Sciences* 32: 259–274.

Domenech-Rodríguez, M. M., A. Baumann, and A. Swartz. 2011. "Cultural Adaptation of an Empirically Supported Intervention: From Theory to Practice in a Latino/a Community Context." *American Journal of Community Psychology,* 47: 170–186.

Dupree, L. W., J. R. Herrera, D. M. Tyson, Y. Jang, and B. L. King-Kallimanis. 2010. "Age Group Differences in Mental Health Care Preferences and Barriers among Latinos: Implications for Research and Practice." *Best Practices in Mental Health* 6: 47–59.

Falicov, J. C. 1998. *Latino Families in Therapy: A Guide to Multicultural Practice.* New York, NY: Guilford Press.

Falicov, J. C. 2009. "Commentary: On the Wisdom and Challenges of Culturally Attuned Treatments for Latinos." *Family Process* 48(2): 292–309.

Finch, B. K. and W. A. Vega. 2003. "Acculturation Stress, Social Support, and self-Rated Health among Latinos in California." *Journal of Immigrant Health* 5(3): 109–117.

Flores, E., J. M. Tschann, J. M. Dimas, E. A. Bachen, L. A. Pasch, and C. L. de Groat. 2008. "Perceived Discrimination, Perceived Stress, and Mental and Physical Health Among Mexican-Origin Adults." *Hispanic Journal of Behavioral Sciences 30*: 401–424.

Garza, Y., and R. Watts. 2010. "Filial Therapy and Hispanic Values: Common Ground for Culturally Sensitive Helping." *Journal of Counseling and Development 88*(1): 108–113.

Gonzalez-Prendes, A. A., C. Hindo, and Y. Pardo. 2011. "Cultural Values Integration in Cognitive-Behavioral Therapy for a Latino with Depression." *Clinical Case Studies 10*(5): 376–394.

Goodkind, J. R., M. Gonzales, L. H. Malcoe, and J. Espinoza. 2008. "The Hispanic Women's Social Stressor Scale: Understanding the Multiple Social Stressors of U.S.- and Mexico-Born Hispanic Women." *Hispanic Journal of Behavioral Sciences 30*: 200–229.

Griner, D., and T. B. Smith. 2006. "Culturally Adapted Mental Health Interventions: A Meta-Analytic Review." *Psychotherapy: Theory, Research, Practice, Training 43*: 531–548.

Guarnaccia, P. J. and I. Martinez. 2002. *Comprehensive In-Depth Literature Review and Analysis of Latino Mental Health Issues.* Report summoned by and property of: Changing Minds, Advancing Mental Health for Latinos. New Jersey Mental Health Institute.

Guarnaccia, P. J, I. Martinez, R. Ramirez, and G. Canino. 2005. "Are Ataques de Nervios in Puerto Rican Children Associated with Psychiatric Disorder?" *Journal of American Academic Child and Adolescent Psychiatry 44*(11): 1184–1192.

Hill, E. N., R. K. Bush, and W. M. Roosa. 2003. "Parenting and Family Socialization Strategies and Children's Mental Health: Low-Income Mexican-American and Euro-American Mothers and Children." *Child Development 74*(1): 189–204.

Holliday, K. V. 2008. "La Limpia de San Lazaro as Individual and Collective Cleansing Rite." In *Latina/o Healing Practices. Mestizo and Indigenous Perspectives,* edited by B. W. McNeill and J. M. Cervantes, 175–193. New York, NY: Routledge.

Interian, A., and A. M. Diaz-Martinez. 2007. "Considerations for Culturally Competent Cognitive-Behavioral Therapy for Depression with Hispanic Patients." *Cognitive and Behavioral Practice 14*: 84–97.

Kessler, R., P. Berglund, O. Demler, R. Jin, and E. Walters. 2005. "Lifetime Prevalence and Age-of-Onset Distributions of DSM-IV Disorders in the National Comorbidity Survey Replication." *Archives of General Psychiatry 62*: 593–602.

Kouyoumdjian, H., B. L. Zamboanga, and D. J. Hansen. 2003. "Barriers to Community Mental Health Services for Latinos: Treatment Considerations." *Clinical Psychology: Science and Practice 10*: 394–422.

Lee, D. L. and S. Ahn. 2012. "Discrimination against Latina/os: A Meta-Analysis of Individual-Level Resources and Outcomes." *The Counseling Psychologist 40*: 28–65.

Lopez, C., M. D. Bergren, and S. G. Painter. 2008. "Latino Disparities in Child Mental Health Services." *Journal of Child and Adolescent Psychiatric Nursing 21*: 137–145.

Marin, H., J. I. Escobar, W.A. Vega. 2005. "Mental Illness in Hispanics: A Review of the Literature." Developing research priorities for Latinos with persistent mental disorders, National Institute of Mental Health. *Focus 4*(1): 361–368.

McNeil, B. W., E. Esquivel, A. Carrasco, and R. Mendoza. 2008. "Santería and the Healing Process in Cuba and the United States." In *Latina/o Healing Practices. Mestizo and Indigenous Perspectives,* edited by B. W. McNeill and J. M. Cervantes, 63–82. New York, NY: Routledge.

Mendelson, T., D. H. Rehkopf, and L. D. Kubzansky. 2008. "Depression among Latinos in the United States: A Meta-Analytic Review." *Journal of Consulting and Clinical Psychology 76*(3): 355–366.

Miranda, J., J. Y. Chung, B. L. Green, J. Krupnick, J. Siddique, D. A. Revicki, et al. 2003. "Treating Depression in Predominately Low-Income Young Minority Women: A Randomized Controlled Trial." *Journal of the American Medical Association 290*: 57–65.

National Alliance for Hispanic Health. 2001. *Quality Health Services for Hispanics: The Cultural Competency Component.* Rockville, MD: Substance Abuse and Mental Health Services Administration.

Organista, K. C. 2000. "Latinos." In *Cognitive Behavioral Group Therapy: For Specific Problems and Populations,* edited by J. R. White and A. Freeman, 281–303. Washington, D. C.: American Psychological Association

Organista, K. C. 2006. "Cognitive-Behavioral Therapy with Latinos and Latinas." In *Culturally Responsive Cognitive-Behavioral Therapy: Assessment, Practice and Supervision,* edited by P. A. Hays and G. Y. Iwamasa, 73–96. Washington D.C.: American Psychological Association.

Organista, K. C. and R. F. Muñoz. 1996. "Cognitive-Behavioral Therapy with Latinos." *Cognitive and Behavioral Practice 3*: 255–270.

Ortega, A. N., R. Rosenheck, M. Alegria, and R. A. Desai. 2000. "Acculturation and the Lifetime Risk of Psychiatric and Substance Use Disorders among Hispanics." *Journal of Nervous and Mental Disorders 188*(11): 728–735.

Ortiz, F. A., K. G. Davis, and B. W. McNeill. 2008. "Curanderismo: Religious and Spiritual Worldviews and Indigenous Healing Traditions." In *Latina/o Healing Practices. Mestizo and Indigenous Perspectives,* edited by B. W. McNeill and J. M. Cervantes, 175–193. New York, NY: Routledge.

Pew Hispanic Center/Kaiser Family Foundation. 2004. *The 2004 National Survey of Latinos: Politics and Civic Participation.* Washington, D.C.: Author.

Prieto, L. R., B. W. McNeill, R. G. Walls, and S. P. Gomez. 2001. "Chicanas/os and Mental Health Services: An Overview of Utilization, Counselor Preference, and Assessment Issues." *The Counseling Psychologist 29*(1): 18–54.

Pumariega, A. 2007. "Stigma of Mental Illness in the Hispanic/Latino Community." *Healthy Minds of the American Psychiatric Association.* http://healthyminds.org/hispanicmh.cfm

Ramos, B., J. Jaccard, and V. Guilamo-Ramos. 2003. "Dual Ethnicity and Depressive Symptoms: Implications for Being Black and Latino in the United States." *Hispanic Journal of Behavioral Sciences* 25: 147–173.

Rios-Ellis, B. 2005. "Critical Disparities in Latino Mental Health: Transforming Research into Action." Institute for Hispanic Health. National Council of La Raza.

Rivera, F. I., P. J. Guarnaccia, N. Mulvaney-Day, J. Y. Lin, M. Torres, and M. Alegria. 2008. "Family Cohesion and Its Relationship to Psychological Distress among Latino Groups." *Hispanic Journal of Behavioral Sciences* 30(3): 357–378.

Rosenbloom, S. R. and N. Way. 2004. "Experiences of Discrimination among African American, Asian American, and Latino Adolescents in an Urban High School." *Youth and Society* 35: 420–451.

Salomon, K. and N. E. Jagusztyn. 2008. "Resting Cardiovascular Levels and Reactivity to Interpersonal Incivility among Black, Latina/o, and White Individuals: The Moderating Role of Ethnic Discrimination." *Health Psychology* 27: 473–481.

Santiago-Rivera, A. L., P. Arredondo, and M. Gallardo-Cooper. 2002. *Counseling Latinos and la Familia: a Practical Guide*. Thousand Oaks, CA: Sage.

Smith, R. A. and S. E. Mannon. 2010. "'Nibbling on the Margins of Patriarchy': Latina Immigrants in Northern Utah." *Ethnic and Racial Studies* 33: 986–1005.

Sue, D. W., C. W. Capodilupo, G. C. Torino, J. M. Bucceri, A. M. B. Holder, L. Kevin, K. L. Nadal, and M. Esquilin. 2007. "Racial Micro-Aggressions in Everyday Life: Implications for Clinical Practice." *American Psychologist* 62: 271–286.

Turner, R. J. and A. G. Gil. 2002. "Psychiatric and Substance Use Disorders in South Florida: Racial/Ethnic and Gender Contrasts." *Archives of General Psychiatry* 59: 43–50.

U. S. Department of Health and Human Services, Substance Abuse, and Mental Health Services Administration. 1999. *Mental Health: A Report of the Surgeon General*. Rockville, MD: U.S. Department of Health and Human Services, National Institute of Mental Health.

U.S. Department of Health and Human Services. 2001. *Mental health: Culture, Race, and Ethnicity—a Supplement to Mental Health: A Report of the Surgeon General*. Rockville, MD: U.S. Department of Health and Human Services, Substance Abuse and Mental Health Services Administration, Center for Mental Health Services.

Varela, R. E., C. F. Weems, S. L. Berman, L. Hensley, and M. C. Rodriguez de Bernal. 2007. "Internalizing Symptoms in Latinos: The Role of Anxiety Sensitivity." *Journal of Youth and Adolescence* 36: 429–440.

Vega, W. A. and S. R. Lopez. 2001. "Priority Issues in Latino Mental Health Services Research." *Mental Health Services Research* 3: 189–200.

Vega, W. A., M. A. Rodriguez, and A. Ang. 2010. "Addressing Stigma of Depression in Latino Primary Care Patients." *General Hospital Psychiatry* 32(2): 182–191.

Vega, W. A., W. M. Sribney, S. Aguilar-Gaxiola, and B. Kolody. 2004. "12-Month Prevalence of DSM-III Psychiatric Disorders among Mexican Americans:

Nativity, Social Assimilation, and Age Determinants." *Journal of Nervous and Mental Disease* 192: 532–541.

Willerton, E., E. M. Dankoski, and S. F. J. Martir. 2008. "Medical Family Therapy: A Model for Addressing Mental Health Disparities among Latinos." *Families, Systems and Health* 26(2): 196–206.

Zhang, W, S. Hong, D. T. Takeuchi, and K. N. Mossakowski. 2012. "Limited English Proficiency and Psychological Distress among Latino and Asian Americans." *Social Science and Medicine* 75: 1006–1014.

CHAPTER FOUR

Stress and Culture

Angela R. Wendorf, Amanda M. Brouwer, and Katie E. Mosack

Stress is often described as a universal experience both in the academic literature and the popular media, yet, cultural nuances in the perception and manifestation of stress are infrequently discussed. Culture has been defined broadly to include the "thoughts, beliefs, practices, and behaviors of a group of people in the areas of history, religion, social organization, economic organization, political organization, and collective production" (Slavin et al. 1991). We present a multicultural perspective to stress and coping as it relates to those with visible as well as less visible minority status and those who identify and who are identified as belonging to a numeric minority or, more frequently, to marginalized groups. Within the United States there exists a sociopolitical structure that influences the experience of being a member of a minority group and is based on the distribution of power, privilege, and resources (Valdez 2006). Disempowered and disenfranchised groups result from such a structure and these groups experience unique stressors both within the group and in the face of more dominant and privileged groups. As such, our approach to understanding a multicultural perspective to stress and coping is one which includes the subjective and objective experiences of stress (e.g., identifying and being identified with a particular cultural group). Furthermore, we will also consider the responses to stress, including coping behaviors and access to coping resources, within this context.

We first review the literature on stress, coping, and health from a multicultural perspective. In so doing, we briefly discuss the major theories of stress, specifically focusing on culture-specific stressors and the sociopolitical and sociocultural contexts in which stress is experienced among groups whose members are more frequently disenfranchised and disempowered. We then briefly review major theories of coping and how individuals from different cultural groups cope with stress. Finally, we examine the extant literature on how cultural identity and resources buffer the deleterious effects of stressors. We conclude with a summary, implications for intervention and future directions in multicultural stress and coping research.

Stress is a dynamic, multidimensional construct involving the cognitive appraisal of external or internal demands and the assessment as to whether the demands exceed one's resources to address and mitigate the source of stress (Lazarus 1976, Lazarus and Folkman 1984). Several theoretical approaches to stress exist, including a focus on biological activity and physiological responses (e.g., fight or flight response, Cannon 1914; e.g., general adaptation syndrome, Selye 1956), the cognitive appraisal model (Lazarus 1966), and sex differences with respect to the stress response (e.g., tend and befriend theory; Taylor et al. 2000). Researchers have explored the sources (Padilla and Correro 2006), outcomes (e.g., physical and mental health, Clark et al. 1999, Gurung and Roethel-Wendorf 2009, Myers 2009, Cochran and Mays 2007, Lehavot and Simoni 2011), and ways of coping with stress (e.g., problem-focused, emotion-focused, and avoidant coping, Lazarus and Folkman 1984), but the approach to understanding stress from a multicultural perspective has not received as much attention (Folkman and Moskowitz 2004, Somerfield and McCrae 2000, Wong, Wong, and Scott 2006). That is, conceptualizing multicultural stress within the framework of current stress theories limits the degree to which we are able to understand how minority groups, (e.g., status as a result of power, privilege and resources) appraise and experience stress (Valdez 2006). Therefore, an examination of the influence of culturally-mediated experiences (e.g. experiences from groups of persons from a variety of multicultural perspectives including but not limited to race, ethnicity, sexual orientation and socioeconomic backgrounds) have on the appraisal, experience, and reaction to stress is needed in order to develop and enrich cross-cultural competence in the understanding, assessment, and management of stress.

Many have argued that current models of stress fail to consider the context in which stress and the coping process occur, omitting core factors which influence both the subjective and objective experience of stress (Chun, Moos, and Cronkite 2006, Slavin et al. 1991). More specifically, researchers have argued that culture is a key aspect affecting the appraisal, experience, and ability and resources to cope with stress from both internal and external sources (Chun et al. 2006, Slavin et al. 1991). Therefore, to better understand stress from a multicultural perspective, one must consider the influence of culture on the individual (e.g., personality, self-construct, values, motivation, etc.), the environment (e.g., neighborhood, group norms and expectations, etc.), and the dynamic relationship between the two.

Minority Status

Understanding the degree to which both external factors (e.g., socio-economic status, lack of access to care and education) and interpersonal factors (e.g., visible minority status) affect the nature and frequency of potentially stressful life events for persons in the cultural minority can aid in addressing the negative outcomes of such events. Membership in a minority group can affect the quality and degree of a potentially stressful event (Slavin et al. 1991, Valdez 2006). That is, having a minority status in a classroom, restaurant, or workplace, for example, could bring about different stressors and consequently bring about more stress than for those in the cultural majority. It may, for instance, be more difficult to find grocery stores that provide ethnically diverse foods, hair salons with skilled professionals to cut different hair types, or social establishments open to one's sexual orientation. Moreover, the experience of heightened visibility and consequently constant threat awareness and lack of anonymity for those in the cultural minority living within a cultural majority setting serves as an additional source of social and interpersonal stress.

Those with minority status tend to be more vulnerable to distressing life events due to lack of political power, lower socio-economic status, limited resources, and poorer health statuses (Chun et al. 2006, Lio et al. 2011). Members of sexual minorities report experiencing more distressing life events too. For example, Corliss and colleagues (2011) found that the odds of being homeless were between 4 and 13 times greater for adolescent lesbian, gay, and bisexual youth compared to their heterosexual peers. Sexual minority persons also report greater risk taking behaviors such as drinking, smoking, and drug use compared to their peers (Hamilton and Mahalik 2009, Hughes et al. 2010). Distressing life circumstances such as lower socio-economic status and greater risk and burden of disease increase the occurrence of perceived and objectively experienced stressful life events and have been consistently associated with poorer health outcomes (Mwachofi and Broyles 2007, Repetti, Taylor, and Seeman 2002).

Illness can be an enduring source of perceived and experienced stress that is directly related to one's cultural status. Comparing heterosexual women with sexual minority women (e.g., lesbian or bisexual), McNair and colleagues (2011) found that women in the sexual minority experienced poorer mental health and greater use of health care services (owing, in large part, to a greater prevalence of depression). In this same study, sexual minority women reported lower satisfaction with their health care providers and less continuity of health care service when compared to heterosexual women. Similar outcomes were reported for persons belonging to ethnic minority groups. Indeed, compared to those in the ethnic majority, those in the minority report poorer health outcomes (American Cancer Society 2012, Centers for Disease Control [CDC] 2011, Institute of Medicine 2002), less access to health care and health insurance (CDC 2011), and more financial barriers to health care (Mwachofi and Broyles 2007, CDC 2011). Some have suggested that the link is directly related to socio-economic status and not merely race alone (Mwachofi and Broyles 2007). However, researchers have demonstrated that at both the individual (e.g., minority status) and environmental (e.g., socio-economic status) levels, those belonging to minority groups experience greater frequencies of these stressful events and consequently must utilize resources and respond to such events more often than those in the cultural majority (Dressler, Bindon, and Neggers 1998, Haas, Krueger, and Rohlfsen 2012, Thorpe et al. 2012). In sum, those marginalized and disenfranchised are likely to have a different experience of stressful life events due to their minority status. As such, a multicultural understanding of stress would therefore take into account the degree to which power, privilege and resources also affect the experience and appraisal of stress.

Cultural Attitudes, Values, and Customs

For people who are marginalized because of minority status intragroup attitudes, values and customs can be a source of additional stress not experienced by those in the cultural majority. One way to more clearly understand these distinctions is through identity rooted in one's ingroup (e.g., family, friends, close social networks)—more specifically differing degrees of collectivism and individualism. Collectivism and individualism represent ways of thinking about and defining one's self in relation to one's ingroup (Baumeister and Bushman 2011, Markus and Kitayama 1991, Triandis 1989). Those with a strong degree of individualistic self-construal tend to emphasize the centrality of self and how the self is different from others. They tend to be more independent and are more likely to give priority to their own motives rather than those of their ingroup. Personal autonomy and self-advancement are often held in high regard for those who think about themselves in more individualistic ways. On the other side of the spectrum, those with more collectivistic tendencies are more likely to focus on the interdependent self. Priority is given to the motives and goals of the ingroup, often at the cost of the individual. Those with an interdependent self-construct tend to value a sense of belonging, and feel a sense of duty and obligation to their ingroup. Although the dichotomy of collectivism and individualism oversimplifies the existing variations of cultural individualism, many have argued that this framework is helpful in determining how culture shapes the self (Markus and Kitayama 1991, Baumeister and Bushman 2011), and consequently how that identity, both in self-identification and identification by others, can influence the degree to which stress is experienced and appraised (Chun et al. 2006, Oysermann, Coon, and Kemmelmeier 2002, Triandis 1989).

Certain cultural customs and the mainstream responses to those cultural customs such as arranged marriages, cultural dress (e.g., burqa, turban, Kippah), and familial practices can be a source of stress that can vary in intensity depending on one's culture. Consider for example the cultural practice and expectation of caring for elderly parents. In cultures that are more collectivist, it is a common practice for parents to live with one or several of their adult children. Conversely, for cultures that are more individualistic, parents usually live alone or in assisted living residences. Individuals in each culture experience stress, but the type and experience can be very different depending on the culture. For those in individualistic cultures the focus is one of independence, but this can often lead to isolation and loneliness. Likewise, having to depend on others is often perceived as negative and may consequently trigger stressful situations (Chun et al. 2006, Slavin et al. 1991). Although those in collectivist cultures may not experience the same sort of stress as a result of dependence, they may, for example, experience stress as a result of interpersonal conflicts. Furthermore, growing new relationships (e.g., a new marriage) in an existing family structure may create stress with respect to the ability to form strong bonds with new members of the group (Chun et al. 2006).

As members of specific cultural groups live among members of the dominant culture group, they may experience culture-specific stress resulting from conformity pressure from their own group (Chavez and French 2007, Contrada et al. 2000). This form of stress has been argued to be recurring and enduring. It occurs because members of one's cultural group have certain expectations for appropriate and inappropriate behaviors which create feelings of pressure or constraint (Contrada et al. 2001). Such expectations can be exemplified in personal interests (e.g., dress, music and food interests), behavior, and social relations (e.g., ethnicity of significant others, language use; Contrada et al. 2001). Pressures to conform to the expectations of one's cultural group, despite conflicts with the dominant group's expectations, are predictive of ill physical and mental health. For example, Chavez and French (2007) found that own-group conformity pressures (e.g., pressures to use native language, date within one's cultural group, dress in accordance with cultural customs) for Latino youths were significantly associated with higher anxiety, depression, and loss of behavioral and emotional control. Contrada and colleagues (2001) investigated whether own-group conformity pressures were associated with mental and physical health outcomes among a group African American, Hispanic, and Asian individuals. The researchers found that own-group conformity pressures significantly predicted negative mood, depression and physical symptoms of illness. Overall, the experience of pressure from one's cultural group to conform to the group's beliefs, attitudes, and behaviors, particularly when the cultural group is not the dominant group, may have important implications for health and wellbeing. Furthermore, stress resulting from in-group conformity pressure is a form of multicultural stress not necessarily considered within traditional stress theories and should be further explored.

Discrimination and Prejudice

The behavioral manifestation of cultural values and beliefs as well as simply belonging to a minority group, particularly if it is a visible group, can often elicit negative attitudes (e.g., prejudice) and behaviors (e.g., discrimination) from others, thereby increasing the frequency of experienced and perceived stressful events. Discrimination can be automatic, unconscious and unintended (e.g., covert) or explicitly enacted toward a group (e.g., overt; Myers 2010). For example, Contrada and colleagues (2000) concluded that ethnic discrimination is enacted in one of at least five different ways:

1. verbal rejection,
2. avoidance,
3. dis-valuation,
4. inequality/exclusion,
5. threat-aggression.

Persons in the minority may experience verbal rejection through insults or ethnic slurs. People may shun those in the minority or give negative evaluations of them. Discrimination can also be experienced through the denial of equal treatment or access to resources. Finally, one may experience actual physical harm or the threat of physical harm. Although Contrada et al.'s (2000), research was specific to racism, it could be generalized to sexism (e.g., negative attitudes and behaviors toward people of a given sex or gender; Myers 2010) or other targeted discrimination based on minority group identification.

Being in the visible minority often causes people to constantly assess, evaluate, and respond to potentially discriminating cues in the environment as a result of microaggressions, brief and commonplace daily verbal, behavioral, and environmental indignities, whether intentional or unintentional that communicate hostile, derogatory, or negative racial slights and insults to a target person or group (Sue et al. 2007, 273). The experience of potentially discriminating cues and microaggressions can consequently cause people in the minority to be more vigilant for potential discriminatory behaviors (e.g., Am I being ignored or is the server just busy? Contrada 2000). Heightened vigilance can increase the perception of threat or harm and consequently result in greater sensitivity to potentially discriminating behaviors. Together, increased sensitivity and vigilance can amplify the perceived nature of the stress and the taxing physiological and emotional stress responses (2000, 2001, Sawyer et al. 2012). Ambiguous and often unresolved social situations such as inequality or avoidance require those in the minority to become hypervigilant to potential instances of discrimination and prejudice.

Chronic stressors based on ethnic, gender, and sexual identities are associated with many adverse consequences, which in turn, compound the intensity with which the discriminatory stress is experienced (Chavez and French 2007, Clark et al. 1999, Lehavot and Simoni 2011, Lewis et al. 2009, Miller et al. 2011, Mossakowski 2003). That is to say, the more prejudice and discrimination is perceived or experienced, the greater likelihood members of these marginalized groups experience consequences of stress such as psychological distress (Chavez and French 2007, Jager, and Davis-Kean 2011, Pieterse et al. 2012) and diminished psychological well-being (Abdou et al. 2010, Diaz et al. 2001, Moradi and Risco 2006). For example, Greene, Way, and Phal (2006) followed a group of African American, Latino, Asian American and Puerto Rican adolescents into adulthood and measured the degree to which discrimination affected self-esteem and rates of depression. Results indicated that the discrimination from both peers and adults was significantly associated with lower self-esteem and higher rates of depression over time. Likewise, Lewis et al. (2009) found that discrimination in the form of violence and harassment was associated with greater emotional distress for bisexual individuals.

Stress as a result of discrimination relating to minority status can also lead to increases in physical health problems (Clark et al. 1999, Myers 2009, Cochran and Mays 2007, Lehavot and Simoni 2011). In their review of studies examining the relationship between racism and hypertension risk, Brondolo and colleagues (2011) found that both institutional (e.g., neighborhood poverty, segregation and incarceration), and interpersonal racism (e.g., negative attitudes and behaviors expressed between individuals) contributed to the increased risk of uncontrolled hypertension. The authors suggested that interpersonal racism was specifically related to increasing the negative perception of the stressor. That is, race-based maltreatment from one individual to another was associated with the perceived increase in frequency, magnitude, and duration of the effects of stress. Institutionalized racism, on the other hand, was the source of stress specifically related to barriers for engaging in health-related behaviors (Brondolo et al. 2011). Discrimination can also be institutional, leading to additional physical health problems. For instance, prejudice and discrimination have been suggested to exist in the health context for some individuals, particularly those in the sexual minority (Mathieson et al. 2002). Such discrimination has implications for the degree and quality of health services received and subsequent stress experienced.

Acculturative Stress

Acculturation, or the process of adopting the values, customs, and beliefs of the dominant culture (Straub 2012) can be stressful. Not all cultural groups or even members within each group experience the process of acculturation similarly nor do they experience the same degree of acculturation to the mainstream culture. Berry (2006) proposes that conflict and acculturative stress can occur at many stages of the acculturation process, particularly at stages where adjustment and changes to fit the dominant culture cannot be easily handled by simply assimilating to them. He states, "acculturative stress is a stress reaction in response to life events that are rooted in the experience of acculturation" (294). When adjusting to a new or dominant culture, various levels of both positive and negative stress exist. For example, a new environment might bring about opportunities for new life developments (e.g., new jobs, better living conditions, less sociopolitical strife, etc.), but negative events may also occur (e.g., discrimination, loneliness, poverty, etc.).

Theoretical models of acculturation differ with respect to explaining how stressful events are experienced. The melting pot model (Griffith 1983) suggests that the quicker those in the minority acculturate to the dominant culture, the less stress they will experience. Conversely, the bicultural theory (LaFramboise, Colman, and Greton 1993) suggests that stress is managed and minimized by keeping traditional values and customs while also adopting the beliefs and systems of the dominant culture. Although research supports both models (Bernstein et al. 2011, Torres and Ong 2010, Jones, Cross, and DeFour 2007), most research demonstrates that acculturation is a stressful process and can have adverse consequences such as increased rates of depression and anxiety (Revollo et al. 2011, Wrobel, Farrag, and Hymes 2009), psychosomatic illness (Greenlan and Brown 2005), and decreased psychological wellbeing (et al. 2012, Jibeen, and Khalid 2010). For example, in a study of acculturative stress factors in Latinos, as the pressure for English language competency increased, the number of depression symptoms reported by participants more than doubled (Torres and Ong 2010). Pressure to acculturate was also significantly associated with depression scores. Although acculturation is historically a process fraught with stress, some suggest that the stress has a more diffuse impact in cases where the move to a new culture is voluntary, when a social support system is already in place and when the new culture tolerates diversity (Straub 2012). Moreover, the acculturation process is one where persons may have the chance to engage in new opportunities and achieve their goals (Berry 2006), a process where the stress experienced may also have positive outcomes.

Coping

As previously discussed, the exposure to and subjective experience of stressful events may vary for individuals who are members of disempowered and disenfranchised minority and cultural groups, compared to exposure to and subjective experience of stressful events among members of the dominant culture. The distribution of power, privilege, and resources affects the multicultural experience of stress. Furthermore, culture (based in part on the visibility and identification of membership within a minority group) influences the appraisal or interpretation of stress, responses to stress, including coping strategies and access to coping resources. To provide a greater context for our discussion on stress appraisal and coping, we refer to the psychological model of stress based on Lazarus and Folkman (1984) and the multicultural model of the stress process adapted from Lazarus and Folkman by Slavin and colleagues (1991).

Appraisal and Coping

Whether or not an individual interprets a potentially stressful event to be a stressor is based on the outcomes of a two-step evaluation process referred to as appraisal. When an individual makes a primary appraisal of the potentially stressful event, one evaluates the harm, threat, or challenge the potentially stressful event poses to oneself. During the secondary appraisal process, the individual evaluates one's available resources to cope with the potentially stressful event (Lazarus and Folkman 1984). If an individual appraises a potentially stressful event to be harmful or threatening and determines that one does not have the resources to cope, the event is appraised as a stressor. If one appraises the event as a challenge and determines that one indeed has the resources to cope, the event is appraised as merely an event and not a stressor.

The process in which one uses strategies to manage perceived stressful or aversive taxing events is referred to as coping (Lazarus and Folkman 1984). Coping strategies have been categorized in the literature as adaptive or maladaptive cognitive, emotional, and behavioral responses. These strategies may be directed toward addressing the stressor head-on (e.g., approach-focused coping, active coping, and problem-focused coping), distancing oneself from the stressor (e.g., avoidant coping), modifying internal psychological states (e.g., emotion-focused coping, Lazarus and Folkman 1984), or by persevering through the experience of the stressful event while trying to find meaning in the occurrence of the event (e.g., existential or transformative coping, Wong, Wong, and Scott 2006).

Culture and the Coping Process

How stress is appraised and which coping strategies are employed is contingent, in part, on one's cultural identity, values, and norms. In this way, culture likely mediates enacted coping strategies (Chun et al. 2006, Slavin et al. 1991). With respect to appraisals, individuals who belong to oppressed groups (particularly those who are visually-identifiable members of oppressed minority groups) may find themselves questioning whether they are the target of an oppressive, discriminative, or otherwise interpersonally stressful action due to their identification with the oppressed group (Slavin et al. 1991). These appraisals may be influenced by actual and vicarious experiences as well as by social norms and expectations. For example, the reference "Driving While Black" refers to the perception of being targeted by police because of race and the belief that this discriminatory practice occurs is widely held among members of the

African American community (Weitzer and Tuch 2002). This type of racial profiling in which African Americans in general and men, in particular, experience a disproportionate amount of searches and arrests is a manifestation of institutionalized racism (Cole 2000, Hacker 2003). Similar concerns have been documented among Latinos who are now the target of anti-immigration legislation (Romero 2006).

The cultural transmission of persecutory beliefs may occur through racial socialization and lived experience; in turn, the lived experience may create feelings of vulnerability due to mistrust in the justice system (Brunson 2007). The subjective nature of the appraisal process requires the individual to evaluate the perceived harm, threat, or challenge associated with a potentially stressful event. The very consideration and evaluation of these events might differ between cultural groups due to systems of privilege and power. For example, a White individual might not think to consider increased police presence in the community as a potentially stressful event that could personally affect him or her. Conversely, those belonging to a racial or ethnic minority group with potential attitudes of mistrust toward the police based on objective and socialized experiences might worry about the increased risk of being wrongfully accused of a crime or subject to police mistreatment. An individual identifying as a member of a sexual majority group might not consider attending a medical appointment and answering questions about marital status, sexual orientation, or sexual behavior necessarily stressful. Similarly, a non-disabled individual might not have to consider the potential stress involved in meeting up with friends after a snowstorm that render sidewalks impassible for someone using a wheelchair. These examples of White, heterosexual, and non-disabled privilege (i.e., majority) are just a few examples of how social status can influence the evaluation of potentially stressful events.

Culture and Coping Goals

Coping goals refer to outcomes that would be the consequence of successful stress resolution (Chun et al. 2006). For instance, if an individual suddenly becomes homeless, a coping goal might be to regain stable housing. These goals for coping may serve to drive and organize one's coping efforts (Chun et al. 2006). Coping goals may be influenced by cultural identity and are also shaped by the contexts of power and privilege. Consider again, the notion of individualistic versus collectivist orientations. As discussed by Chun and colleagues (2006), coping goals may differ in four important ways depending on whether one has a more individualistic or collectivist orientation. For example, those operating from a more individualist orientation likely demonstrate a greater focus on self versus others, autonomy and independence versus cohesiveness and interdependence, changing self versus the environment in which they live, and enhancing gains versus reducing loss. Individuals belonging to collectivistic cultures might be more likely to develop coping goals consistent with focus on others, sustaining interdependence, changing oneself to fit the environmental constraints, and minimizing loss incurred by the experience of the stressful event. Conversely, in response to a stressor, individuals belonging to individualistic cultures may develop coping goals with intentions of self-focus, upholding independence, modifying the environment to reduce the impact of the stressor on oneself, and maximizing gains from the aftermath of the stressful event.

The coping goals that are formulated may also be influenced by the distribution of power and privilege. For example, consider a member of a marginalized ethnic minority group who is the target of discrimination on the basis of ethnicity. Power and privilege may dictate whether an individual may be a target for racism and other forms of discrimination. Furthermore, power and privilege may influence how one perceives his/her vulnerability in terms of anticipated intrapersonal, interpersonal, and societal consequences of racism and other forms of discrimination. This sense of vulnerability can shape the coping goals that are formulated, which often center on regaining control in the situation, enhancing self-esteem, or altering one's identity with respect to the threatened marginalized group (Swim and Thomas 2006). Thus, in response to experiencing discrimination, an individual may formulate a coping goal to regain control and preserve self-esteem by directly challenging or redressing discrimination (which may incur additional costs), attributing discrimination to characterological deficits of the offender, comparing oneself to other members of the discriminated group, devaluing attributes in question that are under attack, or strengthening ties with other aspects of one's non-discriminated identity (c.f., Swim and Thomas 2006).

Coping goals may be tangible (e.g., obtaining material resources) or intangible (e.g., reduction in emotional distress). For example, relief of distress as a primary goal of coping efforts is a widely-held assumption in the extant stress and coping literature, however, reduction of emotional distress may not be a universally-held coping goal (Menaghan 1983). For individuals from a collectivistic culture, protecting the wellbeing of the group or community might usurp a coping goal of enhancing one's personal wellbeing; in fact, immediate psychological distress may increase for these individuals who are placing others' wellbeing above their own (Chun et al. 2006). For individuals who are members of marginalized groups, the focus of coping efforts may be on preventing further marginalization such as concealing stigmatized identities or self-silencing one's reactions to stressors while learning to cope with often inescapable chronic stress (Iwasaki et al., 2008, Swim and Thomas 2006).

Culture and Coping Strategies

Returning to our introductory discussion on coping strategies, coping efforts may be directed toward addressing the stressor directly (e.g., approach-focused coping, active coping, and problem-focused coping; Lazarus and Folkman 1984), distancing oneself from the stressor (e.g., avoidant coping), modifying internal psychological states (e.g., emotion-focused coping; Lazarus and Folkman 1984), or persevering through the experience of the stressful event while trying to find meaning in the occurrence of the event (e.g., existential or transformative coping; Wong et al. 2006). Individuals in cultures oriented toward individualism may be more likely to use a more active approach and problem-focused coping strategies which directly modify the stressors, though the evidence is somewhat mixed, while individuals from collectivistic cultures more often tend to rely on coping strategies such as passive or avoidant coping in which the focus of coping is on distancing oneself from the distress caused by the stressor (Bjorck et al. 2001, Essau and Trommsdorff 1996, Radford et al. 1993, Chun et al. 2006). As mentioned previously, coping strategies have been categorized in the literature to be adaptive and maladaptive, with most adaptive coping strategies being most often utilized by those in individualistically-oriented cultures while coping strategies typically referred to as maladaptive include avoidant coping and other passive strategies which are most often adopted by individuals from collectivistic cultures. This has been said to reflect a Eurocentric bias, which ignores the cultural context that influences the stress process (Chun et al. 2006, Wong et al. 2006). Another coping strategy which is less frequently discussed in the stress and coping literature is existential or transformative coping. Individuals from many marginalized groups have reported turning to a higher power or religious institutions to cope with the stressors they may be experiencing due to individual and societal circumstances. Finding strength in the church and the social structure that it provides is a common coping strategy in the African American community (Chatters et al. 2008). Furthermore, this coping strategy may be often employed as a way of making meaning out of severely stressful circumstances among individuals belonging to cultural groups associated with severe, chronic, or uncontrollable stress.

Culture and Coping Efficacy

When individuals appraise the potential stressor and generate coping goals, they also develop expectations of confidence in their ability to successfully cope with the stressful circumstance (e.g., coping efficacy). A lack of correspondence between coping efficacy and actual outcomes can be stressful in and of itself and may be associated with negative mental and physical health outcomes. For instance, a pervasive message in the United States is that to be successful, one simply needs to "work hard and pull yourself up by your bootstraps." Thus, individuals are socialized to hold a belief that constant striving must pay off eventually in terms of attaining the popularized "American dream" of success, the ethos of our nation which decrees equality of opportunities for all citizens. However, individuals belonging to marginalized groups with limited power and resources and numerous institutional barriers to success may be able to work as diligently as another in a dominant cultural group without ever attaining the same level of success as those in the dominant group. In fact, employing high effort active coping styles such as "John Henryism," which refers to an active coping style categorized by high efforts and persistent striving against adversity and stressful circumstances with expectations of obtaining success as a result of one's vigorous efforts, may have deleterious effects on health such as uncontrolled hypertension particularly for those with limited resources and low socioeconomic status (James 1994). Moreover, racial differences emerge at the same low socioeconomic status, as additional risk conferred by this coping style is seen for African American men but not for low-SES Caucasian men and women (Dressler, Bindon, and Neggers 1998, James 1994).

Culture and Coping Resources

The availability and effectiveness of resources surely influence the coping process and outcomes. Compared to more dominant cultural groups, marginalized groups often have restricted access to institutional and other structural coping resources. Specifically, individuals from non-dominant and marginalized cultural groups may have limited or inadequate social or financial capital, access to services, and institutional assistance. The impact of these limited resources, particularly for those with low SES, may be an increased vulnerability to the effects of stressors which may have deleterious physical and mental health outcomes (Gallo and Matthews 2003). Having inadequate resources may in fact deplete an individual's perceived capacity to cope with stressors (Hobfoll, 2001, Gallo and Matthews 2003).

Despite having limited resources, individuals from non-dominant and marginalized cultural groups must find a way to cope with often chronic and uncontrollable sources of stress. Coping with chronic and uncontrollable stress may be facilitated by utilizing many different resources for coping, which may be categorized into individual coping resources, interpersonal coping resources, and institutional coping resources. Our discussion of these types of coping resources will include a consideration of the definition of coping resources and the perception of availability of coping resources, as different cultures may designate unique resources for coping, may place higher value on certain resources for coping, and may have a differential perspective regarding the availability of coping resources.

Individual coping resources center on personal psychological resources and personality traits. In qualitative research, members from non-dominant cultural groups have endorsed the traits of optimism, having a good sense of humor, and being able to view struggles as opportunities for growth as important personal coping resources to deal with oppression-related stress (Iwasaki et al., 2008). The personality trait of hardiness, or a "pattern of attitudes and skills that facilitates resilience under stressful circumstances" (Maddi and Harvey 2006, 409), has been associated with better outcomes in terms of psychological adjustment across cultures (Maddi and Harvey 2006).

Individuals may also turn to interpersonal coping resources, particularly if they find that utilization of their personal coping resources is not sufficient to deal with their stressors. Family support is a frequently utilized interpersonal resource for coping among members of marginalized cultural groups. For instance, family support has been indicated to be a primary source of coping with stress among Latino Americans, African Americans, Arab Americans, and Asian Americans (Chiang, Hunter, and Yeh 2004, Chilman 1993, Erickson and Al-Timimi 2001, Yeh et al. 2006). Strong connections to family are seen in many marginalized cultural groups as buffering mechanisms for experienced stress (Pierce, Sarason, and Sarason 1992, Treharne, Lyons, and Tupling 2001). Nevertheless, it is important to consider how the definition of family support and identification of members of family networks varies widely between different cultural groups as the perceived support provided for coping may vary between groups. For example, in collectivistic cultures such as many Asian and Latino cultures, the definition of family tends to be more broad and the extended family as a unit is often viewed as an integral source of support for coping with stressors, while for those belonging to individualistic cultures the family is generally defined by the immediate nuclear family members and more distant family members and the extended family is less often involved as a key coping resource for stressful circumstances (Triandis 1989). Among individuals with sexual minority status, the definition of family tends to be more inclusive of peers (e.g., "families of choice"), who are often perceived to provide more support for LGBTQ individuals than biological family members. As such, peers in their community often provide support more often than family members (Peplau 1991).

Relationships with those outside of one's immediate family context but within the marginalized group such as peers, elders, or community leaders in the marginalized communities and cultures are resources that are often utilized to cope with a wide variety of stressors, and may reflect a collective orientation in coping (Yeh, Arora, and Wu 2006). A primary component of collective coping is reliance on social resources within one's family network and ethnic-cultural networks is utilized during the process of coping (Kuo 2012) and has been observed in many cultures within the United States such as Asian Americans (e.g., Yeh and Wang 2000, Yeh et al. 2006), African Americans (e.g., Utsey, Adams, and Bolden 2000), and Latinos (e.g., Chiang, Hunter, and Yeh 2004, Constantine et al. 2005). Having a strong group identity can provide interpersonal social support or serve as a political base from which to effect change and possibly power differentials (Swim and Thomas 2006)

Individuals may also turn to coping resources at the structural or institutional levels to cope with the stress they experience, although those resources can be limited due to marginalization. Institutional resources associated with the marginalized cultural groups, for example the "Black church" or venues or organized groups affiliated with or allied to particular sexual minority groups (e.g., gay-affirming organizations), may serve as coping resources by providing safe environments, sense of belonging, and affiliated social support networks (Iwasaki et al. 2008, Wallace and Bergman 2002). Often within these institutions there exists a shared understanding of the sociopolitical structures that reinforce marginalization and social exclusion of the individuals belonging to the cultural minority groups which may help to foster a sense of trust and reliance on these institutions for coping efforts. However, it is important to acknowledge that some individuals in these cultural minority groups do not necessarily get a sense of belonging from such venues.

More recently, research suggests that within limited resource environments, those in the minority (especially African Americans), use poor health behaviors (e.g., smoking, poor diet, drug, and alcohol use) as coping resources to protect mental health. Given that the environment does not provide opportunities to healthily cope with psychological and physiologically taxing events, individuals living in such environments use what is available to cope (Mezuk et al. 2010). The use of poor health behaviors as a coping resource has been identified among African Americans a moderator between stress and depression with rates of depression being less for those who engaged in more poor health behaviors compared to those who engage in fewer poor health behaviors (Jackson, Knight, and Rafferty 2010, Mezuk et al. 2010). As such, negative health behaviors are theorized to have a buffering effect for mental health among African Americans wherein the status of the environment and institutional resources available affects how those in the minority cope with stress. In the case of African Americans, the approach to mental health is at the cost of physical health states.

Having a greater understanding of the coping resources available to marginalized cultural groups may illuminate psychological, social, and tangible resources to target for increased capacity building and strengthening among marginalized groups and communities in an effort to affect change in individuals and communities. For example, individual change could be affected by generating increased coping efficacy and change could occur at the community level by increasing the available connections to resources for coping with perceived stressors.

Culture, Coping, and Resilience: Protective Effects of Culture

We have discussed several ways in which membership in a marginalized cultural group may influence exposure and vulnerability to stress, but we would be remiss to omit a review of the stress buffering effects associated with culture and one's cultural identification. A strong ethnic identity itself may act as a buffer for deleterious effects of stress on mental and physical health and has been the focus of several studies in the multicultural stress and coping literature. Ethnic identity has been defined as the degree of identification with one's ethnicity, including a sense of commitment to one's ethnic or cultural group, pride in one's belonging and identifying with the ethnic group, and participation in cultural practices (Phinney 1991). Results from a recent meta-analysis examining the relationship between ethnic identity and wellbeing (grouping variable defined as general wellbeing, self-esteem, lack of mental health symptoms such as depression and anxiety) across 184 studies with adolescents and adults in North America demonstrated a modest relationship between the ethnic identity and wellbeing, with an omnibus effect size of $r = 0.17$. On the other hand, the association between ethnic identity and symptoms of impaired mental health such as depression and anxiety were not as strong as the associations between ethnic identity and self-esteem or wellbeing, with an aggregated effect size of $r = 0.79$ (Smith and Silva 2011). Interestingly, the associations of ethnic identity and wellbeing and ethnic identity and self-esteem were not moderated by participant characteristics such as race, gender, level of education, or SES, suggesting that the strength of these relationships do not change based on these categorical participant sociodemographic characteristics (Smith and Silva 2011). However, two important moderating variables of the relationship between ethnic identity and wellbeing were identified, namely, age of participants and acculturation status, such that the relationship was somewhat stronger among adolescents and young adults, and somewhat weaker for those with lower levels of acculturation to the United States. Ethnic identity has been shown to be a significant protective factor for race-related stress and discrimination on wellbeing and mental health among African Americans (Jones, Cross, and DeFour 2007, Tovar-Murray and Munley 2007), among Asian Americans (Mossakowski 2003, Yip, Gee, and Takeuchi 2008), and among Latino Americans (Torres and Ong 2010, Torres, Yznaga, and Moore 2011).

Researchers have posited that disconnection from one's cultural identity (particularly among groups with a history of sociopolitical marginalization and historical trauma) may be associated with poorer psychological adjustment and in some cases with more problematic health behaviors (Sotero 2006). Common examples cited include increased rates of substance use disorders and poor health outcomes in American Indian and Alaskan Native communities (Walters, Simoni, and Evans-Campbell 2002), and poorer physical and mental health status among members of many marginalized and oppressed racial and ethnic groups (Williams, Neighbors, and Jackson 2003). In an effort to foster the renewal of a connection to one's cultural identity to facilitate healing, many prevention and intervention programs have begun to include cultural dimensions and incorporate an enhancement of connection to cultural identity and strengthening of culture, while acknowledging a history of cultural and historical trauma (Sotero 2006).

Conclusion

Viewing stress and coping through a multicultural lens can enhance cross-cultural competence in the understanding, assessment, and management of stress and coping. Culture influences the appraisal, interpretation and responses to stress, as well as coping strategies and access to coping resources. Sociopolitical structures based on the distribution of power, privilege and resources can create differential stressors and differential experiences of those stressors for members of cultural minority groups compared to those in the dominant culture. As such, the process of coping and availability of coping resources also differs among those in the often marginalized minority groups. Therefore, by understanding how the distribution of power and privilege influence the experience of stress and coping, we can begin to address the existing disparities and the approach to stress and coping which has traditionally been focused on the dominant culture. When working with individuals from marginalized cultural groups, an awareness and acknowledgement of the sociopolitical structures associated with differential stress experiences can enhance the process of finding ways to continually cope with the often chronic sources of stress. A greater awareness of differential stress experiences can also illuminate different areas (e.g., individual, interpersonal and environmental) of intervention. Furthermore, by understanding coping within a multicultural context, we are better able to identify and strengthen connections to available and effective coping resources for those in minority groups. Areas of intervention could include enhancing individuals' coping efficacy, strengthening connections to cultural identity, and strengthening cultural communities through capacity building. Continued research, however, is needed to determine how visibility and identification with a minority group can influence coping resources and the degree to which visibility and identification can influence health and wellbeing.

References

Abdou, C. M., C. D. Schetter, F. Jones, D. Roubinov, S. Tsai, L. Jones, C. Hobel. 2010. "Community Perspectives: Mixed-Methods Investigation of Culture, Stress, Resilience, and Health." *Ethnicity and Disease* 20(S2): 41–48. http://www.ishib.org/journal/20-1s2/ethn-20-01s2-s41.pdf.

American Cancer Society. 2012. "Cancer Facts and Figures for African Americans 2011–2012." Atlanta, GA: American Cancer Society. http://www.cancer.org/acs/groups/content/@epidemiologysurveilance/documents/document/acspc-027765.pdf

Baker, A. M., J. A. Soto, C. R. Perez, and E. A. Lee. 2012. "Acculturative Status and Psychological Wellbeing in an Asian American Sample." *Asian American Journal of Psychology* 3(4): 275–285. doi:10.1037/a0026842

Baumeister, R. F. and B. J. Bushman. 2011. *Social Psychology and Human Nature.* Belmont, CA: Wadsworth.

Bernstein, K. D., S. Park, J. Shin, S. Cho, and Y. Park. 2011. "Acculturation, Discrimination and Depressive Symptoms among Korean Immigrants in New York City." *Community Mental Health Journal* 47: 24–34. doi:10.1007/s10597-009-9261-0

Berry, J. W. 2006. "Acculturative Stress." In *Handbook of Multicultural Perspectives on Stress and Coping,* edited by P. T. P. Wong and L. C. J. Wong, 287–298. New York: Springer.

Bjorck, J. P., W. Cuthbertson, J. W. Thurman, and Y. S. Lee. 2001. "Ethnicity, Coping, and Distress among Korean Americans, Filipino Americans, and Caucasian Americans." *Journal of Social Psychology* 141: 421–442. doi:10 .1080/00224540109600563

Brondolo, E., D. D. Love, M. Pencille, A. Schoenthaler, and G. Ogedegbe. 2011. "Racism and Hypertension: A Review of the Empirical Evidence and Implications for Clinical Practice." *American Journal of Hypertension* 24: 518–529. doi:10.1038/ ajh.2011.9

Brunson, R. K. 2007. "'Police Don't Like Black People': African-American Young Men's Accumulated Police Experiences." *Criminology and Public Policy* 6: 71–101. doi:10.1111/j.1745-9133.2007.00423.x

Cannon, W. B. 1914. "The Emergency Function of the Adrenal Medulla in Pain and the Major Emotions." *American Journal of Physiology* 33: 356–372. http:// ajplegacy.physiology.org/content/33/2/356.full.pdf+html

Centers for Disease Control. 2011. "CDC Health Disparities and Inequalities Report—United States—2011." *Morbidity and Mortality Weekly Report* 60. http://www.cdc.gov/mmwr/pdf/other/su6001.pdf.

Chatters, L. M., R. J. Taylor, J. S. Jackson, and K. D. Lincoln. 2008. "Religious Coping among African Americans, Caribbean Blacks, and Non-Hispanic Whites." *Journal of Community Psychology* 36: 371–386. doi:10.1002/jcop.20202

Chavez, N., R. and S. E. French. 2007. "Ethnicity-Related Stressors and Mental Health in Latino Americans: The Moderating Role of Parental Racial Socialization." *Journal of Applied Social Psychology* 37: 1974–1998. doi:10.1111/j.1559 -1816.2007.00246.x

Chiang, L., C. D. Hunter, and C. J. Yeh. 2004. "Coping Attitudes, Sources, and Practices among Black and Latino College Students." *Adolescence* 39: 793–815. http://www.ncbi.nlm.nih.gov/pubmed/15727415

Chilman, C. S. 1993. "Hispanic Families in the United States: Research Perspectives." In *Family Ethnicity: Strength in Diversity,* edited by H. P. McAdoo, 141–163. Newbury Park, CA: Sage Publications.

Chun, C., R. H. Moos, and C. Cronkite. 2006. "Culture: A Fundamental Context for the Stress and Coping Paradigm." In *Handbook of Multicultural Perspectives on Stress and Coping,* edited by P. T. P. Wong and L. C. J. Wong, 29–54. New York: Springer.

Clark, R., N. B. Anderson, V. R. Clark, and D. R. Williams. 1999. "Racism as a Stressor for African Americans: A Biopsychosocial Model." *American Psychologist* 54: 805–816. doi:10.1037/0003-066X.54.10.805

Cochran, S. D., and V. M. Mays. 2007. "Physical Health Complaints among Lesbian, Gay Men, and Bisexual and Homosexually Experienced Heterosexual Individuals: Results from the California Quality of Life Survey." *American Journal of Public Health* 97(11): 2048–2055. doi:10.2105/AJPH.2005.082511

Cole, D. 2000. *No Equal Justice: Race and Class in the American Justice System.* New York: W. W. Norton and Company.

Constantine, M., V. Alleyne, L. Caldwell, M. McRae, and L. Suzuki. 2005. "Coping Responses of Asian, Black, and Latino/Latina New York City Residents Following the September 11, 2001, Terrorist Attacks against the United States." *Cultural Diversity and Ethnic Minority Psychology* 11: 293–308. doi:10.1037/1099–9809.11.4.293

Contrada, R. J., R. D. Ashmore, M. L. Gary, E. Coups, J. D. Egeth, A. Sewell, V. Chasse. 2000. "Ethnicity-Related Sources of Stress and Their Effects on Wellbeing." *Current Directions in Psychological Science* 9: 136–139. doi:10.2307/20182647

Contrada, R. J., R. D. Ashmore, M. L. Gary, E. Coups, J. D. Egeth, A. Sewell, V. Chasse. 2001. "Measures of Ethnicity-Related Stress: Psychometric Properties, Ethnic Group Differences, and Associations with Psychological and Physical Wellbeing." *Journal of Applied Social Psychology* 31: 1775–1820. doi:10.1111/j.1559-1816.2001.tb00205.x

Corliss, H. L., C. S. Goodenow, N. Lauren, and A. S. Bryn. 2011. "High Burden of Homelessness among Sexual-Minority Adolescents: Findings from a Representative Massachusetts High School Sample." *American Journal of Public Health* 101: 1683–1689. doi:10.2105/AJPH.2011.300155

Diaz, R. M., G. Ayala, E. Bein, J. Henne, and B. V. Marin. 2001. "The Impact of Homophobia, Poverty, and Racism on the Mental Health of Gay and Bisexual Latino Men: Findings from Three Cities." *American Journal of Public Health* 91: 927–932. doi:10.2105/AJPH.91.6.927

Dressler, W. W., J. R. Bindon, and Y. H. Neggers. 1998. "John Henryism, Gender, and Arterial Blood Pressure in an African American Community." *Psychosomatic Medicine 60*: 620–624. http://www.psychosomaticmedicine.org/content/60/5/620.short

Erickson, C. D., and N. R. Al-Timimi. 2001. "Providing Mental Health Services to Arab Americans: Recommendations and Considerations." *Cultural Diversity and Ethnic Minority Psychology* 7: 308–327. doi:10.1037/1099-9809.7.4.308

Essau, C. A., and G. Trommsdorff. 1996. "Coping with University-Related Problems: A Cross-Cultural Comparison." *Journal of Cross-Cultural Psychology* 27: 315–328. doi:10.1177/0022022196273004

Folkman, S. and J. T. Moskowitz. 2004. "Coping: Pitfalls, and Promise." *Annual Review of Psychology 55*: 745–774. doi:10.1146/annurev.psych.55.090902.141456

Gallo, L. C. and K. A. Matthews. 2003. "Understanding the Association between Socioeconomic Status and Physical Health: Do Negative Emotions Play a Role?" *Psychological Bulletin 129*: 10–51. doi:10.1037/0033-2909.129.1.10.

Greene, M. L., M. L. Way, and K. Phal, 2006. "Trajectories of Perceived Adult and Peer Discrimination among Black, Latino, and Asian American Adolescents: Patterns and Psychological Correlates." *Developmental Psychology 42*: 218–238. doi:10.1037/0012-1649.42.2.218

Greenland, K. and R. Brown. 2005. "Acculturation and Acculturative Stress Among Japanese Students in the United Kingdom," *Journal of Social Psychology 145*: 373–389, doi: 10.3200/SOCP.145.4.373-390

Griffith, J. 1983. "Relationship between Acculturation and Psychological Impairment in Adult Mexian Americans." *Hispanic Journal of Behavioral Sciences* 5: 431–459. doi:10.1177/07399863830050040

Gurung, R. A. R., and A. Roethel-Wendorf. 2009. "Stress and Mental Health." In *Culture and Mental Health: Sociocultural Influences, Theory, and Practice*, edited by S. Eshun and R. A. R. Gurung, 35–54. Malden, MA: Wiley-Blackwell.

Haas, S. A., P. M. Krueger, and L. Rohlfsen. 2012. "Race/Ethnic and Nativity Disparities in Later Life Physical Performance: The Role of Health and Socioeconomic Status over the Life Course." *The Journals of Gerontology, Series B: Psychological Sciences and Social Sciences* 67: 238–248. doi:10.1093/geronb/gbr155

Hacker, A. 2003. *Two Nations: Black and White, Separate, Hostile, Unequal.* New York: Simon and Schuster.

Hamilton, C. J., and J. R. Mahalik. 2009. "Minority Stress, Masculinity, and Social Norms Predicting Gay Men's Health Risk Behaviors." *Journal of Counseling Psychology* 56: 132–141. doi:10.1037/a0014440

Hobfoll, S. E. 2001. "The Influence of Culture, Community, and the Nested-Self in the Stress Process: Advancing Conservation of Resources Theory." *Applied Psychology* 50: 337–370. doi:10.1111/1464-0597.00062.

Hughes, T. A., L. A. Szalacha, T. P. Johnson, K. E. Kinnison, K. E. Wilsnack, and S. C. C. Young. 2010. "Sexual Victimization and Hazardous Drinking among Heterosexual and Sexual Minority Women." *Addictive Behaviors* 35: 1152–1156. doi:10.1016/j.addbeh.2010.07.004

Iwasaki, Y., J. Bartlett, K. MacKay, J. Mactavish, and J. Ristock. 2008. "Mapping Non-Dominant Voices into Understanding Stress-Coping Mechanisms." *Journal of Community Psychology* 36: 702–722. doi:10.1002/jcop.20251

Jackson, J. S., K. M. Knight, and J. A. Rafferty. 2010. "Race and Unhealthy Behaviors: Chronic Stress, the HPA Axis, and Physical and Mental Health Disparities over the Life Course." *American Journal of Public Health* 100: 933–939.

Jager, J., and P. Davis-Kean. 2011. "Same-Sex Sexuality and Adolescent Psychological Wellbeing: The Influence of Sexual Orientation, Early Reports of Same-Sex Attraction and Gender." *Self and Identity* 10: 417–444. doi:10.1080/15298861003771155

James, S. A. 1994. "John Henryism and the Health of African Americans." *Culture, Medicine, and Psychiatry* 18: 163–182. doi:10.1007/BF01379448

Jibeen, R. and R. Khalid. 2010. "Predictors of Psychological Wellbeing of Pakistani Immigrants in Toronto, Canada." *International Journal of Intercultural Relations* 34: 452–464. doi:10.1016/j.ijintrel.2010.04.010

Jones, H. L., W. E. Cross, Jr., and D. C. DeFour. 2007. "Race-Related Stress, Racial Identity Attitudes, and Mental Health among Black Women." *Journal of Black Psychology* 33: 208–231. doi:10.1177/0095798407299517

Kuo, B. C. H. 2012. "Collectivism and Coping: Current Theories, Evidence, and Measurements of Collective Coping." *International Journal of Psychology* 48: 374–388. doi:10.1080/00207594.2011.640681

LaFramboise, T., H. L. K. Colman, and J. Greton. 1993. "Psychological Impact of Biculturalism: Evidence and Theory." *Psychological Bulletin* 114: 395–412. doi:10.1037/0033-2909.114.3.395

Lazarus, R. S. 1966. *Psychological Stress and the Coping Process.* New York: McGraw-Hill.

Lazarus, R. S. 1976. *Patterns of Adjustment*. McGraw-Hill, New York.

Lazarus, R. S. and S. Folkman. 1984. *Stress, Appraisal and Coping*. New York: Springer.

Lehavot, K. and J. Simoni. 2011. "The impact of minority stress on mental health and substance abuse among sexual minority women." *Journal of Consulting & Clinical Psychology* 79: 159-170. doi:10.1037/a0022839

Lewis, R. J., V. J. Derlega, D. Brown, S. Rose, and J. M. Henson. 2009. "Sexual Minority Stress, Depressive Symptoms, and Sexual Orientation Conflict: Focus on the Experiences of Bisexuals." *Journal of Social and Clinical Psychology* 28: 971–992. doi:10.1037/a0022839

Lio, Y., D. Bang, S. Cosgrove, R. Dulin, Z. Harris, A. Stewart, and W. Giles. 2011. "Surveillance of Health Status in Minority Communities—Racial and Ethnic Approaches to Community Health across the U.S. (REACH U.S.) Risk Factor Survey, United States, 2009." *Morbidity and Mortality Weekly Report* 60: 1–41. http://www.cdc.gov/mmwr/preview/mmwrhtml/ss6006a1.htm

Maddi, S. R., and R. H. Harvey. 2006. "Hardiness Considered across Cultures." In *Handbook of Multicultural Perspectives on Stress and Coping*, edited by P. T. P. Wong, and L. C. J. Wong, 418–426. New York: Springer.

Markus, H. R., and S. Kitayama. 1991. "Culture and the Self: Implications for Cognition, Emotion, and Motivation." *Psychological Review* 98: 224–253. doi:10.1037/0033-295X.98.2.224

Mathieson, C. M., N. Bailey, and M. Gurevich. 2002. "Health Care Services for Lesbian and Bisexual Women: Canadian Data." *Health Care for Women International* 23: 185–196. doi:10.1080/073993302753429059

McNair, R., L. A. Szalacha, T. L. Hughes, and R. O. Straub. 2011. "Health Status, Health Service Use, and Satisfaction According to Sexual Identity of Young Australian Women." *Women's Health Issues* 21: 40–47. doi:10.1016/j.whi.2010.08.002

Menaghan, E. G. 1983. "Individual Coping Efforts: Moderators of the Relationship between Life Stress and Mental Health Outcomes" In *Psychosocial Stress: Trends in Theory and Research*, edited by H. B. Kaplan, 157–191. New York: Academic Press.

Mezuk, B., J. A. Rafferty, K. N. Kershaw, D. Hudson, H. L. Abdou, W. W. Eaton, and J. S. Jackson. 2010. "Reconsidering the Role of Social Disadvantage in Physical and Mental Health: Stressful Life Events, Health Behaviors, Race, and Depression." *American Journal of Epidemiology* 172: 1238–1249. doi:10.1093/aje/kwq283

Miller, M. J., M. Yang, J. A. Farrell, and L. L. Lin. 2011. "Racial and Cultural Factors Affecting the Mental Health of Asian Americans." *Journal of Orthopsychiatry* 81: 489–497. doi:10.1111/j.1939-0025.2011.01118.x

Moradi, B. and C. Risco. 2006. "Perceived Discrimination Experiences and Mental Health of Latino/a American Persons." *Journal of Counseling Psychology* 53: 411–421. doi:10.1037/0022-0167.53.4.411

Mossakowski, K. N. 2003. "Coping with Perceived Discrimination: Does Ethnic Identity Protect Mental Health?" *Journal of Health and Social Behavior* 44: 318–331. http://www.jstor.org/stable/10.2307/1519782

Mwachofi, A. K. and R. W. Broyles. 2007. "Consistency of Minority and Socioeconomic Status as Predictors of Health." *Journal of Health Disparities Research and Practice* 2: 103–118. http://chdr.unlv.edu/JHDRPpercent20V2_1percent20Fall07.pdf

Myers, D. G. 2010. *Social psychology* (10th ed.). New York: McGraw-Hill.

Myers, F. H. 2009. "Ethnicity- and Socio-Economic Status-Related Stresses in Context: An Integrative Review and Conceptual Model." *Journal of Behavioral Medicine* 32: 9–19. doi:10.1007/s10865-08-9181-4

Oyserman, D., H. M. Coon, and M. Kemmelmeier. 2002. "Rethinking individualism and collectivism: Evaluation of Theoretical Assumptions and Meta-analysis." *Psychological Bulletin* 128: 3–72. doi:10.1037/0033-2909.128.1.3

Padilla, A. M., and N. E. Correro. 2006. "The Effects of Acculturative Stress on the Hispanic Family." In *Handbook of Multicultural Perspectives on Stress and Coping,* edited by P. T. P. Wong and L. C. J. Wong, 299–318. New York: Springer.

Peplau, L. A. 1991. "Lesbian and Gay Relationships." In *Homosexuality: Research Implications for Public Policy,* edited by J. C. Gonsiorek and J. D. Weinrich, 177–196. Newbury Park, CA: Sage.

Phinney, J. S. 1991. "Ethnic Identity and Self-Esteem: A Review and Integration." *Hispanic Journal of Behavioral Sciences* 13: 193–208. doi:10.1177/07399863910132005

Pierce, G. R., B. R. Sarason, and I. G. Sarason. 1992. "General and Specific Support Expectations and Stress as Predictors of Perceived Supportiveness: An Experimental Study." *Journal of Personality and Social Psychology* 63: 297–307. doi:10.1037/0022-3514.63.2.297

Pieterse, A. L., N. R. Todd, H. A. Neville, and R. T. Carter. 2012. "Perceived Racism and Mental health among Black American Adults: A Meta-Analytic Review." *Journal of Counseling Psychology* 59: 1–9. doi:10.1037/a0026208

Radford, M. H., L. Mann, Y. Ohta, and Y. Nakane. 1993. "Differences between Australian and Japanese Students in Decisional Self-Esteem, Decisional Stress, and Coping Styles." *Journal of Cross-Cultural Psychology* 24: 284–297. doi:10.1177/0022022193243002

Repetti, R. L., S. E. Taylor, and T. E. Seeman. 2002. "Risky Families: Family Social Environments and the Mental and Physical Health of Offspring." *Psychological Bulletin* 128: 330–366. doi:10.1037/0033-2909.128.2.330

Revollo, H., A. Qureshi, F. Collazos, D. Valero, and M. Casa. 2011. "Acculturative Stress as a Risk Factor of Depression and Anxiety in the Latin American Immigrant Population." *International Review of Psychiatry* 23: 84–92. doi:10.3109/09540261.2010.545988

Romero, M. 2006. "Racial Profiling and Immigration Law Enforcement: Rounding up of Usual Suspects." *Critical Sociology* 32: 447–473. doi:10.1163/156916306777835376

Sawyer, P. J., B. Major, B. J. Casad, S. S. Townsend, and W. B. Mendes. 2012. "Discrimination and the Stress Response: Psychological and Physiological Consequences of Anticipating Prejudice and Interethnic Interactions." *American Journal of Public Health* 102: 1020–1026. doi:10.2105/AJPH.2011.300620

Selye, H. 1956. *The Stress of Life.* McGraw-Hill, New York.

Slavin, L. A., K. L. Rainer, M. L. McCreary, and K. K. Gowda. 1991. "Toward a Multicultural Model of the Stress Process." *Journal of Counseling and Development* 71: 156–163. doi:10.1002/j.1556-6676.1991.tb01578.x

Smith, T. B. and L. Silva. 2011. "Ethnic Identity and Personal Wellbeing of People of Color: A Meta-Analysis." *Journal of Counseling Psychology* 58: 42–60. doi:10.1037/a0021528

Somerfield, M. R. and R. R. McCrae. 2000. "Stress and Coping Research: Methodological Challenges, Theoretical Advances, and Clinical Applications." *American Psychologist* 55: 620–625. doi:10.1037/0003-066X.55.6.620

Sotero, M. M. 2006. "A Conceptual Model of Historical Trauma: Implications for Public Health Practice and Research." *Journal of Health Disparities Research and Practice* 1: 93–98. http://www.ressourcesactuarielles.net/EXT/ISFA/1226.nsf/7 69998e0a65ea348c1257052003eb94f/bbd469e12b2d9eb2c12576000032b2 89/$FILE/Sotero_2006.pdf

Straub, R. O. 2012. *Health Psychology: A Biopsychosocial Approach* (3rd ed.). New York: Worth Publisher.

Sue, D. W., C. Capodilupo, G. C. Torino, J. M. Bucceri, A. M. B. Holder, K. L. Nadal, and M. E. Esquilin. 2007. "Racial Microaggressions in Everyday Life: Implications for Clinical Practice." *American Psychologist* 62: J 271–286. doi: 10.1037/0003066X.62.4.271

Swim, J. K., and M. A. Thomas. 2006. "Responding to Everyday Discrimination: A Synthesis of Research on Goal-Directed, Self-Regulatory Coping Behaviors." In *Stigma and Group Inequality,* edited by S. Levin and C. Van Laar, 105–128. Mahwah, NJ: Erlbaum.

Taylor, S. E., L. C. Klein, B. Lewis, T. Gruenewald, R. A. R. Gurung, and J. Updegraff. 2000. "The Female Stress Response: Tend and Befriend not Fight or Flight." *Psychological Review* 107: 411–429. doi:10.1037/0033-295X.107.3.411

Thorpe, R. J. Jr., A. Koster, H. Bosma, T. B. Harris, E. M. Simonsick, J. T. van Eijk, and S. B. Kritchevsky. 2012. "Racial Differences in Mortality in Older Adults: Factors beyond Socioeconomic Status." *Annals of Behavioral Medicine* 43: 29–38. doi:10.1007/s12160-011-9335-4

Torres, L., and A. D. Ong. 2010. "A Daily Diary Investigation of Latino Ethnic Identity, Discrimination, and Depression." *Cultural Diversity and Ethnic Minority Psychology* 16: 561–568. doi:10.1037/a0020652

Torres, L., S. Yznaga, and K. Moore. 2011. "Discrimination and Latino Psychological Distress: The Moderating Role of Ethnic Identity Exploration and Commitment." *American Journal of Orthopsychiatry* 81: 498–506. doi:10.1111/j.1939 -0025.2011.01117.x

Tovar-Murray, D. T. and P. H. Munley. 2007. "Exploring the Relationship between Race-Related Stress, Identity, and Wellbeing among African Americans." *The Western Journal of Black Studies* 31: 58–71. http://public.wsu.edu/~wjbs/vol311a .html

Treharne, G. J., A. C. Lyons, and R. E. Tupling. 2001. "The Effects of Optimism, Pessimism, Social Support, and Mood on the Lagged Relationship between

Daily Stress and Symptoms." *Current Research in Social Psychology* 7: 60–81. http://www.uiowa.edu/~grpproc/crisp/crisp.7.5.htm

Triandis, H. C. 1989. "The Self and Social Behavior in Differing Cultural Context." *Psychological Review* 96: 506–520. doi:10.1037/0033-295X.96.3.506

Utsey, S. O., E. P. Adams, and M. Bolden. 2000. "Development and Initial Validation of the Africultural Coping Systems Inventory." *Journal of Black Psychology* 26: 194–215. doi:10.1177/0095798400026002005

Valdez, J. 2006. "Stress." In *Encyclopedia of Multicultural Psychology*, edited by Y. Jackson, 446–451. Thousand Oaks, CA: SAGE Publications, Inc.

Wallace, K. A. and C. S. Bergeman. 2002. "Spirituality and Religiosity in a Sample of African American Elders: A Life Story Approach." *Journal of Adult Development* 9: 141–154. doi:10.1023/A:1015789513985

Walters, K. L., J. M. Simoni, and T. Evans-Campbell. 2002. "Substance Use among American Indians and Alaska Natives: Incorporating Culture in an "Indigenist" Stress-Coping Paradigm." *Public Health Reports* 117: S104-S117. http://www.ncbi .nlm.nih.gov/pmc/articles/PMC1913706/pdf/pubhealthrep00207-0109.pdf

Weitzer, R. and S. A. Tuch. 2002. "Perceptions of Racial Profiling: Race, Class, and Personal Experience." *Criminology* 40:435–456. doi:10.1111/j.1745-9125.2002. tb00962.x

Williams, D. R., H. W. Neighbors, and J. S. Jackson. 2003. "Racial/Ethnic Discrimination and Health: Findings from Community Studies." *American Journal of Public Health* 93: 200–208. http://ajph.aphapublications.org/doi/ pdf/10.2105/AJPH.93.2.200

Wong, P. T. P., L. C. J. Wong, and C. Scott. 2006. "Beyond stress and coping: The positive psychology of transformation." In *Handbook of Multicultural Perspectives on stress and Coping*, edited by P. T. P. Wong and L. C. J. Wong, 1–28. New York: Springer.

Wrobel, N. H., M. F. Farrag, and R. W. Hymes. 2009. "Acculturative Stress and Depression in an Elderly Arabic Sample." *Journal of Cross-Cultural Gerontology* 24: 273–290. doi:10.1007/s10823-009-9096-8

Yeh, C. J., A. K. Arora, and K. A. Wu. 2006. "A new theoretical model of collectivistic coping." In *Handbook of Multicultural Perspectives on stress and Coping*, edited by P. T. P. Wong and L. C. J. Wong, 56–72. New York: Springer.

Yeh, C. J., A. G. Inman, A. B. Kim, and Y. Okubo. 2006. "Asian American Families' Collectivistic Coping Strategies in Response to 9/11." *Cultural Diversity and Ethnic Minority Psychology* 12: 134–148. doi:10.1037/1099-9809.12.1.134

Yeh, C. J., and Y. W. Wang. 2000. "Asian American Coping Attitudes, Sources, and Practices: Implications for Indigenous Counseling Strategies." *Journal of College Student Development* 41: 94–103. ISSN 1543-3382

Yip, T., G. C. Gee, and D. T. Takeuchi. 2008. "Racial Discrimination and Psychological Distress: The Impact of Ethnic Identity and Age among Immigrant and United States-Born Asian Adults." *Developmental Psychology* 44: 787–801. doi:10. 1037/0012-1649.44.3.787

Mood and Anxiety Disorders across Ethnic Minority Groups in the United States

Sussie Eshun

Being a part of any minority group often comes with challenges that have a deeper impact than others in the majority group could accurately imagine or understand. In general, society tends to communicate that majority is either right or acceptable without seriously considering views and perceptions of the minority. There exists push and pull factors in each society that more or less force (or expect) ethnic minority people to assimilate and fit in with the norms of the majority through enculturation and acculturation. Ethnic minorities in the United States are no exception: they have a long history of prejudice and discrimination, which influences their perception of themselves, perception of others, as well as how others perceive them (Ayalon and Young 2005, Mills and Edwards 2002, Williams and Williams-Morris 2000). These influences have a significant impact on their lives in general, including health, socioeconomic, political, religious and explanatory style in general (Menke and Flynn 2009, Kleinmann (1988a).

This chapter focuses on issues pertaining to mental health among ethnic minorities in the United States, which include African-Americans, Asian-Americans, Latino or Hispanic-Americans, and Native American Indians. Specifically I begin by reviewing literature on prevalence and incidence rates and symptom presentation. I follow this section with a review and analyses of literature on conceptualization and perception of mental illness among ethnic minorities. Finally, I review information about health seeking behaviors and recommended treatment approaches.

Prevalence and Incidence Rates

Mood Disorders

Mood disorders (also known as affective disorders) refer to disturbance in an individual's mood. In general they are divided into two broad diagnostic categories: Depressive and Bipolar Disorders. According to the *Diagnostic and Statistical Manual-IV Text Revised (DSM-IV-TR)*, a diagnosable depressive episode represents experiencing five or more symptoms that have caused a change in an individual's functioning over a two-week period. The symptoms must include either depressed mood and/or loss of interest or pleasure, as well as others, such as appetite disturbance, sleep disturbance, fatigue or loss of energy, feelings of worthlessness, psychomotor agitation or retardation, concentration difficulties, and recurrent suicidal ideation (American Psychiatric Association 2000). Bipolar disorders (formerly manic-depression) consist of cycling between depressive and manic episodes. A manic episode is characterized by a period of unrelenting elevated and/or irritable mood that lasts for one week or more. The period of elevated/irritable mood is typically accompanied by three or more other symptoms, including grandiosity, pressured speech, flight of ideas, diminished need for sleep, and distractibility (American Psychiatric Association 2000).

Mood disorders are common worldwide as well as in the United States. Reports from the World Health Organization indicate that depression is the third leading cause of disease globally, and is expected to be the second (only to cardiovascular disease) by 2020 (World Health Organization 2008). According to the National Institutes of Mental Health (2010), approximately 9.5 percent of American adults age 18 and older have a mood disorder (Kessler et al. 2005). Furthermore, depression is the leading cause of disability for American adults ages 18–44 (World Health Organization 2008). A review of information from Morbidity and Mortality Weekly Report (Gonzalez et al. 2010) showed that in 2006 and 2008, approximately 9 percent of a national sample reported symptoms of depression in the preceding two-week period. These statistics reflect that depression is common, regardless of ethnicity, age, and other demographic factors.

Reports of ethnic variations in mood disorders are somewhat inconsistent. For instance, compared to non-Hispanic Whites, Non-Hispanic

Blacks, Hispanics, and other minority races reported significantly higher levels of major depression (Gonzalez et al. 2010). Other studies have also found elevated levels of major depression among minorities (Dunlop et al. 2003). In contrast, higher prevalence rates among non-Hispanic Whites have been reported. In a study of results of the National Survey of American Life, lifetime prevalence estimates for major depression was found to be highest for Whites (17.9 percent), compared to that for Caribbean Blacks (12.9 percent) and African Americans (10.4 percent). However, further analyses indicated that regardless of prevalence rates, the level of chronicity and severity was higher for both African American and Caribbean Blacks (Williams et al. 2007). Similar findings were reported among African American, Black Caribbean, and non-Hispanic White mothers (Boyd et al. 2011).

Ethnic variations in prevalence, symptom presentation, and illness characteristics also exists for Bipolar disorder. In a study of symptom presentation, severity, and treatment of Bipolar disorder among a sample of patients in the Stanford University Bipolar Clinic, Asian and Latino patients had higher prevalence rates of Bipolar I disorder than White patients (Hwang et al. 2010). Specifically, Asian and Latino patients' prevalence rates were approximately 58 percent and 60 percent respectively, While whites had rates of about 37 percent. Other studies comparing symptoms of bipolar disorder reported that of all the symptoms, Latino and African American respondents presented with significantly higher levels of excessive restlessness and inflated self-esteem (Perron et al. 2010). Furthermore, some investigators found that compared to Whites, African Americans diagnosed with bipolar disorder tended to report psychotic symptoms, particularly auditory hallucinations and delusions (Kennedy et al. 2004). The latter findings may explain the increased risk of misdiagnosis of bipolar disorder with schizophrenia among African Americans (Kilbourne et al. 2004).

It is noteworthy mentioning that even though there is a paucity of research on the mental health of ethnic/racial minorities, there is a stark lack of research on mood disorders among Native American Indians. A review of the limited studies available has shown that compared to national comorbidity rates, major depression was one of the most common psychological disorders among a sample of tribal members in the southwest and northern plains of the United States (Beals et al. 2005). Some researchers have found different types of mood disorders more prevalent among certain ethnic groups. Riolo, Nguye, Greden, and King (2005) reported significantly higher prevalence rates of major depression among Whites (compared with African-Americans and Mexican-Americans), but highest for dysthymic disorder among African-Americans in a nationally representative sample.

The general consensus seems to be that ethnic and racial minorities have higher prevalence rates for mood disorders (especially major depression), and that their increased risk for this disorder is related to negative experiences associated with prejudice, discrimination, poverty, education, and some other factors that make it hard for them to meet their basic needs (Riolo et al. 2005, Plants and Sachs-Ericsson 2004).

Anxiety Disorders

Anxiety disorders are characterized by excessive rumination and/or worrying, apprehension, fear of future uncertainties, persistent phobias with associated avoidant behaviors, and generalized physiological symptoms, such as increased heart rate, sweating, and gastrointestinal discomfort. The DSM-TR categorizes anxiety disorders into generalized anxiety, phobias, panic, obsessive-compulsive, and post-traumatic stress disorders (American Psychiatric Association 2000). Generalized anxiety disorder involves excessive worrying about different situations to the point that the worry causes significant problems in daily functioning. It is associated with several physiological symptoms, including edginess, fatigue, irritability, muscle tension, sleep disturbance, and concentration difficulties. Phobias refer to persistent irrational fear of either a specific object or situation (Specific Phobia), being in a place in which help or escape may be difficult (Agoraphobia) or fear of performance or exposure to an unfamiliar environment or audience (Social Phobia). Panic disorders are characterized by an unexpected experience of intense fear for a brief period (up to 10 minutes), with symptoms including palpitations, sweating, shaking, chest pain, dizziness, nausea, and fear of losing control. The DSMIV-TR defines Obsessive-Compulsive Disorder as typified by persistent, recurring, intrusive, thoughts, images, and impulses (i.e., obsession) that cause significant distress to the sufferer, and thus drives the compulsion (repetitive behaviors or mental acts) in an effort to reduce the distress. Last, Posttraumatic Stress Disorder is characterized by exposure to a significant threat with a response of intense fear and helplessness, followed by persistent re-experiencing of the trauma in diverse ways (e.g., nightmares, reliving experience, etc.), and avoidance of the situations associated with the trauma (American Psychiatric Association 2000).

Prevalence rates for anxiety disorders have also been found to be influenced by ethnicity. Similar to mood disorders, many studies have concluded that anxiety disorders are less prevalent in ethnic minorities than in

Whites (Grant et al. 2005), with the exception of Native American Indians who have been reported to have higher rates of anxiety and anxiety/depression comorbidity (Duran et al. 2004). Findings of lower rates of Generalized Anxiety Disorder have been confirmed in numerous studies, with lifetime risk higher for non-Latino Whites compared with African-Americans, Asian-Americans, Caribbean Blacks, and Latinos (Himle et al. 2009, Breslau et al. 2006). Others have reported an increased risk for Social Anxiety Disorder among Native American Indians (Breslau et al. 2006, Grant et al. 2005) and concluded that "in the United States, being American Indian, young, and having low income increases the risk for Social Anxiety Disorder, whereas being Asian, Latino, African American, or Caribbean Black race/ethnicity, male, or living in urban or populated regions reduces this risk" (Lewis-Fernandez et al. 2010).

In a study that examined lifetime prevalence rates of anxiety disorders among a sample of over 16,000 Americans, Asnaani and colleagues reported that different ethnic groups were more likely to be diagnosed with specific anxiety disorders (Asnaani et al. 2010). The authors found that compared to African-Americans, Asian-Americans, and Hispanics, White Americans were more likely to endorse symptoms that met the diagnostic criteria for social anxiety, generalized anxiety disorder, and panic disorder, but African-Americans were more likely to be diagnosed with post-traumatic stress disorder (PTSD). The latter findings have been confirmed by a more recent study of a larger sample of over 34,000 people, with lifetime prevalence rates of PTSD being highest in Blacks (8.7 percent), followed by Whites (7.4 percent) and Hispanics (7.0 percent), and then Asian-American with the lowest (4.0 percent) (Roberts et al. 2011). Similarly, Beals et al. (2005) reported that according to data from the National Comorbidity Survey, Native American Indians were more likely to have higher rates of PTSD and alcohol dependence but lower rates of depression.

Other studies have reported different rates of Post-Traumatic Stress Disorder, with Hispanics having the highest prevalence rates of the disorder (Pole, Gone, and Kulkarni 2008). Some national studies have confirmed higher rates of PTSD in Blacks (Himle et al. 2009), while others found no significant differences across ethnic groups (Breslau et al. 2006). Even more interesting are studies that indicate variations in prevalence rates for anxiety among U.S.-born and non-U.S. born ethnic minorities. Alegria, Mulvaney-Day, Torres, Polo, Cao, and Canino (2007) found prevalence rates of psychiatric disorders among U.S.-born Latinos to be higher than among foreign (or non U.S.) born Latinos. Similar findings have been reported among U.S.-born and foreign born Caribbean Blacks as well as U.S.-born and foreign-born Asians (National Institute for Mental Health 2012).

Symptom Presentation, Conceptualization, and Perception of Mental Illness

While reviewing studies that point to differences in prevalence rates among ethnic minority groups, it is also important to focus on the fact that culture may influence how and what symptoms are presented. For instance Roberts et al.'s (2011) study of PTSD prevalence rates revealed that compared to Whites, Blacks and Hispanics were more likely to have experienced childhood maltreatment and witnessed domestic violence, and Asians, Black men, and Hispanic women were more likely to have experienced war-related trauma. Other studies have reported that although African Americans reported higher rates of depression than White Americans, African Americans tended to suffer from more severe forms of depression as well as more specific symptoms (Jackson and Knight 2006, Williams et al. 2007). Even more specific are studies that have indicated that African Africans and Hispanics tend to report somatic symptoms more than non-Hispanic Whites (Ayalon and Young 2003, Myers 2002). It has been speculated that among some ethnic minority groups, unlike the negative stigma associated with clinical depression, somatization of depression is a more acceptable way of presenting one's stress (Nadeem, Lange, and Miranda 2009).

Similar to Hispanics and non-Hispanic Blacks, Asian-Americans have been found to emphasize somatic symptoms of depression (Kleinman 2004, Ryder, Yang, and Heine 2002, Ryder et al. 2008). These symptoms include appetite disturbance, sleep disturbance, bodily pains or weakness, and fatigue (Kleinman 1996). However, other recent studies have found evidence of both affective and somatic complaints among Asian-Americans (Yang and Wonpat-Borja 2007). A review of literature on the somatization of depression suggests that unlike western medicine that considers the mind and body as different entities, eastern practice tends to emphasize an integration of mind and body, and hence the seemingly higher rate of somatic complaints (Kalibatseva and Leong 2011). All in all, these studies point to the important role of culture in mental illness and symptom perception, presentation, and treatment.

Given the relevance of culture in psychopathology, it is important to review some basic tenets in this section. Culture is defined as a general way of life or behaviors of a group of people, which reflects their shared social experiences, values, attitudes, norms, and beliefs; culture is transmitted from generation to generation and changes over time (Eshun and

Gurung 2009). In general, culture has many characteristics in that it is learned, changes over time, is cyclical or self-reinforcing, consists of tangible and intangible behaviors, and most important of all, is crucial for survival and adaptation. Thus, cultural traits and norms do influence how we think, how we respond to distress, and how comfortable we are expressing our emotions. This means that an understanding of one's culture is crucial to fully understanding the precedents of mental illness, as surmised in a statement by the U.S. Surgeon General (1999) on mental health that a patient's culture shapes their perceptions about mental health and ultimately affects their decision about the types of mental health services they use. Similarly, the clinician's culture, training and the service system affect diagnosis and treatment as well as how services are organized and financed.

Culture influences how individuals present their symptoms and illness behaviors through verbal and non-verbal communication, how they cope with psychological challenges, their diagnosis, and also their willingness to seek treatment. It has been argued that culture and mental illness are more or less embedded in each other and that understanding the role of culture in mental health is crucial to comprehensive and accurate diagnoses and treatment of illnesses (Castillo 1997, Sam andMoreira 2002). Specifically, Castillo (1997) identified that culture influences mental health in many ways, including:

1. The individual's own personal experience of the illness and associated symptoms.
2. How the individual expresses his or her experience or symptoms within the context of his or her cultural norms.
3. How the symptoms expressed are interpreted and hence diagnosed.
4. How the mental illness is treated and ultimately the outcome.

Overall, there seem to be negative beliefs about depression and mental illness in general among ethnic minority groups (Menke and Flynn 2009). As discussed earlier, such negative beliefs tend to influence symptom presentation. In a study of beliefs, attitudes, stigma, and treatment preference for depression, ethnic minorities (specifically, African-Americans, Asian/Pacific Islanders, and Hispanics) were less likely to believe that depression had a biological basis, and thus also less likely to perceive antidepressant medication as an effective treatment for depression (Givens et al. 2007).

A group's perception of an illness and cultural worldview also influences how well the individual and close relatives cope with mental illness. People from cultures in which mental illness is linked with supernatural causes (e.g., sorcerer, witchcraft, evil eye), such as Native American

Indians, Caribbean Blacks, and others of African descent are less likely to seek help from a mental health professional, more likely to seek help from a traditional healer or medicine man (Mateus, dos Santos, and de Jesus Mari 2005). They also tend to view mental illness as a reflection of dysfunction in the larger social group and thus require healing "for the collective, as well as the individual" (James et al. 2003). Thus, to be able to build a trusted relationship with ethnic minority clients, health practitioners need to demonstrate some knowledge as well as show respect for their traditions (Broome and Broome 2007, Foster 2006).

Even beyond cultural factors, other sociodemographic factors do influence the likelihood of ethnic minorities reporting or seeking help for psychological disorders. These factors include perceived racial discrimination and prejudice, stigmatization, socioeconomic status, and educational attainment. Studies of PTSD have concluded that the reported higher rates among Blacks may be associated with racial discrimination (Ellis et al. 2008), low educational attainment and low income (DeNavas-Walt, Proctor, and Smith 2008). These studies have also linked lower rates of PTSD among Asian-Americans to higher educational attainment and higher income.

Health Seeking Behaviors

Although mood disorders such as Major Depression are treatable conditions, less than two-thirds of adults and about one-half of children diagnosed with the disorder seek treatment (U.S. Department of Health and Human Services 1999). As mentioned earlier in this chapter, although the chronicity and severity of major depressive disorder was higher in Blacks than Whites, less than half of African Americans and less than a quarter of Caribbean Blacks who met criteria received treatment for their condition (Williams et al. 2007). Furthermore, Black mothers, particularly African American mothers with bipolar disorder, tend to underutilize treatment (Boyd et al. 2011). Similarly, ethnic minorities are less likely to receive treatment for serious anxiety disorders such as PTSD (Roberts et al. 2011). According to Roberts and colleagues, less than half of their minority sample sought treatment for their PTSD symptoms.

Stigmatization is one of the factors that have been associated with the reluctance of minorities to seek help for mental illness (Yamoshiro and Matsuoka 1997). The stigma (and/or shame) associated with mental illness has been confirmed among Native American Indians (Grandbois 2005), Asian Americans (Loya, Reddy, and Hinshaw 2010, Yang, Phelan, and Link 2008), African-Americans (Ward, Clark, and Heidrich 2009), and

Latinos (Guarnaccia, Martinez, and Acosta 2005). Overall, it has been established that an individual's own perceived stigma about mental illness, as well as the stigma from society in general both have a significant impact on help-seeking behaviors for mental illness (Grandbois 2005, Vogel, Wade, and Hackler 2007).

Among Native American Indians, mental health stigmas have been associated with differences in their worldview and that of the majority culture, such as the unity of the mind, body and spirit, importance of spirituality, balance, interconnectedness, and cooperation. In general, mental illness is viewed as a "form of supernatural possession . . . disharmony between inner and outer natural forces . . . a hopeless state . . . [and] the terminal phase . . ." (Grandbois 2005, 1005). Such views may influence the individual's decisions for healthcare; whereas western medicine may recommend psychotherapy and medication, a Native American Indian with a traditional perspective may appreciate alternate treatments such us herbs and spirituality or body-mind-soul connections.

Similarly, a comparative study of older African American and Caucasian samples indicated that African Americans viewed depression as a personal weakness, and were less likely to see depression as a medical condition (Mills, Alea, and Cheong 2004). Among the explanations offered, Mills et al pointed out that the racial differences in beliefs about depression "may be due to [reports of] African Americans' strongly held religious attitudes suggesting that through faith one can endure and overcome life's burdens. Accordingly, if you are depressed, then your faith is not strong (e.g., you have a character flaw)" (Mills et al. 2004, 324). Other more recent studies have confirmed the negativity associated with mental illness among African Americans. For instance, they have been found to view mental illness as chronic and also associate it with stigmas (Ward et al. 2009). Furthermore, a study of the extent to which stigmatization of mental health was associated with underutilization of mental health services among a sample of low income Black and Latina women confirmed the negative impact of stigmas on help-seeking behaviors (Nadeem et al. 2007). Specifically, Nadeem, et al. reported that respondent's concerns about stigma decreased their likelihood of seeking treatment for mental illness.

For Latino or Hispanic Americans, Guarnaccia, Martinez, and Acosta (2005) summarized that "The stigma of mental illness is particularly powerful as a barrier to seeking care. In particular, the label of *locura* or madness carries strong negative connotations. Someone who is *loco* is seen as severely mentally ill, potentially violent and incurable" (36). Other studies point to an attitude of self-reliance— *ponerse de su* parte, a feeling that one should contribute one's part or be able to cope with their problems—tends to strongly influence whether or not an individual seeks psychological help (Guarnaccia et al. 2005, 37, Ortega and Alegria 2002). Furthermore, it has been argued that the concept of *familismo*— the extended family network—as a crucial source of social support may be a barrier to seeking help for mental illness, in that, it serves as a buffer and lengthens the time before actually seeking help.

The picture is no different for Asian Americans, who have also been found to have negative attitudes about psychotherapy and are therefore less likely to seek help for mental illness. Loya et al. (2010) investigated the role of personal and public stigma about mental illness in health seeking behaviors; their findings indicated that higher levels of personal stigma (e.g., concerns about social distance from sufferers of mental illness) accounted for a significant proportion of the variance in attitudes towards counseling. Other studies have confirmed associations between concerns about stigmatization and likelihood of seeking help from an appropriate health professional. For instance, Chinese Americans reported significantly more shame with accessing western psychiatric services compared with traditional Chinese medicine as a treatment option (Yang, Phelan, and Link 2008). Furthermore, compared to European American samples, Asian Americans tend to have less favorable attitudes about seeking help for mental illness and hold more mental health stigmas (Masuda and Boone 2011). In general, holding on to Asian values of shame avoidance, loss of face, and not disgracing the family name are all negatively related to likelihood of seeking help (Kim 2007, David 2010).

Other factors are mostly related to attitudes and perceptions of healthcare workers, such as mistrust of health professionals and personal biases on the part of healthcare professionals. Cultural mistrust of professionals has been associated with a history of oppression, prejudice, and discrimination against ethnic minority groups (Williams and Williams-Morris 2000, Rajakumar et al. 2009, David 2010). For instance, among African Americans, the long, painful history of slavery, segregation (Whaley 2001), and unfortunate examples of discrimination in the medical field such as the Tuskegee syphilis study (Centers for Disease Control and Prevention 2013) have contributed to their mistrust of health professionals. Other studies have demonstrated a positive relationship between familiarity and assimilation into the main U.S. culture (which may decrease mistrust of professionals) and mental health service utilization (Abe-Kim et al. 2007, Shea and Yeh 2008). All in all, health seeking behaviors among ethnic minorities are related to immigration, acculturation, alienation and the long history of prejudice and discrimination, all of which strongly influence trust in healthcare workers or the health system in general (Rodenhauser 1994).

Treatment Approaches – Multimodal Approach

Preferences and Biases in Treatment among Ethnic Minorities

Review of research suggests that although certain mood and anxiety disorders tend to be more chronic and severe among ethnic minorities, the illnesses are more likely to remain untreated, compared to Whites. This fact was emphasized by the U.S. Surgeon General in his report on race, culture, ethnicity, and mental health (U.S. Department of Health and Human Services 2001). A combination of factors on the part of health seekers (in this case ethnic minorities) as well as healthcare providers often influence whether or not help would be sought, an accurate diagnosis would be made, the appropriate treatment would be selected, and last (and equally important), whether or not the patient would comply with treatment. From the patient's perspective some crucial questions determine potential treatment success. For instance, when immigrants and members of ethnic minority groups ask for references from relatives, it is typical that they inquire about medical expertise as well as comfort level, based on cultural knowledge and acceptance (American Psychological Association 2003, 382).

Members of ethnic minority groups have been reported to show bias towards counseling and psychotherapy. Even when no differences in prevalence rates were found in comparing Mexican Americans, Puerto Ricans, African Americans, Caribbean Blacks, and non-Latino Whites, Mexican Americans and African Americans reported lower rates of depression therapy utilization (Gonzalez et al. 2010). This may be because African Americans tend to use alternative treatment approaches such as church and the extended family (Thompson, Bazile, and Akbar 2004) and some Latinos may prefer to use traditional resources such as Espiritismo, Santeria, and Curanderos (Guarnaccia et al. 2005). Similarly, Asian Americans tend to have less favorable attitudes towards counseling services and are less likely to use them (Masuda et al. 2009). The latter may be associated with a general Asian cultural worldview of avoiding shame, maintaining one's family name, and presenting oneself as emotionally resilient, which more or less discourages self-disclosure, a crucial part of counseling and psychotherapy (Kim 2007).

In working with ethnic minorities, health practitioners are strongly encouraged to be aware of their own personal biases. They are "encouraged to recognize that, as cultural beings, they may hold attitudes and beliefs that can detrimentally influence their perceptions of and interactions with individuals who are ethnically and racially different from themselves" (American Psychological Association 2003, 382). Awareness of such individual biases is crucial, as it entails a recognition of, and understanding that such biases may influence their assessment, diagnosis, and treatment of minority patients, and could negatively impact their wellbeing. Mental health practitioners ought to be "aware of their own attitudes and values," and make every effort to change the "automatically favorable perceptions of the in-group," and make every effort to change the "automatically . . . negative perceptions of the out-group" (American Psychological Association, 384).

Ethnic minorities are even less likely to utilize psychopharmacological treatment: Mexican American and African Americans used psychotherapy significantly more than the other ethnic minority groups, but they were less likely to utilize psychopharmacology (Gonzalez et al. 2010). Similarly, compared to a White sample, African Americans and Latinos were less likely to accept antidepressants for treating depression, but more open to counseling as a treatment option (Cooper et al. 2003). In a study of psychopharmacologic treatment success, African American and Latino members were less successful with antidepressant medication only, compared to Whites, and emphasized a need for more comprehensive treatment protocol to include psychotherapy (Lesser et al. 2007). Other studies have also found a preference for counseling and prayer over antidepressant medication among African American, Asian/Pacific Islander, and Hispanic samples (Givens et al. 2007, Ward, Clark, and Heidrich 2009).

Research studies point to the fact that some ethnic minority groups tend to prefer treatments that are in sync with their own traditional values and norms. Native American Indians, for example, believe in the important link between mind-body-spirit, as well as the social collective in their psychological wellbeing (Manson 2000); they may thus prefer to seek help from a traditional healer (Beals et al. 2005). Furthermore, based on anecdotal observations and a review of historical and political information, some authors have pointed to the importance of respect (as perceived by Native American Indians) and concluded that to be able to build a trusted relationship with ethnic minority clients, health practitioners need to demonstrate some knowledge as well as show respect for their traditions (Broome and Broome 2007, Foster 2006). These reports suggest that in lieu of seeking help from a traditional healer, Native Americans are more likely to trust and comply with treatment from a health professional who seriously considers their world view about mind-body-spirit, respect for others and nature, and the importance of the collective (family and community elders).

Biases in Diagnosis and Treatment among Health Practitioners

Similar to the general population, health practitioners have their own attitudes, values, and beliefs that have been shaped by their own unique cultural experiences. Thus, in interacting with patients, their worldview is likely to influence their perception of the patient in issues pertaining to diagnosis, treatment selection, and cost involved in treatment (Snowden, 2003). Race plays an important role in diagnosis of psychological disorders: studies have shown that Asian-Americans and Whites are more likely to be diagnosed with a mood disorder, while African-Americans are more likely to be diagnosed with schizophrenia (Flaskerud and Hu 1992).

According to the American Psychological Association's *Guidelines on Multicultural Education, Training, research, Practice, and Organizational Change for Psychologists* (2003), it is important that health professionals promote an environment conducive to patients seeking help, complying with, and following up with treatment by becoming familiar with diverse cultural groups. Specifically, APA suggests that mental health practitioners build trust and increase patient help-seeking and compliance behaviors by:

1. Becoming aware of their own attitudes, stereotypes, and expectations of minorities
2. Changing their "automatically favorable perception of in-group" and
3. Changing "automatically negative perception of out-group"

Biases in quality and type of treatment have also been reported (see Snowden 2003). For instance, in a study of Medicaid recipients, African Americans were less likely to be prescribed antidepressants even if needed (Melfi et al.1997). Other studies have confirmed that ethnic minorities are less likely to use antidepressants than Caucasians (Delaney et al. 2009). Still, some researchers have suggested African Americans are more likely to be prescribed older types of antidepressant medication (e.g., Tricyclic antidepressants and MAO inhibitors) (Chen and Rizzo 2008), and less likely to be prescribed antidepressants in general compared to Whites (Lin, Erickson, and Balkrishnan 2011)

Even after an individual agrees to pharmacologic treatment, their cultural norms and diet could have a significant impact on the effectiveness of the medication. For instance, fava beans (very common in Mediterranean diets), has been found to have high levels of dopamine, which could cause "severe hypertensive reactions in individuals taking monoamine oxidase inhibitors (see Foulks 2004 for review). Other observations have shown that grapefruit juice could cause increases in the blood levels of certain drugs, including Zoloft, Prozac, Buspar, and Trazedone (Foulks 2004). Such nutritional information is important knowledge for health practitioners, and emphasizes the need to include some level of inquiry into the patient's diet and common food preferences before prescribing some of these psychotropic medications.

In Conclusion

In general, life experiences shape one's worldview and may influence illness behaviors such as symptom presentation, meaning and attributions of illness, likelihood to seek treatment, treatment compliance, and ultimately treatment effectiveness (APA 2003). This is even much so for psychological disorders like depression and anxiety, which are often diagnosed based on subjective symptom descriptions. It is worth mentioning that rates of professional service use for treatment of mental health challenges among Latinos (in general) has improved in the last two decades (Alegria et al. 2007). Researchers hope to see similar trends among other ethnic minority groups. However, the large differences in percentage of untreated mood and anxiety disorders among ethnic minorities call for "investment in accessible and culturally sensitive treatment options" (Roberts et al. 2011).

In spite of their high prevalence rates for mood and anxiety disorders, ethnic minorities seem to have strong social networks stemming from a history and culture of collectivism and interdependence. This strong sense of social support tends to have a buffering effect on stress, which may help decrease the potential impact of depression and anxiety (for review, see Plant and Sachs-Ericsson 2004). As summarized by the National Alliance on Mental Illness (NAMI), "sensitivity to African American cultural differences, such as differences in medication metabolization rates, unique views of mental illness and propensity towards experiencing certain mental illnesses, can improve African Americans' treatment experiences and increase utilization of mental health care services." Mental healthcare workers should seriously consider the following in working with ethnic minority populations:

1. Knowledge of the individual's culture and level of acculturation.
2. Perceptions and stigma associated with mental illness and be ready to provide educational material.

3. Pay close attention to symptom presentation and consider individual and ethnic group's sociopolitical history of oppression, racial prejudice, and continued discrimination.
4. Comprehensive treatment planning to include psychotherapy and medication (if indicated).
5. If medication is needed, be mindful to select ones that are newer, more effective (considering possible ethnic differences in metabolic rates), and with fewer side effects in an effort to increase medication compliance.

References

Abe-Kim, J., D. T. Takeuchi, S. Hong, N. Zane, S. Sue, M. S. Spencer, and M. Alegria. 2007. "Use of Mental Health-Related Services among Immigrant and U.S.-Born Asian Americans: Results from the National Latino and Asian American Study." *American Journal of Public Health* 97: 91–98.

Alegria, M., N. Mulvaney-Day, M. Torres, A. Polo, Z. Cao, and G. Canino. 2007. "Prevalence of Psychiatric Disorders across Latino Subgroups in the United States." *American Journal of Public Health* 97(1): 68–75.

Alegria, M., N. Mulvaney-Day, M. Woo, M. Torres, S. Gao. and V. Oddo. 2007. "Correlates of Past-Year Mental Health Service Use among Latinos: Results of National Latino and Asian-American Study." *American Journal of Public Health* 97(1): 76–83.

American Psychiatric Association. 2000. *Diagnostic and Statistical Manual* (4th ed., text rev.). Washington, DC: Author.

American Psychological Association—APA. 2003. *Guidelines on Multicultural Education, Training, Research, Practice, and Organizational Change for Psychologists.* American Psychologist 58(5): 377–402.

Asnaani, A., A. Richey, R. Dimaite, D. E. Hinton, and S. G. Hoffman. 2010. "A Cross-Ethnic Comparison of Lifetime Prevalence Rates of Anxiety Disorders." *Journal of Nervous and Mental Disease* 198(8): 551–555.

Ayalon, L., and M. A. Young. 2003. "A Comparison of Depressive Symptoms in African Americans and Caucasian Americans." *Journal of Cross-Cultural Psychology* 34: 111–124.

Ayalon, L. and M. A. Young. 2005. "Racial Group Differences in Help-Seeking Behaviors. *Journal of Social Psychology* 145: 391–403.

Beals, J., D. K. Novins, N. R. Whitesell, P. Spicer, C. M. Mitchell, and S. M. Manson. 2005. "Prevalence of Mental Disorders and Utilization of Mental Health Services in Two American Indian Reservation Populations: Mental Health Disparities in a National Context." *American Journal of Psychiatry* 162(9): 1723–1732.

Boyd, R. C., L. Michalopoulos, E. Davis, and J. S. Jackson. 2011. "Prevalence of Mood Disorders and Service Use among U.S. Mothers by Race and Ethnicity: Results from the National Survey of American Life." *Journal of Clinical Psychiatry* 72(11): 1538–1545.

Breslau, J., S. Aguilar-Gaxiola, K. S. Kendler, D. Williams, and R. C. Kessler. 2006. "Specifying Race-Ethnic Differences in Risk for Psychiatric Disorder in a USA National Sample." *Psychological Medicine 36*: 57–68.

Broome, B and R. Broome. 2007. "Native Americans: Traditional Healing." *Urologic Nursing 27*(2): 161–163.

Carrasco, M. and J. Weiss. 2005. "Asian American and Pacific Islander Outreach Manual, National Alliance on Mental Illness (NAMI)." http://www.nami.org/Tem plate.cfm?Section=MIOandTemplate=/ContentManagement/ContentDisplay .cfmandContentID=24476.

Castillo, R. J. 1997. *Culture and Mental Illness.* Pacific Grove, CA: ITP.

Centers for Disease Control and Prevention. 2013. *U.S. Public Health Service Syphilis Study at Tuskegee,* Atlanta, GA: Centers for Disease Control. http://www.cdc.gov/ tuskegee/timeline.htm

Chen, J. and J. A. Rizzo. 2008. "Racial and Ethnic Disparities in Antidepressant Drug Use." *Journal of Mental Health Policy and Economics 11*(4): 155–165.

Cooper, L. A., J. J. Gonzales, J. J. Gallo, K. M. Rost, L. S. Meredith, J. V. Rubenstein, N. Y. Wang, and D. E. Ford. 2003. "The Acceptability of Treatment for Depression among African-American, Hispanic, and White Primary Care Patients." *Medical Care 41*(4): 479–489.

David, E. J. R. 2010. "Cultural Mistrust and Mental Health Help-Seeking Attitudes Among Filipino Americans." *Asian American Journal of Psychology 1*(1): 57–66.

Delaney, J. A. C., B. E. Oddson, R. L. McClelland, and B. M. Psaty. 2009. "Estimating Ethnic Differences in Self-Reported New Use of Antidepressant Medications: Results from the Multi-Ethnic Study of Atherosclerosis, Pharmacoepidemiology and Drug Safety." doi: 10.1002/pds.1751.

DeNavas-Walt, C., B. D. Proctor, and J. C. Smith. 2008. "Current Population Reports: Consumer Income." United States Census Bureau and United States Department of Commerce; Washington, DC: 2008. Income, Poverty, and Health Insurance Coverage in the United States: 2007, 1–71.

Dunlop, D. D., J. Song, J. S. Lyons, L. M. Manheim, and R. W. Chang. 2003. "Racial/Ethnic Differences in Rates of Depression among Preretirement Adults." *American Journal of Public Health 93*(11): 1945–1952.

Duran, B., M. Sanders, B. Skipper, H. Waitzkin, L. H. Malcoe, S. Paine, and J. Yager. 2004. "Prevalence and Correlates of Mental Disorders among Native American Women in Primary Care." *American Journal of Public Health 94*(1): 71–77.

Ellis, B. H., H. Z. MacDonald, A. K. Lincoln, and H. J. Cabral. 2008. "Mental Health of Somali Adolescent Refugees: The Role of Trauma, Stress, and Perceived Discrimination." *Journal of Consulting and Clinical Psychology 76*: 184–193.

Eshun, S. and R. A. R. Gurung. 2009. "Introduction to Culture and Psychopathology." In *Culture and Mental Health: Sociocultural Influences, Theory and Practice.* Boston, MA: Wiley-Blackwell.

Flaskerud, J. H. and L. T. Hu. 1992. "Relationship of Ethnicity to Psychiatric Diagnosis." *Journal of Nervous and Mental Disease 180*(5): 296–303.

Foster, C. H. 2006. "What Nurses Should Know when Working in Aboriginal Communities." *Canadian Nurse 102*(4): 28–31.

Foulks, E. F. 2004. "Cultural Variables in Psychiatry." *Psychiatric Times Global Watch 21*: 28–30.

Givens, J. L., T. K. Houston, B. W. Van Voorhees, D. E. Ford, and L. A. Cooper. 2007. "Ethnicity and Preference for Depression Treatment." *General Hospital Psychiatry 29*(3): 182–191.

Gonzalez, H. M., W. A. Vega, D. R. Williams, W. Tarraf, B. T. West, and H. W. Neighbors. 2010. "Depression Care in the United States: Too Little for Too Few." *Archives of General Psychiatry 67*(1): 37–46.

Gonzalez, O., J. T. Berry, L. R. McKnight-Eily, T. Strine, V. J. Edwards, H. Lu, and J. B. Croft. 2010. "Current Depression among Adults, United States 2006 and 2008." *Morbidity and Mortality Weekly Report 59*(38). National Center for Chronic Disease Prevention and Health Promotion, CDC.

Grandbois, D. 2005. "Stigma of Mental Illness among American Indian and Alaska Native Nations: Historical and Contemporary Perspectives." *Issues in Mental Health Nursing 26*(10): 1001–1024.

Grant, D. F., D. S. Hasin, C. Blanco, F. S. Stinson, P. Chou, R. B. Goldstein, B. Huang. 2005. "The Epidemiology of Social Anxiety Disorders in the United States: Results from the National Epidemiological Survey on Alcohol and Related Conditions." *Journal of Clinical Psychiatry 66*: 1351–1361.

Guarnaccia, P. J., I. Martinez, and H. Acosta. 2005. "Mental Health in the Hispanic Immigrant Community: An Overview." *Journal of Immigrant and Refugee Services* (The Haworth Social Work Practice Press, an imprint of The Haworth Press, Inc.) 3(1/2):21–46.

Himle, J. A., R. E. Baser, R. J. Taylor, R. D. Campbell, and J. S. Jackson. 2009. "Anxiety Disorders among African Americans, Blacks of Caribbean Descent, and Non-Hispanic Whites in the United States." *Journal of Anxiety Disorders 23*: 578–590.

Hwang, S. H. J., M. E. Childers, P. W. Wang, J. Y. Nam, K. L. Keller, S. J. Hill, and T. A. Ketter. 2010. "Higher Prevalence of Bipolar I Disorder among Asian and Latino Compared to Caucasian Patients Receiving Treatment." *Asia-Pacific Psychiatry 2*(3): 156–165. DOI: 10.1111/j.1758-5872.2010.00080.x

Jackson, J. S. and K. M. Knight. 2006. "Race and Self-Regulatory Health Behaviors: The Role of the Stress Response and the HPA Axis in Physical and Mental Health Disparities." In *Social Structure, Aging, and Self-Regulation in the Elderly,* edited by L. L. Cartensen and K. W. Schaie. New York: Springer.

James Myers, L., A. Young, E. Obasi, and S. Speight. 2003. "Recommendations for the Psychological Treatment of Persons of African Descent (Chapter 3)." *Psychological Treatment of Ethnic Minority Populations, Council of National Psychological Associations for the Advancement of Ethnic Minority Interests.* Washington, D.C.: Association of Black Psychologists.

Kalibatseva, Z. and F. T. L. Leong. 2011. "Depression among Asian Americans: Review and Recommendations." *Depression Research and Treatment.* doi: 10.1155/2011/320902.

Kennedy, N., J. Boydell, J. van Os, R. M. Murray. 2004. "Ethnic Differences in First Clinical Presentation of Bipolar Disorder: Results from an Epidemiological Study." *Journal of Affective Disorders* 83: 161–168.

Kessler, R. C., W. T. Chiu, O. Demler, and E. E. Walters. 2005. "Prevalence, Severity, and Comorbidity of Twelve-Month DSM-IV Disorders in the National Comorbidity Survey Replication (NCS-R)." *Archives of General Psychiatry* 62(6): 617–27.

Kilbourne, A. M., G. L. Haas, B. H. Mulsant, M. S. Bauer, and H. A. Pincus. 2004. "Concurrent Psychiatric Diagnoses by Age and Race among Persons with Bipolar Disorder." *Psychiatric Services* 55: 931–933.

Kim, B. S. K. 2007. "Adherence to Asian and European American Cultural Values and Attitudes toward Seeking Professional Psychological Help among Asian American College Students." *Journal of Counseling Psychology* 54: 474–480.

Kleinman, A. 1988a. "Do Psychiatric Disorders Differ in Different Cultures?" In *Understanding and Applying Medical Anthropology*, edited by P. Brown,185–196, CA: Mayfield Publishing Company.

Kleinman, A. 1988b. *Rethinking Psychiatry.* New York, NY: Free Press.

Kleinman, A. 1996. "How is culture important for DSM-IV?" In *Culture and Psychiatric Diagnosis: A DSM-IV Perspective,* edited by J.E Mezzich, A. Kleinman, H. Fabrega, and D. L. Parrons, 15–25. Washington DC: American Psychiatric Press.

Kleinman, A. 2004. "Culture and Depression." *The New England Journal of Medicine* 351(10): 951–953.

Lesser, I. M., D. B. Castro, B. N. Gayes, J. Gonzalez, A. J. Rush, J. E. Alpert, and S. R. Wisniewski. 2007. "Ethnicity/Race and Outcome in the Treatment of Depression: Results from STAR*D." *Medical Care* 45(11): 1043–1051.

Lewis-Fernandez, R., D. E. Hinton, A. J. Laria, E. H. Patterson, S. G. Hoffman, M. G. Craske, and B. Liao. 2010. "Culture and the Anxiety Diorders: Recommendations for DSM-IV." *Depression and Anxiety* 27(2): 212–229.

Lin, H. C., S. R. Erickson, and R. Balkrishnan. 2011. "Physician Prescribing Patterns of Innovative Antidepressants in the United States: The Case of MDD Patients 1993–2007." *The International Journal of Psychiatry in Medicine* 42(4): 353–368.

Loya, F., R. Reddy, and S. P. Hinshaw. 2010. "Mental Illness Stigma as a Mediator of Differences in Caucasian and South Asian College Students' Attitudes toward Psychological Counseling." *Journal of Counseling Psychology* 57(4): 484–490.

Manson, S. M. 2000. "Mental Health Services for American Indians and Alaska Natives Need, Use, and Barriers to Effective Care." *Canadian Journal of Psychiatry* 45(7): 617–626.

Masuda, A., P. L. Anderson, M. P. Twohig, A. B. Fenstein, Y. Y. Chou, J. W. Wendell, and A. R. Stormo. 2009. "Help-Seeking Experiences and Attitudes among African American, Asian American, and European American College Students." *International Journal for Advancement of Counseling* 31: 168–180.

Masuda, A and M. S. Boone. 2011. "Mental Health Stigma, Self-Concealment, and Help-Seeking Attitudes among Asian American and European American College Students with No Help-Seeking Experience." *International Journal for the Advancement of Counselling* 33(4): 266–279.

Mateus, M. D., J. Q. dos Santos, and J. de Jesus Mari. 2005. "Popular Conceptions of Schizophrenia in Cape Verde, Africa." *Revista Brasileira de Psiquiatria* 27(2): 101–107.

Melfi, C., T. Croghan, M. Hanna, and R. Robinson. 1997. "Racial Variation in Antidepressant Treatment in a Medicaid Population." *Journal of Clinical Psychiatry* 61: 16–21.

Menke, R. and H. Flynn. 2009. "Relationships between Stigma, Depression, and Treatment in White and African American Primary Care Patients." *The Journal of Nervous and Mental Disease* 197(6): 407–411.

Mills, T. L. and C. A. Edwards. 2002. "A Critical Review of Research on the Mental Health Status of older African Africans." *Ageing and Society* 22(3): 273–304.

Mills, T. L., N. L. Alea, and J. A. Cheong. 2004. "Differences in the Indicators of Depressive Symptoms among a Community Sample of African-American and Caucasian Older Adults." *Community Mental Health Journal* 40(4): 309–331.

Moscicki, E. K., D. Rae, D. A. Regier and B. Z. Locke. 1987. "The Hispanic Health and Nutrition Examination Survey: Depression among Mexican-Americans, Cuban-Americans, Puerto Ricans." In *Health and Behavior: Research Agenda for Hispanics*, edited by M. Gaviria and J. D. Arana. Chicago: University of Chicago at Illinois.

Myers, H. F., I. Lesser, N. Rodriguez, C. B. Mira, W. C. Hwang, C. Camp, and M. Wohl. 2002. "Ethnic Differences in Clinical Presentation of Depression in Adult Women." *Cultural Diversity and Ethnic Minority Psychology* 8(2): 138–156.

Nadeem, E., J. M. Lange, D. Edge, M. Fongwa, T. Belin, and J. Miranda. 2007. "Does Stigma Keep Poor Young Immigrants and U.S.-Born Black and Latina Women from Seeking Mental Health Care?" *Psychiatric Services* 58(12): 1547–1554.

Nadeem, E., J. M. Lange, and J. Miranda. 2009. "Perceived Need for Care among Low-Income Immigrant and U.S. Born Black and Latina Women with Depression." *Journal of Women's Health* 18(3): 369–375. doi: 10.1089/jwh.2008.0898

The National Alliance on Mental Illness (NAMI). "African American Community Mental Health, Fact Sheet." www.nami.org

National Institutes of Mental Health. 2010. "Mood Disorders—Fact Sheet." http://www.nimh.nih.gov/statistics/1ANYMOODDIS_ADULT.shtml

National Institute of Mental Health. 2012. "U.S.-Born Children of Immigrants May Have Higher Risk for Mental Disorder than Parents." http://www.nimh.nih.gov/science-news/2007/us-born-children-of-immigrants-may-have-higher-risk-for-mental-disorders-than-parents.shtml.

Ortega, A. and M. Alegria. 2002. "Self-Reliance, Mental Health Need and Use of Mental Healthcare among Island Puerto Ricans." *Mental Health Services Research* 4: 131–140.

Perron, B. E., L. E. Fries, A. M. Kilbourne, M. G. Vaughn, and M. S. Bauer. 2010. "Racial/Ethnic Group Differences in Bipolar Symptomatology in a Community Sample of Persons with Bipolar 1 Disorder." *The Journal of Nervous and Mental Disease* 198: 16–21.

Plant, E. A. and N. Sachs-Ericsson. 2004. "Racial and Ethnic Differences in Depression: The Roles of Social Support and Meeting Basic Needs." *Journal of Consulting and Clinical Psychology* 72: 41–52.

Pole, N., J. P. Gone, and M. Kulkarni. 2008. "Posttraumatic Stress Disorder among Ethnoracial Minorities in the United States." *Clinical Psychology: Science and Practice* 15(1): 35–61.

Rajakumar K., S. B. Thomas, D. Musa, D. Almario, and M. A. Garza. 2009. "Racial Differences in Parents' Distrust of Medicine and Research." *Archives of Pediatric and Adolescent Medicine* 163: 108–114.

Riolo, S., T. A. Nguyen, J. F. Greden, and C. A. King. 2005. "Prevalence of Depression by Race/Ethnicity: Findings from the National Health and Nutrition Examination Survey III." *American Journal of Public Health* 95(6): 998–1000.

Roberts, A. L., S. E. Gilman, J. Breslau, N. Breslau, and K. C. Koenen. 2011. "Race/Ethnic Differences in Exposure to Traumatic Events, Development of Post-Traumatic Stress Disorder, and Treatment Seeking for Post-Traumatic Stress Disorder in the United States." *Psychological Medicine* 41(1): 71–83.

Rodenhauser, P. 1994. "Cultural Barriers to Mental Health Care Delivery in Alaska." *Journal of Mental Health Administration* 21(1): 60–70.

Ryder, A. G., J. Yang, and S. J. Heine. 2002. "Somatization vs. Psychologization of Emotional Distress: a Paradigmatic Example for Cultural Psychopathology." In *Online Readings in Psychology and Culture,* Unit 9, Chapter 3, International Association for Cross-Cultural Psychology. http://orpc.iaccp.org/index.php?option=com_contentandview=articleandid=68 percent3Aandrew-d-ryderandcatid=28 percent3Achapterandltemid=15/.

Ryder, A. G., J. Yang, X. Zhu, S. Yao, J. Yi, S. J. Heine, and M. R. Bagby. 2008. "The Cultural Shaping of Depression: Somatic Symptoms in China, Psychological Symptoms in North America?" *Journal of Abnormal Psychology* 117(2): 300–313.

Sam, D. L. and V. Moreira. 2002. "The Mutual Embeddedness of Culture and Mental Illness." In *Online Readings in Psychology and Culture,* edited by W. J. Lonner, D. L. Dinnel, S. A. Hayes, and D. N. Sattler (Unit 9, chapter 1). Center for Cross-Cultural Research, Western Washington University, Bellingham, Washington, U.S.A.

Shea, M., and C. J. Yeh. 2008. "Asian American Students' Cultural Values, Stigma, and Relational Self-Construal: Correlates of Attitudes toward Professional Help Seeking." *Journal of Mental Health Counseling* 30: 157–172.

Snowden, L. R. 2003. "Bias in Mental Health Assessment and Intervention: Theory and Evidence." *American Journal of Public Health* 93(2): 239–243.

Thompson, V. L. S., A. Bazile, and M. Akbar. 2004. "African Americans' Perceptions of Psychotherapy and Psychotherapists." *Professional Psychology: Research and Practice* 35: 19–26.

U.S. Department of Health and Human Services. 2001. *Mental Health: Culture, Race, and Ethnicity—A Supplement to Mental Health: A Report of the Surgeon General, U.S. Dept. of Health and Human Services.* Rockville, MD: Author.

U.S. Department of Health and Human Services. 1999. "Mental Health: A Report of the Surgeon General. Rockville, MD." U.S. Department of Health and Human Services, Substance Abuse and Mental Health Services Administration, Center for Mental Health Services, 408–409, 411.

Vogel, D. L., N. G. Wade, and A. H. Hackler. 2007. "Perceived Public Stigma and the Willingness to Seek Counseling: The Mediating Roles of Self-Stigma and Attitudes toward Counseling." *Journal of Counseling Psychology* 54: 40–50.

Ward, E. C., O. Clark, and S. Heidrich. 2009. "African American Women's Beliefs, Coping Behaviors and Barriers to Seeking Mental Health Services." *Qualitative Health Research* 19(11): 1589–1601.

Whaley, A. 2001. "Cultural Mistrust: An Important Psychological Construct for Diagnosis and Treatment of African Americans." *Professional Psychology: Research and Practice* 32(6): 555–562.

Williams, D. R., H. M. Gonzalez, H. Neighbors, R. Neese, J. M. Abelson, J. Sweetman, and J. S. Jackson. 2007. "Prevalence and Distribution of Major Depressive Disorder in African Americans, Caribbean Blacks, and Non-Hispanic Whites: Results from the National Survey of American Life." *Archives of General Psychiatry* 64(3): 305–315.

Williams, D. R. and R. Williams-Morris. 2000. "Racism and Mental Health: The African American Experience." *Ethnicity and Health* 5(314): 243–268.

World Health Organization. 2008. *The Global Burden of Disease: 2004 Update,* Table A2: Burden of Disease in DALYs by Cause, Sex, and Income Group in WHO Regions, Estimates for 2004. Geneva, Switzerland: WHO http://www.who.int/healthinfo/global_burden_disease/GBD_report_2004update_AnnexA.pdf

Yamashiro, G. and J. K. Matsuoka. 1997. "Help-seeking among Asian and Pacific Americans: A Multiperspective Analysis." *Social Work* 42(2): 176–186.

Yang, L. H., J. C. Phelan, and B. G. Link. 2008. "Stigma and Beliefs of Efficacy Towards Traditional Chinese Medicine and Western Psychiatric Treatment among Chinese-Americans." *Cultural Diversity and Ethnic Minority Psychology* 14: 10–18.

Yang, L. H. and Wonpat-Borja. 2007. "Psychopathology among Asian Americans." In *Handbook of Asian American Psychology,* edited by F. T. L. Leong, A. Ebreo, L. Kinoshita, A. G. Inman, and L. H. Yang, 379–405. Thousand Oaks, CA: Sage.

CHAPTER SIX

Religion and Health: Ideological Contexts and Their Influences on Health-Associated Behaviors

Dean D. VonDras

A person's religious background, activities, and associated faith beliefs can be powerful influences on health perceptions and resultantly on health behavior (Koenig 2005, Koenig, King, and Carson 2012, Koenig, McCullough, and Larson 2001, Miller and Thoreson 2003). However, health perceptions are often biased and incomplete (Klein and Helweg-Larsen 2002, Weinstein 1980, 1983, 1987). As Jung (1964) instructs, there are unconscious aspects of our perceptions and behavior, and a number of unknown factors that are operative, so that "Man . . . never perceives anything fully, or comprehends anything completely" (4). Moreover, as advanced by the construct of perceptual readiness (Bruner 1957), the way the person views their health or illness reflects previous experience, characteristic habits, and present need states. As the ancient understanding expressed in the *Talmud* makes clear: "We do not see things the way they are, rather, we see things the way we *are*." The impetus for this chapter is to gain a deeper understanding and greater discernment of these factors, exploring prominent religious contexts and examining how their various beliefs, idealized practices, and rituals may influence health perceptions and behaviors. Following in accord with the orientations of Smith (1991) and Barzun (2000), a primary focus of discussion is to understand the built-up system of ideas surrounding different religions, that is to say their respective ideologies. Thus this selective review offers a glimpse of the various ideologies found within different religions that, while prescribing a way of meaning-making and seeking of a transcendent force beyond the individual, also express a system of cultural values that direct behavior and promote health and well-being.

Religion as an Aspect of Cultural and Psychological Life

Religions and spiritual practices have existed since ancient times, and in all cultures there have been narratives constructed involving the deepest meanings of life, existence, and death (Campbell 1968, 1972, Malinowski 1954). Thus as Nord (2010) postulates, religion is "embedded in broader cultural and intellectual traditions, narratives, and worldviews" (203-204). Certainly, in all cultures people speak about faith and articulate various forms of spirituality, again illustrating religion to be an important interest and dimension of human experience. Common in these articulations of faith and beliefs are the particular values and virtues that take on a distinct significance for the individual and the community.

Religion is also perhaps one of the most basic and universal aspects of psychological life (Norenzayan and Heine 2005). As the renowned anthropologist Margaret Mead (1955) noted in describing cultural patterns and emerging technological changes, it is impossible to describe the life of a people, without speaking of their religion. Indeed, when we look for a common psychological element across cultures, we find religious beliefs as a central characteristic and point of reference (Taylor 2011). Even at a time in history when secular and materialistic orientations have supplanted traditional worldviews (Smith 2001), and when there is greater faith in science to offer ways of preventing illness and in attaining positive health outcomes than ever before (Taylor 2011), across many cultures religion is still recognized as an as essential framework of thought and action, "providing an order by which to live" (Taylor 2011, 151). For example, within the United States, as reported in the *U.S. Religious Landscape Survey—Religious Beliefs and Practices: Diverse and Politically Relevant* (Pew Forum 2008), 92 percent of Americans from diverse religious backgrounds express a belief in God, 75 percent report praying at least once weekly, and 61 percent characterize themselves as formal church members. Thus, culturally and psychologically, religion is noted as a central aspect and concern of the person.

At this point it might be useful to clarify somewhat what is meant by *religion*. It should be noted that religion has many dimensions, and may also be reflected in one's spirituality. Religion offers and describes a cumulative history, a communal connection, the holding of shared values, and a way of defining meaning for the person. Further, religion may be reflected in the person's attending religious services and following specific theological texts (e.g., the Bible in Christianity, the Bhagavad-Gita in Hinduism, the Koran in Islam) that contain narrative stories that express and convey explanations, interpretations, and prescriptions for living and life-experiences. Moreover, religion describes a history of traditions and rituals (e.g., christening and baptism, wedding, healing prayer, days of sacred observance, fasting), forms of art (e.g., architecture, music, paintings, sculptures), and exclusive terminologies by which to characterize and guide behavior.

In contrast, *spirituality* has a somewhat broader definition, but like religion is understood as having many different aspects (Armatowski 2001, Moberg 2001). As suggested by Sulmasy (2002), spirituality describes and expresses a person's ultimate concerns in life, their faith, or religious beliefs, or relation to nature, or one's relation to others. These expressions of ultimate concern may overlap with theological doctrine, but also may be devoid of connection to a specific theology. Thus, everyone may express a spirituality (Nelson 2010). For example, spirituality could reflect one's philosophy of life, or religious practices, or adherence to theological principles, or sensitivity to nature and people, or being present in the moment. Thus, while being defined in somewhat different ways, religion and spirituality are recognized as interwoven constructs that may include expression of specific beliefs, customs, language, and rituals that involve the search for transcendent meaning (Moberg 2001, Nelson 2010). Therefore, within this discussion, religion will be considered to be synonymous with spirituality, so that the diversity of beliefs and behaviors found in different traditions are considered and respected (Hill et al. 2000, Moberg 2002).

Interpretive Challenges

As noted above, the faith beliefs and ritual practices of various religions allude to cultural differences but also to a universal aspect of psychological life. These faith beliefs and practices also implicitly tell of contextual influences found in different religious orientations. However, when we consider possible causal or correlative relationships involving religion and health, we confront an interpretive barrier. That is, as Watts (1951) characterizes, "science and religion are talking about the same universe, but using different kinds of language" (135-136). Further, as Smith (2001) notes, empirical questions about religion, and frequently our desire to understand the critical influence of religion on behavior, often fall outside the scope of scientific investigation. Therefore discerning a precise means by which religious beliefs and actions may impact upon an individual's health may lie well beyond the immediate concerns of health psychology and medical science. In addition, when considering religious beliefs as a parameter of illness prevention and disease management, as Freedland (2004) suggests: "Even if there were solid evidence for these tenuous mechanisms, it would relegate religious beliefs to a distal node in the causal pathways . . . one far removed from the dominion of the physicians, surgeons and nurses in charge of preventing and managing illness" (240). Yet as Bruner (1990) has indicated, to gain a complete understanding of behavior, there must also be a comprehension of the context in which it occurs (see also Lewin 1951). Indeed, the social norms, expectations, and powers of suggestion found within various social contexts have a powerful influence on health-associated behaviors (e.g., Bandura 1998, D'Blasi et al. 2010, Reid, Cialdini, and Aiken 2010). Thus, to gain insight into how religious beliefs may shape health perceptions and behaviors, it is important to understand the ideological features found within the different contexts of religions, and how these features may influence thought and actions.

The Ideological Contexts of Religion

Health care professionals often lack understanding of the religious traditions that they wish to investigate and comprehend more in depth. (Nelson 2010). Further, the needed understanding is not a quantitative type of scrutiny, but rather of a deeper qualitative awareness and knowledge of the ideological features and associated characteristics they contain. Thus throughout this discussion, the reviews of Smith (1991), Feiser and Powers (2008), Nelson (2010) and others are employed as a point of departure to develop this template of awareness and understanding.

With further regard to the influence of ideological context on health behavior, it is important to note that religious beliefs are suggested to, "endow the person with a perspective (and a goal) that goes far beyond their limited existence . . . and offers them a full life . . . infinitely more satisfactory than that of a man . . . with no inner meaning to his life" (Jung 1964, 76). Moreover, much like the multiple levels of meaning found within language (Grice 1989), religion contains a deeper, more complex meaning to understand. That is, both verbal (e.g., scripture, theological text) and non-verbal (e.g., ritual behavior, architecture, art, music) aspects of religion reflect an *implicature* (Grice 1989), an interpretive meaning beyond the literal statement, that expresses a mutual dependence of participants, and which is intended to inspire belief and compel the person to action.

Thus discussed below are the perspectives and goals that represent the ideological contexts of prominent world religions, which, while prescribing ways of meaning-making and transcendental union, also express systems of cultural values that promote illness prevention, health management, and wellbeing.

Hinduism

In Hinduism we discover an ideological context with many images of an Ultimate Authority, and like other religious traditions, the individual's beliefs and practices provide a psychological framework for life. As Smith (1991) describes (see also, Burtt 1957, Feiser and Powers 2008, Flood 2003, Nelson 2010), Hinduism presents a basic ideology concerning human nature that is described in its description of the four major goals in life. Each goal references the human condition and ways to be happy, as well as instruction on how to better understand life via the adoption of life-style orientations that underlie positive health outcomes. The first goal describes our primal psychological characteristic, to seek pleasure and escape pain. Relevant health-behavior analogues of this ideological feature to consider are the various therapeutic understandings and approaches used to prevent and treat over-eating, anorexia or bulimia, or drug addiction (e.g., Berthoud 2011, Finlayson, King, and Blundell 2007, Keating et al. 2012, Kelly 2011). A second goal of life suggested in Hinduism is to be successful in terms of gaining wealth, or fame, or power, but while these are more public endeavors, they are also recognized as having limitations in that they lead to competitive modes of behavior with uncertain outcomes. Relevant health-behavior analogues to consider for this goal are the overwhelming ego-expectations or work-stress individuals endure that increase risk for disease and illness (e.g., Dittner, Rimes, and Thorpe 2011, Jenkins 1978, Schulz et al. 2011).

A third goal suggests happiness is to be found in the transition from the desire to get, to the desire to give, and from the desire to succeed to the desire to serve. While a fourth goal is liberation from the finite world. So that a sense of the infinite and eternal is realized in the Infinite Self or Atman (God) within (Smith 1991). Combined, these four goals of how happiness may be attained and the promotion of a self-detached, mind-over-matter orientation, suggest elements of a cognitive schema that influences self-regulation and personal-control, and which may positively or negatively impact upon health behaviors and risk for disease and illness (Dull and Skokan 1995, Himle et al. 2011, McCullough and Willoughby 2009).

While a growing self- and spiritual-awareness may serve to promote illness-prevention behaviors, the different yogas, or methods of spiritual training in Hinduism further suggest methods for cultivating positive health habits (see Chapters 6 and 7 in volume 1 for more on yoga and Ayurveda). Similar to other research reporting positive effects of spiritual practices on health (e.g., Campbell, Yoon, and Johnstone 2010), these life-style values and physical exercises also are suggested to lead to positive health outcomes. For example, yoga postures and breathing techniques have been found to reduce dypsnea-related distress, and increase walking distance and self-rated functionality in older adults with chronic obstructive pulmonary disorder (Donesky-Cuenco et al. 2009). Yogic breathing techniques have also been shown to help reduce stress, anxiety, and depression (Brown and Gerbarg 2005a, 2005b), and use of yogic postures have shown benefit beyond other exercise regimes in preventing and managing illness (Jayasinghe 2004, Ross, and Thomas 2010). Further, as reviewed by Raub (2002), yogic postures and breathing techniques have been suggested to improve strength and flexibility, as well as aid in the control of blood pressure, heart rate, respiration, and metabolic rate for individuals with musculosketal and cardiopulmonary disease.

Other key ideological features of Hinduism include a system of social castes, reincarnation, and Karma. The caste system refers to social classes that range from the homeless and very poor, the Untouchables (outcastes), to the most affluent, the Brahmins (seers). The significance of class in considering health behavior is that economic status is noted as an important factor of concern in illness prevention and health education programs. Indeed, low socio-economic status and poverty are found to be associated with higher risk for disease, reduced life-expectancy, lower rates of maternal health care, childhood vaccinations, and utilization of health services (Adler and Rehkopt 2008, Kaplan 1996, Nayar 2007), as well as variation in how prevention information is perceived (Viswanath and Ackerson 2011). Reincarnation, as Smith (1991) describes, involves the belief that each soul entered the world mysteriously by God's power, and that we outgrow our bodies as we grow in a positive spiritual way. Closely associated with reincarnation is Karma. As Smith (1991) notes, Karma has two dimensions and refers to a doctrine concerning the moral law of cause and effect. The first dimension of Karma expresses a belief that each person is responsible for his or her present condition and fate in the future. The second dimension expresses a belief that while each decision and action has deterministic consequences, the person has free-choice in the decisions and actions he or she take. This second dimension has great significance for illness-prevention, as one makes choices in selecting his or her lifestyle and in enacting behaviors that lead to positive or negative health outcomes.

In Hinduism, as in many traditions, a person's health and religious concerns are intertwined and seen as one (Koenig, McCullough, and Larson 2001). Thus both reincarnation and karma beliefs may introduce unique challenges with regard to how the causes of illness are perceived and understood (e.g., Spiro 2005), and in mental health interventions (e.g., Juthani 2001). Yet, as Chattapodhyay (2007) suggests, religious beliefs and spiritual practices may also offer physicians opportunities to help patients better achieve health outcomes, for example, by suggesting to a follower of Krishna that abstinence from alcohol or tobacco addiction is a way to grow in closer union with God. Similarly, when considering dietary and nutritional practices and their effect on health outcomes, the vegetarianism practiced by many Hindus is also a way of expressing a devotion and seeking of a closer union with God (Nath 2010), and may have useful cross-cultural application in the prevention of heart-disease (e.g., Sticher, Smith, and Davidson 2010), obesity (Farmer et al. 2011), and other illnesses (American Dietetic Association 2009). Other research investigating the belief in Karma and its inherent pessimism for negative events (Cartwright 2010, Johnstone, Glass, and Oliver 2007) has reported greater risk for post-traumatic stress disorder, and poorer health in survivors of a natural disaster who expressed belief in Karma (Levy, Slade, and Ranasinghe 2009). However, both positive and negative coping orientations are suggested by Karma beliefs, and positively vectored interpretations may make it easier to accept disability (Johnstone et al. 2007), follow treatment regimens (Sandhu 2009), and lead to more affirming experiences as death is encountered at the end of life (Bulow et al. 2008). Thus taken as a whole, the ideological context of Hinduism, its descriptions of human nature, mind-body connection, and methods of spiritual enlightenment, offer and present powerful frameworks of social norms and motives that influence health-associated behaviors.

Buddhism

Buddhism also characterizes a spiritual context that influences health perceptions and behaviors. Buddhism is an outgrowth of Hinduism and the seeking of the *Atman* (God) within so as to attain enlightenment and experience nirvana in the present life (Smith 1991). Buddhism follows the life of Siddhartha Gautama, the man who awoke and attained enlightenment and thus became the Buddha. The basic ideological features of Buddhism are found in the four noble truths and eight-fold path (Feiser and Powers 2008, Nelson 2010, Paonil and Sringernyuang 2002, Smith 1991, Walshe 1999, Watts 1957). The four noble truths, like the four goals in Hinduism, describe a psychological framework of human nature and existence. If the person understands these truths, they begin on the path to attain enlightenment. Indeed, to practice Buddhism is to accept and embrace the Four Noble Truths: life is suffering (*dukkha*), our suffering is due to our selfish craving or desire (*tanha*), the cure to *tanha* is in overcoming this selfish craving, and the way out of the captivity of our suffering is through the *Eightfold Path*. The Eightfold Path prescribes the adoption of specific attitudes, behaviors, and use of meditation or mindfulness training so as to overcome human desires and cravings, and thus reflects corollaries of illness-prevention and health behaviors. Indeed, as suggested by Paonil and Sringernyuang (2002), "the Eightfold Path, in its broader meaning, is a way to prevent all diseases" (99). Again, it should be noted that Buddhism grows out of Hinduism, so the notion that one undergoes a "training" designed to involve the person in an inner discovery that leads to enlightenment is a basic feature of this orientation. Further, like Jnana yoga of Hinduism, Buddhism incorporates the cultivation of meditation as a method to develop inner peace, to express an outward behavior of pacifism, and to find enlightenment. The goal of this search for enlightenment is to become better able to understand basic life truths, to overcome our selfish nature, and to ultimately reach nirvana.

Beyond the attainment of spiritual enlightenment, Buddhist meditation and life-style habits (e.g., practice of vegetarianism) have been noted to be correlates of positive health-outcomes (Wisst et al. 2010). For example, even brief instruction in meditation techniques is suggested to reduce stress and enhance mood (Lane, Seskevich, and Pieper 2007), however, these outcomes may be more effortlessly achieved by individuals who already have experience with meditation (Lutz et al. 2009) or possess the trait for mindfulness (Shapiro et al. 2011). Meditation has also been indicated as a technique to manage chronic pain (e.g., Kabat-Zinn 1982, Kabat-Zinn, Lipworth, and Burney 1985). Indeed, the original purpose of meditation in Buddhism was "to alleviate suffering and cultivate compassion" (Ludwig and Kabat-Zinn 2008, 1350). Thus, as an illness management tool, mindfulness training is a way to learn how to self-regulate attention from moment to moment, and to treat all thoughts similarly by just noting that they have arisen. Moreover, mindfulness training is suggested to promote a greater participation by the individual in their health care by strengthening "internal resources for optimizing health in both prevention and recovery from illness" (Ludwig and Kabat-Zinn 2008, 1351). For example, as reported by Kabat-Zinn (1982), after a 10-week training program, 65 percent of patients with chronic pain showed a reduction of 1/3 or more in pain rating, along with similar reductions in the amount of pain medication used, mood disturbances, and psychiatric symptoms, suggesting meditation is a useful intervention tool for patients with chronic pain.

Further, as reported in a meta-review by Baer (2003), mindfulness training has been suggested as an efficacious intervention in the treatment of individuals with anxiety disorder, fibromyalgia, and psoriasis. Research has also suggested mindfulness training to be helpful in treating bulimia nervosa (Proulx 2008), sleep disorder (Carlson and Garland 2008), and in reducing blood pressure in cardiovascular disease patients and blood glucose levels in individuals with diabetes (Dhar 2009). Other research (Teasdale et al. 2000) reports prevention of relapse and recurrence in patients with three or more episodes of major depression following mindfulness-based cognitive therapy. The key feature of this intervention program to treat chronic depression is training patients during remission to become more aware of and relate differently to their thoughts, feelings, and bodily sensations. This intervention approach also cultivates an awareness of being in the present moment and one's freedom of choice to engage or disengage with different thoughts and feelings. The therapeutic goal is that the individual will learn and be able to use this training to disengage from habitual and automatic cognitive-affective routines that are dysfunctional and thereby avoid and lower risk for relapse and recurrence of depression.

The values inherent in Buddhism such as pacifism may function as preventative deterrents of disease, and the practice of meditation has been suggested as a primary, secondary, and tertiary prevention strategy for chronic illness (Bonadonna 2003). For example, the Buddhist teaching of not causing harm to other human beings has been suggested as a way to instruct about safe sexual practices in the context of HIV transmission (Loue et al. 1999). From a caregiving perspective, the notion of following the compassionate caring concern of Buddhism is suggested to provide an essential framework for the caregiver, as well as support and meaning to life of those who face terminal illness (McGrath 1998); that is, an understanding that death is part of living and dying is part of rebirth, that leads to acceptance and peace of mind (Mok, Wong and Wong 2010). Overall, mindfulness training and other ideological features of Buddhism are noted to reflect positive health practices and have shown efficacy in illness-prevention and disease management.

Confucianism and Taoism

Confucianism and Taoism are spiritual orientations influenced by the ideological descriptions of human nature found in Hinduism (e.g., self-oriented and pleasure seeking) and in Buddhism (e.g., life is suffering).

Reflecting the collectivism of eastern societies, the teaching of Confucius centers on creating a cohesive society, and an honorable and honoring social order. Ideologically, as Smith (1991, see also Feiser and Powers 2008, Nelson 2010) describes, in Confucianism there is a noted reference to the selfish concerns of human nature, and the promotion of the Golden Rule in describing the Way of becoming fully human via Confucian doctrine. Reflecting great psychological insight, Confucius considered the mind to function within the framework of attitudes and emotions, and held that this framework of attitudes and emotions is learned from the person's interaction and involvement with the family and community. Thus, with concern for health behavior, the Confucian instruction to respect and follow tradition becomes a way to direct society and guide the person in illness prevention and the attainment of positive health outcomes.

The consideration of instilling a focus on tradition and a guide for living are noted by the following five key principles in Confucianism (Feiser and Powers 2008, Nelson 2010, Smith 1991). The first principle, *Jen,* refers to the ideal relation that should exist between people. There should be respect for others and for one's self. In terms of health behavior, Jen may be realized in the precaution taken not to spread influenza germs (e.g., wearing of gloves or a mask) as well as in the unselfishness and empathic awareness of caregiving. A second related principle is *Chun tzu,* which refers to the ideal reflection of Jen. In this regard, the person acts selflessly and graciously in serving and accommodating the needs of others.

The third principle, *Li,* refers to the way things should be done, and suggests following the best practices of the finest models. With regard to health behaviors, these best practices provide a prescription for doing things in moderation, acting with compassion, expressing care, and being ethical. Another meaning of Li is a ritual respectfulness in relations, and the honor and reverence held and expressed towards parents and elders. This second meaning reflects a positive parameter of social control that has significance for reducing negative behaviors (e.g., to follow parents' instruction not to eat or drink to excess) and for filial piety, a practice that venerates the elders of a society. The fourth principle, *Te,* refers to the power of moral example. The idea here as applied to behavior may again be health-protective, as the individual may reduce consumption of food or drink, maintain exercise regimens etc., as they model the positive health behaviors and thereby lead by example. The fifth principle, *Wen* refers to the practicing of "peace" as opposed to the practicing of "war." The directive here is that by practicing "peace" there is a transformation to a more virtuous style of living, and to a higher moral character. Like Buddhism then, Confucianism may be regarded as perhaps not so much a "religion" as a philosophy for living (Smith 1991).

In Taoism the master that teaches and provides spiritual direction is Lao Tzu, whose instruction is found in the *Tao Te Ching*. As noted by Smith (1991, see also, Feiser and Powers 2008, Nelson 2010, Watts 1957), Taoism emphasizes a perspective on living in which the person is in harmony with nature. Embedded within this perspective is the duality in the yin/yang principle, as well as three meanings of Tao, that refer to the way of the ultimate reality, the way of the universe, and the way of human life (see Chapter 9, volume 1). The Taoist emphasis on the person being in harmony with nature recognizes prescriptions for living and ways of being that have direct influence on health behavior.

As a behavioral guide then, Taoism engages the individual in training to seek and attain the Tao's vitality and the Tao's energy for living the harmonious or "loved life" (Smith 1991, 201). In this framework, Tao refers to a vital power beyond the person that can be maximized via matter, movement, and mind. Like Buddhism and Hinduism, there is the instruction "to reverse all self-seeking and cultivate perfect cleanliness of thought and body" (Smith 1991, 202). Thus, Taoism has long promoted a holistic understanding of the mind-body connection, and emphasized self-diagnosis, as well as the use of folk medicines and acupuncture (Purnell 2008, Zaccarrini 2011). The Taoist perspective also includes the practice of shamanism and faith healing, and emphasizes proper nutrition, personal hygiene and exercise as important behavioral practices to gain the energy and vitality of Tao. With regard to mind, Taoism incorporates the Raja-style of yoga and its psychophysical exercises to discover a greater and more vital consciousness.

Again, with concern for health behaviors, the establishment and reliance on Confucian and Taoist principles are suggested to influence community-wide health improvements and prevention concerns (Berzruchka, Namekata, and Sistrom 2008, Yip 2004). Further, adherence to Confucian doctrine, with its subscribed social order and dynamic of approval, is suggested to inhibit rates of alcohol abuse in women (Kim and Kim 2008) and sexually transmitted disease (Tang 2008, Xiao, Mehrotra, Zimmerman 2011). However, the gender stereotypes embedded in Confucianism may also prevent men from seeking health care (Tung 2010), and its patriarchal tradition that has placed women in an inferior position with regard to demanding self-autonomy, especially with regard to heterosexual relations, may increase risk for sexually transmitted disease in women (e.g., Tang 2008).

In a related manner, Taoist beliefs and the explanation of physical and mental maladies as due to evil-spirits, as well as reliance on self-diagnosis and use of folk medicines, may counteract public health prevention initiatives (Chen 2001, Muecke 1983, Ng et al. 2011, Visscher 2006). Further, rather than following prescribed western medical therapies, there is often a reliance on the folk practices of skin rubbing or pinching, cup suctioning, and acupuncture, as well as the ingestion of herbal concoctions and special foods or meats, that may constrain the attainment of optimal health, illness prevention, and maintenance goals (Chen 2001, Purnell 2008). Confucian and Taoist mores may also influence perceptions of healthcare workers and the seeking of information in a way that limits positive health outcomes, especially when the discussion of health issues and concerns occur within the bounds of the superior-physician and subordinate-patient relational framework, where the patient dutifully listens but does not assertively ask questions about relevant and important health concerns or prescribed health regimens (Chen 2001, Muecke 1983, Visscher 2006, Weitzman, Ballah, and Levkoff 2008). In the area of transplantation research, Confucian, Taoist, and Buddhist orientations of filial piety and returning of one's body to the ancestors in the same condition it was received may also influence perceptions of organ transplants from dead persons, with transplantations from the deceased donor viewed as corpse mutilation, as opposed to the Christian ideal of a self- sacrificing and thoughtful giving (e.g., LaFleur 2002, Lam and McCullough 2000). Similarly, in caregiving for those with chronic and terminal illnesses, research suggests that the filial piety and familism orientations of Confucianism may reduce the emotional distress of caregiving (Mok, Wong and Wong 2010, Tang, Li, and Liao 2007). Further, as encountered in Buddhism, Confucian and Taoist meditation is recognized as a way to manage stress. Similar to Buddhism, Taoist meditation concerns escaping the artificial distinction of self and the separation between the human being and nature, so as to repose in a mindfulness that avoids the egocentric and dysfunctional thinking that characterizes and encompasses "stress" (Santee 2008). In summary then, as also shown in Hinduism and Buddhism, Confucianism and Taoism constitute ideological contexts that have important significance for health perceptions and behavior.

Islam, Judaism, and Christianity

Islam, Judaism, and Christianity share common historical roots, with each religion recognizing Abraham, Moses, and Jesus as important prophetic figures (Nelson 2010, Smith 1991). All are also monotheistic religions, expressing a personification of the Other as a "God above all others." In terms of ideological orientation, the shared historical narrative describes a creation by an all-powerful God, thus humankind and all creatures are subordinates of God.

Similar to beliefs in other religions, in Islam, Judaism, and Christianity, health and spirituality are interwoven. For example, dietary restrictions and fasting during the month-long holy time of Ramadan are prescribed ways of practicing one's spirituality and maintaining compliance with Koranic teachings; yet there are variations in and exceptions to these practices (Pathy et al. 2011). The dietary restrictions in Islam include eating foods that are *halal,* therefore abiding by approved methods for ritual slaughter of animals, and abstaining from foods that are *halam* or forbidden, thus the eating of pork, blood, and meat sacrificed to idols, as well as use of alcohol is prohibited (Eliasi and Dwyer 2002, Leung and Stanner 2011). There are similar dietary restrictions practiced by Jews who follow the laws of Kashrut that prescribe which foods may be eaten and how foods must be prepared and eaten (Romaguera et al. 2009). Similarly, within Christianity, various sects such as the Seventh-Day Adventist Church encourage vegetarianism, as well as the avoidance of alcohol, tobacco, illicit drugs, coffee, and other beverages containing caffeine (Jenkins et al. 2010). The dietary restrictions followed by devotees of Islam, Judaism, or Christianity suggest a more careful selection in food choices and avoidance of alcohol and restaurant foods, all of which are suggested to have positive health benefit (U.S. Department of Agriculture, U.S. Department of Health and Human Services 2010). Further, fasting during Islamic, Judaic, or Christian holy periods also reflects the interweaving of religion and health-associated practices. As a health-behavior analogue, clinical investigation has suggested health benefits of fasting during Ramadan, showing decreases in blood glucose and HDL cholesterol levels, and increases in LDL cholesterol (Ziaee et al. 2006), as well as decrease of waist circumference, body mass index, fasting blood sugar, and mean arterial pressure, all modifiable cardiovascular risk factors (Almutairi et al.2012).

Other research has pointed to religious values as an influence on health behavior. For example Christian values are suggested to endorse a worldview and inculcate a virtue of social responsibility that promotes HIV/AIDS prevention as well as compassionate care giving for those afflicted (Kang, Chin, and Behar 2011). A similar prevention perspective is suggested to be possible within Islamic teaching (Maulana, Krumich, and Van Den Borne 2009). Yet, worldwide, there is controversy involving interpretation of theological doctrine and positions expressed by Christian and Islamic religious leaders that have been suggested to obfuscate and undermine the implementation of condom use as preventative behavior (Maulana et al. 2009, Muula 2010). Nevertheless, the teachings of Islam, Judaism, and Christianity hold great power as models for social justice and for application within community psychology (Canning 2011). For example, Imams are noted to play a key role in promoting healthy behaviors through their scripture-based sermons (Padela et al. 2011), and recent public health advertisement directed at followers of Islam promoted the prevention of tobacco use through the belief-inspired advertisement catch-phrase, "Whatever harms the body or another person in sinful" (Maulana et al. 2009, 566, see also Morrow and Barraclough 2003). In a related way, experimentation with tobacco is noted to be less likely in adolescents who express higher adherence, commitment and practice of Islamic teachings (Islam and Johnson 2003). In a similar way, other research has suggested the regular and more frequent attendance at Christian church services to be associated with lower risk for HIV/AIDS (Gillum and Holt 2010), and involvement of church leaders is seen as essential in promoting accurate information about HIV transmission and in dispelling stigma (Kang, Chin, and Behar 2011). Further, lower usage rates for both alcohol and tobacco have been reported in church members with greater religious adherence (e.g., the importance of religion in one's life), religious service attendance, and participation in religious activities (Benjamin and Buck 2008). Correspondingly, another study indicated that new immigrants from Korea who self-identified as Christians were less likely to be tobacco users (Kim et al. 2000). Further, it is increasingly common that information about risk for illness and prevention behaviors is disseminated through Christian faith-based programs for self-management of diabetes (Krisberg 2012) and screening for blood pressure, cardiovascular disease and stroke (Frank and Grubbs 2009). Research with Jewish populations also reflects this interweaving of religious belief with health perceptions and behavior (Coleman-Brueckheimer and Dein 2011). For example, discussion of moral dilemmas in the Torah and spiritual support have been suggested to be key aspects of recovery for Jewish alcoholics and drug addicts, and in their rebuilding of integrity, i.e., ability to be aware of moral dilemmas, conflicts, and make positive choices (Blakeney, Blakeney, and Reich 2005). The study and understanding of the Torah has also been proposed to have a generally positive influence on brain plasticity and the development of self (Drubach 2002).

Ritual practices also are noted to have a positive effect on health behavior. For example, prayer, meditation, use of amulets, and other religious rituals are suggested to carry sacred meaning and are considered a source from which to take hope and expect healing (e.g., Bertrand 2005, Campion and Bhugra 1998, Dane 2000, Muecke 1983). For example, prayers and other expressions of spirituality are noted to be positively associated with greater optimism (e.g., Carver, Scheier, and Weintraub 1989), and lower levels of trait-anxiety (Harris, Schoneman, and Carrera 2002), and indicated as a method for reframing life challenges in a positive way (e.g., Fredrickson 2000, Shapiro et al. 2011). Further, the Christian centering prayer, much like Buddhist or Taoist meditation, has been suggested to have positive benefit in reducing stress (Ferguson, Willemsen, and Casteneto 2010). While sharing many of the attributes of mindfulness meditation, such as sitting comfortably with eyes closed and redirecting thoughts to a beginning point or mantra, the focus in centering prayer is on a sacred word or symbol, with the intention of becoming aware of God's presence and action within the person (Ferguson et al. 2010). Thus, attending worship or prayer services, private prayer or meditation, Bible reading, and expression of living in God's presence have all been suggested to enhance the self-management of health (Arcury et al. 2000), and provide inspiration to overcome and transcend the challenges of the moment (Maddi et al. 2006).

Further, religious beliefs and practices are suggested to activate cognitive schemata that support positive coping and health behaviors such as accepting the challenges of illness and disease processes, framing illness and end-of-life events in a positive way, and being optimistic and open toward the future (Ahmad, Muhammad, and Abdullah 2011, Jones 2006, Koenig 2002, 2005, McCullough and Willoughby 2009, McIntosh, Silver, and Wortman 1993). For example, as one Islamic woman expressed while enduring breast cancer, "God has the best reason for me. I never give up," (Ahmad et al. 2011, 53). Religious beliefs are also noted to influence the selection and use of coping strategies, as well as health-behavior outcomes (e.g., Chatters 2000, Gorsuch 1995, Maynard, Gorsuch, and Bjorck 2001, Murray, Malcarne, and Goggin 2003, Smith, McCullough, and Poll 2003, Stylianou 2004). Indeed, research has suggested religious beliefs to influence cognitive or attitudinal mechanisms in such a way as to inhibit alcohol and drug use (e.g., Dunn 2005, Hazel and Mohatt 2001). For example, greater endorsement of religious statements such as, "I believe that God loves me and cares about me," "I have a personally meaningful relationship with God," "My relationship with God contributes to my well-being" from the Spiritual Well-Being Scale developed by Ellison (1983) were found to be inversely associated with rates of alcohol use, as well as beliefs about the social effects of alcohol in college students (VonDras, Schmitt, and Marx 2007). Further, as noted in various recovery programs such as Alcoholics Anonymous, a belief in a Higher Power is noted as an essential component in successful treatment of addiction to alcohol and maintenance of sobriety (e.g., Brown, Peterson, Cunningham 1988, Johnsen 1993, Pullen et al.

1999). In summary then, the ideological contexts represented by Islam, Judaism, and Christianity are noted to shape behavior and impact upon health behaviors and outcomes.

Conclusion

Religion is an important aspect of life in all cultures, and as suggested in this selective review, represents an ideological context that powerfully influences health-associated behaviors. However, while an aid for many people, religious beliefs and practices may also reinforce emotional states of anxiety, guilt, and shame, along with transcendental beliefs that negatively impact upon physical and mental health (Chatters 2000, Fitchett et al. 1999, Koenig 2002, 2009). Further, excessive religious activities such as prayer or ritual fasting may also have negative health effects, exacerbating morbid conditions (e.g., Cangiano et al. 2011) or psychological disorder (e.g., Bonchek and Greenberg 2009, Taylor 2002). In addition, negative types of religious coping (e.g., spiritual discontent, punishing God reappraisals, interpersonal religious discontent, demonic reappraisal and reappraisal of God's power) have been found to be associated with higher emotional distress and psychosomatic symptoms (Pargament et al. 1998, Table 3).

Nevertheless, it is important to note the psychological benefits of religious belief for the individual. For example, research examining end-of-life despair in patients with advanced cancer found that individuals who reported a belief in an afterlife also expressed greater spiritual wellbeing (e.g., being able to find inner peace and comfort), and lower levels of hopelessness, desire for death, and suicidal ideation (McClain-Jacobson et al. 2004). Correspondingly, in partners of men with AIDS who were HIV-positive, higher spiritual beliefs and practices of caregivers were negatively correlated with caregiver burden (Folkman et al. 1994), and, at the time of death, caregivers of persons who lived with HIV-AIDS who reported spiritual beliefs were found to engage in more positive coping than caregivers who did not express spiritual beliefs (Richards and Folkman 1997). Thus, there are many benefits of religious beliefs, both for those who confront and manage illness and for caregivers who provide assistance.

While there are different orientations found within the religious ideological contexts presented, there are also many commonalities. For example, all religions provide a powerful form of connection to an Ultimate Other as well as to community (Yalom 2002). This connectivity instills an awareness and relationship to shared beliefs and communal values that offers hope of holding in abeyance illness and disease, and provides motivations to live healthfully and to seek positive health outcomes. Further, each religion expresses two key health-associated values for parents and community to teach young people: respect for self, and concern for others.

As suggested throughout this discussion, it has been noted that "religious and spiritual dimensions of culture are among the most important factors that structure human experience, beliefs, values, behavior, and illness patterns" (Turner et al. 1995, 435). But beyond the provision of social support resources that impact upon preventative behaviors and health-outcomes (George, Ellison, and Larson 2002, Krause 2008), religious and spiritual communities are also recognized as access points to a wide array of social and health services (Chatters, Levin, and Ellison 1998, Ellison and Levin 1998, Cnaan, Sinha, and McGrew 2004). Therefore noting these important aspects of the person, culture, and community, there is a need to accommodate religion and spirituality in illness-prevention and wellness programs.

Speaking to this concern, in the argument for the need of collaboration between physicians and chaplains in assisting patients as they encounter illness (Friburg 2001, Thiel and Robinson 1997) is found three reasons to accommodate religious and spiritual dimensions in illness-prevention and wellness programs. The first reason is to embrace a holistic orientation in prevention and wellness interventions, that is, to recognize the religious and spiritual orientation of the person as an important aspect of his/her life, and to use this aspect as a grounds to begin discussion of particular faith beliefs that may direct behavior in such a way so that the individual will be most successful in the attainment of positive health outcomes. A second reason is to affirm the value of the person's religious and spiritual practices as worthwhile ways of living, and their utility in illness-prevention and maintenance of health. A third reason is to "facilitate connection to the spiritual world of wellbeing" (Thiel and Robinson 1997, 95), where there can be greater understanding of one's spirituality and the address of existential concerns of living. An explicit goal of this holistic prevention and wellness approach then, as described in the research discussed above, is to offer support for religious worldviews that are beneficial to the individual as well as the broader community, and that lead to positive health outcomes. Indeed, this accommodation of religious orientation and spiritual practices in prevention and wellness programs may provide a greater sense of control that helps the person live a more fulfilled and healthful life (Neeleman and Persaud 1995).

While often regarded as a foundation of thought and action (Nelson 2010), religion and spirituality have been long ignored by psychology (Rhi 2001). Yet, for the person, the uncertainty of illness often calls to mind one's spiritual need of divine assistance and reconciliation (e.g., Koenig 1998, 2005). In response, healthcare professionals have recognized an obligation to provide a dignity-conserving style of care (Chochinov 2002) and a means to incorporate spirituality in the delivery of medical care and associated health services (e.g., Daaleman 2004, Daaleman and VandeCreek 2000, Koenig 2005, Mytko and Knight 1999, Shea 2000, Sulmasy 2002). Indeed, religious beliefs are key concerns of medical decision-making (Silvestri et al. 2003), and various spiritual activities, while adjunctive of medical therapies, are noted to be associated with good or enhanced health (Sloan et al. 2000). Further, special accommodations should be made to respect different cultural and spiritual practices of the person (Baker 2006). For example, within the Buddhist tradition, providing health and counseling services that relate to Buddhist teachings (Koenig 2005) and respecting the individual and families, wish to pray and chant as a part of finding healing (Chan and Kayser-Jones 2005). In general then, as emphasized by researchers and clinicians (e.g., Koenig 2002, 2005, Shea 2000), there is need to make available to the person opportunities to express, relate to, and explore his or her spirituality and spiritual concerns in the various illness prevention and wellness programs that may be offered to them. Furthermore, while the focus of this discussion was to enhance awareness of the ideological contexts of religion, and to recognize that "all religions include theological and ethical dimensions, which provide a framework for understanding the divine and for leading a good life" (Blanch 2007, 258), there is still much more to learn and understand—particularly, as conceptualized by the term *implicature* (Grice 1989), that religion is more than an ideological context, or "a collection of views and practices . . . it is a spiritual way of being in the world" (Sloan et al. 2000, 1916).

References

Adler, N. F., and D. H. Rehkopf. 2008. "U.S. Disparities in Health: Descriptions, Causes, and Mechanisms." *Annual Review of Public Health* 29: 235–252.

Ahmad, F., M. Muhammad, and A. A. Abdullah. 2011. "Religion and Spirituality in Coping with Advanced Breast Cancer: Perspectives from Malaysian Muslim Women." In *Journal of Religion and Health 50*: 36–45.

Almutairi, H., M. H. Alhendi, B. Alhelal, and M. Mouro. 2012. "The Effect of Ramadan Fasting on Waist Circumference (WC), Body Mass Index (BMI), C-Reactive Protein (CRP), Mean Arterial Pressure (MAP), and Fasting Blood Sugar (FBS) in Type 2 diabetic Kuwaiti patients." *Middle East Journal of Family Medicine 10*: 33–40.

American Dietetic Association. 2009. "Position of the American Dietetic Association: Vegetarian Diets." *Journal of the American Dietetic Association 109*: 1266–1282.

Arcury, T. A., S. A. Quandt, J. McDonald, and R. A. Bell. 2000. "Faith and Health Self-Management of Rural Older Adults." *Journal of Cross-Cultural Gerontology 15*: 55–74.

Armatowski, J. 2001. "Attitudes toward Death and Dying among Persons in the Fourth Quarter of Life." In *Aging and Spirituality: Spiritual Dimensions of Aging Theory, Research, Practice, and Policy*, edited by D. O. Moberg, 71–83. New York: Haworth Pastoral Press.

Baer, R. A. 2003. "Mindfulness Training as a Clinical Intervention: A Conceptual and Empirical Review." *Clinical Psychology: Science and Practice 10*: 125–143.

Baker, F. M. 2006. "Ethnic Elders and Caregiving." In *Supporting the Caregiver in Dementia: A Guide for Health Care Professionals*, edited by S. M. LoboPrabhu, V. A. Molinari, and J. W. Lomax, 237–260. Baltimore, MD: Johns Hopkins University Press.

Bandura, A. 1998. "Health Promotion from the Perspective of Social Cognitive Theory." *Psychology and Health 13*: 623–649.

Barzun, J. 2000. *From Dawn to Decadence*. New York, NY: HarperCollins.

Benjamin, M. B., and A. C. Buck. 2008. "Religion: A Sociocultural Predictor of Health Behaviors in Mexico." *Journal of Aging and Health 20*: 290–305.

Berthoud, H. 2011. "Metabolic and Hedonic Drive in Neural Control of Appetite: Who is the Boss?" *Current Opinion in Neurobiology 21*: 888–896.

Bertrand, D. 2005. "The Therapeutic Role of Khmer Mediums (Kru Boramei) in Contemporary Cambodia." *Mental Health, Religion and Culture 8*: 309–327.

Berzruchka, S., T. Namekata, and M. G. Sistrom. 2008. "Interplay of Politics and Law to Promote Health: Improving Economic Equality and Health: The Case of Postwar Japan." *American Journal of Public Health 98*: 589–594.

Blakeney, C. D., R. F. Blakeney, and H. Reich. 2005. "Leaps of Faith: The Role of Religious Development in Recovering Integrity among Jewish Alcoholics and Drug Addicts." *Mental Health, Religion, and Culture 8*: 63–77.

Blanch, A. 2007. "Integrating Religion and Spirituality in Mental Health: The Promise and the Challenge." *Psychiatric Rehabilitation Journal 30*: 251–260.

Bonadonna, R. 2003. "Meditation's Impact on Chronic Illness." *Holistic Nursing Practices 17*: 309–319.

Bonchek, A., and D. Greenberg. 2009. "Compulsive Prayer and its Management." *Journal of Clinical Psychology 65*: 396–405.

Brown, H. P., J. H. Peterson, and O. Cunningham. 1988. "Rationale and Theoretical Basis for Behavioral/Cognitive Approach to Spirituality." *Alcohol Treatment Quarterly 5*(2): 47–59.

Brown, R. P., and P. L. Gerbarg. 2005a. "Sudarshan Kriya Yogic Breathing in the Treatment of Stress, Anxiety, and Depression. Part I—Neurophysiologic Model." *Journal of Alternative and Complementary Medicine 11*: 189–201.

Brown, R. P., and P. L. Gerbarg. 2005b. "Sudarshan Kriya Yogic Breathing in the Treatment of Stress, Anxiety, and Depression. Part II—Clinical Applications and Guidelines." *Journal of Alternative and Complementary Medicine 11*: 711–717.

Bruner, J. S. 1957. "On Perceptual Readiness." *Psychological Review* 64: 123–152.

Bruner, J. 1990. *Acts of Meaning*. Cambridge, MA: Harvard University Press.

Bulow, H. H., C. L. Sprung, K. Reinhart, S. Prayag, B. Du, F. Abroug, and M. M. Levy. 2008. "The World's Major Religions' Points of View on End-of-Life Decisions in the Intensive Care Unit." *Intensive Care Medicine* 34: 423–430.

Burtt, E. A. 1957. *Man Seeks the Divine*. New York: Harper.

Campbell, J. 1968. *The Hero with a Thousand Faces (2nd Edition)*. New York: Princeton University.

Campbell, J. 1972. *Myths to Live By*. New York: Viking.

Campbell, J. D., D. P. Yoon, and B. Johnstone. 2010. "Determining Relationships between Physical Health and Spiritual Experience, Religious Practices, and Congregational Support in a Heterogeneous Medical Sample." *Journal of Religion and Health* 49: 3–17.

Campion, J. and D. Bhugra. 1998. "Religious and Indigenous Treatment of Mental Illness in South India—A Descriptive Study." *Mental Health, Religion, and Culture* 1: 21–29.

Cangiano, M., M. J. Chisti, M. A. C. Pietroni, and J. H. Smith. 2011. "Extending Prayer Marks as a Sign of Worsening Chronic Disease." *Journal of Health, Population, and Nutrition* 29: 290–291.

Canning, S. S. 2011. "Core Assumptions and Values in Community Psychology: A Christian Reflection." *Journal of Psychology and Theology* 39: 186–199.

Carlson, L. E. and S. N. Garland. 2005. "Impact of Mindfulness-Based Stress Reduction (MVSR) on Sleep, Mood, Stress, and Fatigue Symptoms in Cancer Outpatients." *International Journal of Behavioral Medicine* 12: 278–285.

Carpenter-Song, E. A., M. N. Schwallie, and J. Longhofer. 2007. "Cultural Competence Reexamined: Critique and Directions for the Future." *Psychiatric Services* 58: 1362–1365.

Cartwright, B. Y. 2010. "Understanding Health Beliefs about Illness: A Culturally Responsive Approach." *Journal of Rehabilitation* 76: 40–45.

Carver, C. S., M. F. Scheier, and J. K. Weintraub. 1989. "Assessing Coping Strategies: A Theoretically Based Approach." *Journal of Personality and Social Psychology* 56: 267–283.

Chan, J. and J. Kayser-Jones. 2005. "The Experience of Dying for Chinese Nursing Home Residents: Cultural Considerations." *Journal of Gerontological Nursing* 31: 26–33.

Chattapodhyay, S. 2007. "Religion, Spirituality, Health and Medicine: Why Should Indian Physicians Care?" *Journal of Post Graduate Medicine* 53: 262–266.

Chatters, L. M. 2000. "Religion and Health: Public Health Research and Practice." *Annual Review of Public Health* 21: 335–367.

Chatters, L. M., J. S. Levin, and C. G. Ellison. 1998. "Public Health and Health Education in Faith Communities." *Health Education and Behavior* 25: 689–699.

Chen, Y. 2001. "Chinese Values, Health, and Nursing." *Journal of Advanced Nursing* 36: 270–273.

Chochinov, H. M. 2002. "Dignity-Conserving Care—a New Model of Palliative Care: Helping the Patient Feel Valued." *Journal of the American Medical Association* 287: 2253–2261.

Cnaan, R. A., J. W. Sinha, and C. C. McGrew. 2004. "Congregations as Social Service Providers: Services, Capacity, Culture, and Organization." *Administration in Social Work* 28: 47–68.

Coleman-Brueckheimer, K., and S. Dein. 2011. "Health Care Behaviours and Beliefs in Hasidic Jewish Populations: A Systematic Review of the Literature." *Journal of Religion and Health* 50: 422–436.

Daaleman, T. P. 2004. "Religion, Spirituality, and the Practice of Medicine." *Journal of the American Board of Family Practice* 17: 370–376.

Daaleman, T. P., and L. VandeCreek. 2000. "Placing Religion and Spirituality in End-of-Life Care." *Journal of the American Medical Association* 284: 2514–2517.

Dane, B. 2000. "Thai Women: Meditation as a Way to Cope with AIDS." *Journal of Religion and Health* 39: 5–21.

D'Blasi, Z., E. Harkness, E. Ernst, A. Georgiou, and J. Kleijnen. 2010. "Influence of Context Effects on Health Outcomes: A Systematic Review." *Lancet* 357: 757–762.

Dhar, H. L. 2009. "Meditation Therapy in Cardiovascular and Metabolic Disorders Special Reference to Coronary Artery Disease and Diabetes." *Bombay Hospital Journal* 51: 472–475.

Dittner, A. J., K. Rimes, and S. Thorpe. 2011. "Negative Perfectionism Increases Risk of Fatigue Following a Period of Stress." *Psychology and Health* 26: 253–268.

Donesky-Cuenco, D., H. Q. Nguyen, S. Paul, and V. Carrieri-Kohlman. 2009. "Yoga Therapy Decreases Dypsnea-Related Distress and Improves Functional Performance in People with Chronic Obstructive Pulmonary Disease: A Pilot Study." *Journal of Alternative and Complementary Medicine* 15: 225–234.

Drubach, D. A. 2002. "Judaism, Brain Plasticity and the Making of the Self." *Journal of Religion and Health* 41: 311–322.

Dull, V. T., and L. A. Skokan. 1995. "A Cognitive Model of Religion's Influence on Health." *Journal of Social Issues* 51: 49–64.

Dunn, M. S. 2005. "The Relationship between Religiosity, Employment, and Political Beliefs on Substance Use among High School Seniors." *Journal of Drug and Alcohol Education* 49: 73–88.

Eliasi, J. R., and J. T. Dwyer. 2002. "Kosher and Halal: Religious Observance affecting Dietary Intakes." *Journal of the American Dietetic Association* 102: 911–913.

Ellison, C. 1983. "Spiritual Wellbeing: Conceptualization and Measurement." *Journal of Psychology and Theology* 11(4): 330–340.

Ellison, C. G, and J. S. Levin. 1998. "The Religion-Health Connection: Evidence, Theory, and Future Directions." *Health Education and Behavior* 25: 700–720.

Farmer, B., B. T. Larson, V. L. Fulgoni, A. J. Rainville, and G. U. Liepa. 2011. "A Vegetarian Dietary Pattern as a Nutrient-Dense Approach to Weight Management:

An Analysis of the National Health and Nutrition Examination Survey 1999–2004." *Journal of the American Dietetic Association* 111: 819–827.

Feiser, J. and J. Powers. 2008. *Scriptures of the World's Religions.* New York, NY: McGraw Hill.

Ferguson, J. K., E. W. Willemsen, and M. V. Casteneto. 2010. "Centering Prayer as a Healing Response to Everyday Stress: A Psychological and Spiritual Process." *Pastoral Psychology* 59: 305–329.

Finlayson, G., N. King, and J. E. Blundell. 2007. "Liking vs. Wanting Food: Importance for Human Appetite Control and Weight Regulation." *Neuroscience and Biobehavioral Reviews* 31: 987–1002.

Fitchett, G., B. D. Rybarczyk, G. A. DeMarco, and J. J. Nicholas. 1999. "The Role of Religion in Medical Rehabilitation Outcomes: A Longitudinal Study." *Rehabilitation Psychology* 44: 333–353.

Flood, G. D. 2003. *Introduction to Hinduism.* New York: Cambridge University Press.

Folkman, S., M. A. Chesney, M. Cooke, A. Boccellari, and L. Collette. 1994. "Caregiver Burden in HIV-Positive and HIV-Negative Partners of Men with AIDS." *Journal of Consulting and Clinical Psychology* 62: 746–756.

Frank, D. and L. Grubbs. 2009. "A Faith-Based Screening/Education Program for Diabetes, CVD, and Stroke in Rural African Americans." *The ABNF Journal* 19: 96–101.

Fredrickson, B. L. 2000. "Cultivating Positive Emotions to Optimize Health and Wellbeing." *Prevention and Treatment* 3: 1–25.

Freedland, K. E. 2004. "Religious Beliefs Shorter Hospital Stay? Psychology Works in Mysterious Ways. Comments on Contrada, et al. (2004)." *Health Psychology* 29: 239–242.

Friburg, N. 2001. "The Role of the Chaplain in Spiritual Care." In *Aging and Spirituality: Spiritual Dimensions of Aging Theory, Research, Practice, and Policy,* edited by D. O. Moberg, 177–190. New York: Haworth Pastoral Press.

George, L. K., C. G. Ellison, and D. B. Larson. 2002. "Explaining the Relationships between Religious Involvement and Health." *Psychological Inquiry* 13: 190–200.

Gillum, R. F. and C. L. Holt. 2010. "Associations between Religious Involvement and Behavioral Risk Factors for HIV/AIDS in American Women and Men in a National Health Survey." *Annals of Behavioral Medicine* 40: 284–293.

Gorsuch, R. L. 1995. "Religious Aspects of Substance Abuse and Recovery." *Journal of Social Issues* 51: 65–83.

Grice, P. 1989. *Studies in the Way of Words.* Cambridge, MA: Harvard University Press.

Harris, J. I., S. W. Schoneman, and S. R. Carrera. 2002. "Approaches to Religiosity Related to Anxiety among College Students." *Mental Health, Religion, and Culture* 5: 253–265.

Hazel, K. W. and G. V. Mohatt. 2001. "Cultural and Spiritual Coping in Sobriety: Informing Substance Abuse Prevention for Alaska Native Communities." *Journal of Community Psychology* 29: 541–562.

Hill, P. C., K. I. Pargament, R. W. Jr. Hood, M. E. McCullough, J. P. Swyers, D. B. Larson, and B. J. Zinnbauer. 2000. "Conceptualizing Religion and Spirituality: Points of Commonality, Points of Departure." *Journal of the Theory of Social Behavior 30*: 51–77.

Himle, J. A., L. M. Chatters, R. J. Taylor, and A. Nguyen. 2011. "The Relationship between Obsessive-Compulsive Disorder and Religious Faith: Clinical Characteristics and Implications for Treatment." *Psychology of Religion and Spirituality 3*: 241–258.

Islam, S. M. S. and C. A. Johnson. 2003. "Correlates of Smoking Behavior among Muslim Arab-American Adolescents." *Ethnicity and Health 8*: 319–337.

Jayasinghe, S. R. 2004. "Yoga in Cardiac Health (a Review)." *Journal of Cardiovascular Prevention and. Rehabilitation 11*: 369–375.

Jenkins, C. D. 1978. "Behavioral Risk Factors in Coronary Artery Disease." *Annual Review of Medicine 29*: 543–562.

Jenkins, E. D., M. Yips, L. Melman, M. M. Frisella, and B. D. Matthews. 2010. "Informed Consent: Cultural and Religious Issues Associated with the Use of Allogenic and Xenogenic Mesh Products." *Journal of the American College of Surgeons 210*: 402–410.

Johnsen, E. 1993. "The Role of Spirituality in Recovery from Chemical Dependency." *Journal of Addictions and Offender Counseling 13*(2): 58–61.

Johnstone, B., B. A. Glass, and R. E. Oliver. 2007. "Religion and Disability: Clinical, Research and Training Considerations for Rehabilitation Professional." *Disability and Rehabilitation 29*: 1153–1163.

Jones, S. H. 2006. "Self-Care in Caregiving." *Journal of Human Behavior in the Social Environment 14*: 95–115.

Jung, C. G. 1964. *Man and His Symbols.* New York, NY: Dell.

Juthani, N. V. 2001. "Psychiatric Treatment of Hindus." *International Review of Psychiatry, 13*: 125–130.

Kabat-Zinn, J. 1982. "An Outpatient Program in Behavioral Medicine for Chronic Pain Patients Based on the Practice of Mindfulness Meditation." *General Hospital Psychiatry 4*: 33–47.

Kabat-Zinn, J., L. Lipworth, and R. Burney. 1985. "The Clinical Use of Mindfulness Meditation for the Self-Regulation of Chronic Pain." *Journal of Behavioral Medicine 8*: 163–190.

Kang, E., J. J. Chin, and E. Behar. 2011. "Faith-Based HIV Care and Prevention in Chinese Immigrant Communities: Rhetoric or Reality?" *Journal of Psychology and Theology 39*: 268–279.

Kaplan, G. A. 1996. "People and Places: Contrasting Perspectives on the Association between Social Class and Health." *International Journal of Health Services 26*: 507–519.

Keating, C., A. J. Tilbrook, S. L. Rosell, P. G. Enticott, and P. B. Fitzgerald. 2012. "Reward Processing in Anorexia Nervosa." *Neuropsychologia 50*: 567–575.

Kelly, P. 2011. "Common Cellular and Molecular Mechanisms in Obesity and Drug Addiction." *Nature Review Neuroscience 12*: 638–651.

Kim, K. K., E. S. H. Yu, E. H. Chen, J. Kim, and R. Brintnall. 2000. "Smoking Behavior, Knowledge, and Beliefs among Korean Americans." *Cancer Practice* 8: 223–230.

Kim, W. and S. Kim. 2008. "Women's Alcohol Use and Alcoholism in Korea." *Substance Use and Misuse* 43: 1078–1087.

Klein, C. T. F. and M. Helweg-Larsen. 2002. "Perceived Control and the Optimistic Bias: A Meta-Analytic Review." *Psychology and Health* 17: 437–446.

Koenig, H. G. 1998. "Religious Attitudes and Practices of Hospitalized Medically Ill Older Adults." *International Journal of Geriatric Psychiatry* 13: 213–224.

Koenig, H. G. 2002. "A Commentary: The Role of Religion and Spirituality at the End of Life." *The Gerontologist* 42, *Special Issue 3*: 20–23.

Koenig, H. G. 2005. *Faith and Mental Health: Religious Resources for Healing.* Philadelphia, PA: Templeton Foundation Press.

Koenig, H. G. 2009. "Research on Religion, Spirituality, and Mental Health: A Review." *Canadian Journal of Psychiatry* 54: 283–291.

Koenig, H. G., D. E. King, and V. B. Carson. 2012. *Handbook of Religion and Health.* New York, NY: Oxford University Press.

Koenig, H. G., M. E. McCullough, and D. B. Larson. 2001. *The Handbook of Religion and Health.* New York, NY: Oxford University Press.

Krause, N. M. 2008. *Aging in the Church.* West Conshohocken, PA: Templeton Press.

Krisberg, K. 2012. "Bronx Diabetes Program Reaching Residents with Spiritual Message." *The Nation's Health* 42(5): 9.

LaFleur, W. R. 2002. "From Agape to Organs: Religious Difference between Japan and America in Judging the Ethics of the Transplant." *Journal of Religion and Science* 37: 623–642.

Lam, W. A., and L. B. McCullough. 2000. "Influence of Religious and Spiritual Values on the Willingness of Chinese-Americans to Donate Organs for Transplantation." *Clinical Transplantation* 14: 449–456.

Lane, J. D., J. E. Seskevich, and C. F. Pieper. 2007. "Brief Meditation Training Can Improve Perceived Stress and Negative Mood." *Alternative Therapies in Health and Medicine* 13: 38–44.

Leung, G., and S. Stanner. 2011. "Diets of Minority Ethnic Groups in the UK: Influence on Chronic Disease Risk and Implications for Prevention." *Nutrition Bulletin* 36: 161–198.

Levy, B. R., M. D. Slade, and P. Ranasinghe. 2009. "Causal Thinking after a Tsunami Wave: Karma Beliefs, Pessimistic Explanatory Style and Health among Sri Lankan Survivors." *Journal of Religion and Health* 48: 38–45.

Lewin, K. 1951. *Field Theory in Social Science.* New York: Harper.

Loue, S., S. D. Lane, L. S. Lloyd, and L. Loh. 1999. "Integrating Buddhism and HIV Prevention in U.S. Southeast Asian Communities." *Journal of Health Care for the Poor and Underserved* 10: 100–122.

Ludwig, D. S. and J. Kabat-Zinn. 2008. "Mindfulness in Medicine." *Journal of the American Medical Association* 300: 1350–1352.

Lutz, A., L. L. Greischan, D. Perlman, and R. J. Davidson. 2009. "Bold Signal in Insula is Differentially Related to Cardiac Functioning during Compassion Meditation in Experts vs. Novices." *Neuroimage 47*: 1038–1046.

Maddi, S. R., M. Brow, D. M., Khoshaba, and M. Vaitkus. 2006. "Relationship of Hardiness and Religiousness to Depression and Anger." *Consulting Psychology Journal: Practice and Research 58*: 148–161.

Malinowski, B. 1954. *Magic, Science, and Religion.* New York, NY: Doubleday.

Maulana, A. O., A. Krumich, and B. Van Den Borne. 2009. "Emerging Discourse: Islamic Teaching in HIV Prevention in Kenya." *Culture, Health, and Sexuality 11*: 559–569.

Maynard, E. A., R. L. Gorsuch, and J. P. Bjorck. 2001. "Religious Coping Style, Concept of God, and Personal Religious Variables in Threat, Loss, and Challenge Situations." *Journal for the Scientific Study of Religion 40*: 65–74.

McClain-Jacobson, C., B. Rosenfeld, A. Kosinski, P. Haley, J. E. Cimino, and W. Breitbart. 2004. "Belief in an Afterlife, Spiritual Well-Being and End-of-Life Despair in Patients with Advanced Cancer." *General Hospital Psychiatry 26*: 484–486.

McCullough, M. E. and B. L. B. Willoughby. 2009. "Religion, Self-Regulation, and Self-Control: Associations, Explanations, and Implications." *Psychological Bulletin 135*: 69–93.

McGrath, P. 1998. "Buddhist Spirituality—a Compassionate Perspective on Hospice Care." *Mortality 3*: 251–263.

McIntosh, D. N., R. C. Silver, and C. B. Wortman. 1993. "Religion's Role in Adjustment to a Negative Life Event: Coping with the Loss of a Child." *Journal of Personality and Social Psychology 65*: 812–821.

Mead, M., ed. 1955. *Cultural Patterns and Technical Change.* New York, NY: United Nations Educational, Scientific and Cultural Organization.

Miller, W. R., and C. E. Thoresen. 2003. "Spirituality, Religion, and Health. An Emerging Research Field." *American Psychologist 58*: 24–35.

Moberg, D. O. 2001. "The Reality and Centrality of Spirituality." In *Aging and Spirituality: Spiritual Dimensions of Aging Theory, Research, Practice, and Policy,* edited by D. O. Moberg, 3–20. New York: Haworth Pastoral Press.

Moberg, D. O. 2002. "Assessing and Measuring Spirituality: Confronting Dilemmas of Universal and Particular Evaluative Criteria." *Journal of Adult Development 9*: 47–60.

Mok, E., F. Wong, and D. Wong. 2010. "The Meaning of Spirituality and Spiritual Care among the Hong Kong Chinese Terminally Ill." *Journal of Advanced Nursing 66*: 360–370.

Morrow, M., and S. Barraclough. 2003. "Tobacco Control and Gender in South-East Asia. Part II Singapore and Vietnam." *Health Promotion International 18*: 373–380.

Muecke, M. A. 1983. "Caring for Southeast Asian Refugee Patients in the USA." *American Journal of Public Health 73*: 431–438.

Muhammad, D. 2009. *Challenges to Native American Advancement: The Recession and Native America.* Washington, DC: Institute for Policy Studies.

Murray, T. S., V. L. Malcarne, and K. Goggin. 2003. "Alcohol-Related God/Higher Power Control Beliefs, Locus of Control, and Recovery within the Alcoholics Anonymous Paradigm." *Alcoholism Treatment Quarterly* 21(3): 23–39.

Muula, A. S. 2010. "'I can't Use a Condom, I Am a Christian:' Salvation, Death, and . . . Naivety in Africa." *Croatian Medical Journal* 51: 468–471.

Mytko, J. J., and S. J. Knight. 1999. "Body, Mind, and Spirit: Towards the Integration of Religiosity and Spirituality in Cancer Quality of Life Research." *Psycho-Oncology* 8: 439–450.

Nath, J. 2010. "'God is a Vegetarian': The Food, Health and Biospirituality of Hare Krishna, Buddhist and Seventh-Day Adventist Devotees." *Health Sociology Review* 19: 356–368.

Nayar, K. R., 2007. "Social Exclusion, Caste, and Health: A Review Based on the Social Determinants Framework." *Indian Journal of Medical Research* 126: 355–363.

Nebelkopf, E. and S. Wright. 2011. "Holistic System of Care: A Ten-Year Perspective. *Journal of Psychoactive Drugs* 43: 302–308.

Neeleman, J. and R. Persaud, R. 1995. "Why do Psychiatrists Neglect Religion?" *British Journal of Medical Psychology* 68: 169–178.

Nelson, J. M. 2010. *Psychology, Religion, and Spirituality.* New York, NY: Springer.

Ng, T. P., M. S. Z. Nyunt, P. C. Chiam, and E. H. Kua. 2011. "Religion, Health Beliefs, and the Use of Mental Health Services by the Elderly." *Aging and Mental Health* 15: 143–149.

Nord, W. A. 2010. *Does God Make a Difference? Taking Religion Seriously in Our Schools and Universities.* New York: Oxford University Press.

Norenzayan, A. and S. J. Heine. 2005. "Psychological Universals: What Are They and How Can We Know." *Psychological Bulletin* 131: 763–784.

Padela, A. I., A. Killawi, M. Heisler, S. Demonner, and M. D. Fetters. 2011. "The Role of Imams in American Muslim Health: Perspectives of Muslim Community Leaders in Southeast Michigan." *Journal of Religion and Health* 50: 359–373.

Paonil, W. and L. Sringernyuang. 2002. "Buddhist Perspectives on Health and Healing." *The Chulalongkorn Journal of Buddhist Studies* 1(2): 93–105.

Pargament, K. I., B. W. Smith, H. G., Koenig, and L. Perez. 1998. "Patterns of Positive and Negative Religious Coping with Major Life Stressors." *Journal for the Scientific Study of Religion* 37: 710–724.

Pathy, R., K. E. Mills, S. Gazeley, A. Ridgley, and T. Kiran. 2011. "Health is a Spiritual Thing: Perspectives of Health Care Professional and Female Somali and Bangladeshi Women on the Health Impacts of Fasting During Ramadan." *Ethnicity and Health* 16: 43–56.

Pew Forum on Religion and Public Life. 2008. *U.S. Religious Landscape Survey— Religious Beliefs and Practices: Diverse and Politically Relevant.* Washington, DC: Pew Research Center.

Proulx, K. 2008. "Experiences of Women with Bulimia Nervosa in a Mindfulness-Based Eating Disorder Treatment Group." *Eating Disorders* 16: 52–72.

Pullen, L., M. A. Modrcin-Talbott, W. R. West, and R. Muenchen. 1999. "Spiritual High vs. High on Spirits: Is Religiosity Related to Adolescent Alcohol and Drug Use?" *Journal of Psychiatric and Mental Health Nursing* 6: 3–8.

Purnell, L. D. 2008. "Traditional Vietnamese Health and Healing." *Urologic Nursing* 28: 63–67.

Raub, J. S. 2002. "Psychophysiologic Effects of Hatha Yoga on Musculoskeletal and Cardiopulmonary Function: A Literature Review." *Journal of Alternative and Complementary Medicine* 6: 797–812.

Reid, A. E., R. B. Cialdini, and L. S. Aiken. 2010. "Social Norms and Health Behavior." In *Handbook of Behavioral Medicine: Methods and Applications,* edited by K. E. Freedland, J. R. Jennings, M. M. Llabre, S. B. Manuck, and E. J. Susman, 263–274. New York, NY: Springer.

Rhi, B. 2001. "Culture, Spirituality, and Mental Health: The Forgotten Aspect of Religion and Health." *Psychiatric Clinics of North America* 24: 569–579.

Richards, T. A. and S. Folkman. 1997. "Spiritual Aspects of Loss at the Time of a Partner's Death from AIDS." *Death Studies* 21: 527–552.

Romaguera, D., C. Bamia, A. Pons, J. Tur, and A. Trichopoulou. 2009. "Food Patterns and Mediterranean Diet in Western and Eastern Mediterranean Islands." *Public Health Nutrition* 12: 1174–1181.

Ross, A., and S. Thomas. 2010. "The Health Benefits of Yoga and Exercise: A Review of Comparison Studies." *Journal of Alternative and Complementary Medicine* 16: 3–12.

Sandhu, J. S. 2009. "A Sikh Perspective on Alcohol and Drugs: Implications for Treatment of Punjabi-Sikh Patients." *Sikh Formations* 5(1): 23–37.

Santee, R. 2008. "Stress Management Using the Zhuangi." *Journal of Daoist Studies* 1: 93–123.

Schulz, M., A. Damkroger, E. Voltmer, B. Lowe, M. Driessen, M. Ward, and K. Wingenfeld. 2011. "Work-Related Behavior and Experience Pattern in Nurses: Impact on Physical and Mental Health." *Journal of Psychiatric and Mental Health Nursing* 18: 411–417.

Shapiro, S. L., K. W. Brown, C. Thorensen, and T. G. Plante. 2011. "The Moderation of Mindfulness-Based Stress Reduction Effects by Trait Mindfulness: Results from a Randomized Controlled Trial." *Journal of Clinical Psychology* 67: 267–277.

Shea, J. 2000. *Spirituality and Health Care: Reaching toward a Holistic Future.* Chicago, IL: Park Ridge Center.

Silvestri, G. A., S. Knittig, J. S. Zoller, and P. J. Nietert. 2003. "Importance of Faith in Medical Decisions Regarding Cancer Care." *Journal of Clinical Oncology* 21: 1379–1382.

Sloan, R. P., E. Bagiella, L. VandeCreek, M. Hover, C. Casalone, T. J. Hirsch, Y. Hasan, R. Krieger, and P. Poulos. 2000. "Should Physicians Prescribe Religious Activities?" *New England Journal of Medicine* 342: 1913–1916.

Smith, H. 1991. *The World's Religions.* New York: HarperCollins.

Smith, H. 2001. *Why Religion Matters.* New York, NY: Harper-Collins.

Smith, T. B., M. E. McCullough, and J. Poll. 2003. "Religiousness and Depression: Evidence for a Main Effect and the Moderating Influence of Stressful Life Events." *Psychological Bulletin* 129: 614–636.

Spiro, A. M. 2005. " Najar or Bhut—Evil Eye or Ghost Affliction: Gujarati Views about Illness Causation." *Anthropology and Medicine* 12: 61–73.

Sticher, M., C. B. Smith, and S. Davidson. 2010. "Reducing Heart Disease through Vegetarian Diet Using Primary Prevention." *Journal of American Academy of Nursing* 22: 134–137.

Stylianou, S. 2004. "The Role of Religiosity in the Opposition to Drug Use." *International Journal of Offender Therapy and Comparative Criminology* 48: 429–448.

Sulmasy, D. P. 2002. "A Biopsychosocial-Spiritual Model of the Care of Patients at the End of Life." *The Gerontologist* 42(Special Issue 3): 24–33.

Tang, C. S. 2008. "Gendered Economic, Social, and Cultural Challenges to HIV/AIDS Prevention and Intervention for Chinese Women." *Journal of Human Behavior in the Social Environment* 17: 339–360.

Tang, S. T., C. Li, and Y. Liao. 2007. "Factors Associated with Depressive Distress among Taiwanese Family Caregivers of Cancer Patients at the End of life." *Palliative Medicine* 21: 249–257.

Taylor, C. 2011. *Dilemmas and Connections*. Cambridge MA: Harvard University Press.

Taylor, C. Z. 2002. "Religious Addiction: Obsession with Spirituality." *Pastoral Psychology* 50: 291–315.

Teasdale, J. D., Z. V. Segal, J. M. G. Williams, V. A. Ridgeway, J. M. Soulsby, and M. A. Lau. 2000. "Prevention of Relapse/Recurrence in Major Depression by Mindfulness-Based Cognitive Therapy." *Journal of Consulting and Clinical Psychology* 68: 615–623.

Thiel, M. M. and M. R. Robinson. 1997. "Physician's Collaboration with Chaplains: Difficulties and Benefits." *Journal of Clinical Ethics* 8: 94–103.

Turner, R. P., D. Lukoff, R. T. Barnhouse, and F. G. Lu. 1995. "Religious or Spiritual Problem: A Culturally Sensitive Diagnostic Category in the DSM-IV." *The Journal of Nervous and Mental Disease* 183: 435–444.

Tung, W. 2010. "Asian American's Confucianism-Based Health-Seeking Behavior and Decision-Making Process." *Home Health Care Management and Practice* 22: 536–538.

U.S. Department of Agriculture, U.S. Department of Health and Human Services. 2010. *Dietary Guidelines for Americans (7th Edition)*. Washington, DC: U.S. Government Printing Office.

Visscher, C. 2006. "Eye on Religion: Understanding the Cultural/Religious Mélange in Treating Chinese Patients." *Southern Medical Journal* 99: 683–684.

Viswanath, K. and L. K. Ackerson. 2011. "Race, Ethnicity, Language, Social Class, and Health Communication Inequalities: A Nationally-Representative Cross-Sectional Study." *PLoS ONE* 6(1): 1–8.

VonDras, D. D., R. R. Schmitt, and D. Marx. 2007. "Associations between Aspects of Spiritual Wellbeing, Alcohol Use and Related Social-Cognitions in Female College Students." *Journal of Religion and Health* 46(4): 500–515.

Walshe, M. 1999. *The Long Discourses of the Buddha.* Boston: Wisdom.

Watts, A. W. 1951. *The Wisdom of Insecurity.* New York, NY: Pantheon.

Watts, A. W. 1957. *The Way of Zen.* New York, NY: Pantheon.

Weinstein, N. D. 1980. "Unrealistic Optimism about Future Life Events." *Journal of Personality and Social Psychology* 39: 806–820.

Weinstein, N. D. 1983. "Reducing Unrealistic Optimism about Illness Susceptibility." *Health Psychology* 2: 11–20.

Weinstein, N. D. 1987. "Unrealistic Optimism about Susceptibility to Health Problems: Conclusions from a Community-Wide Sample." *Journal of Behavioral Medicine* 10: 481–500.

Weitzman, P. F., K. Ballah, and S. E. Levkoff. 2008. "Native-Born Chinese Women's Experiences in Medical Encounters in the U.S." *Ageing International* 32: 128–139.

Wisst, W. H., B. M. Sullivan, H. A. Wayment, and M. Warren. 2010. "A Web-Based Survey of the Relationship between Buddhist Religious Practices, Health, and Psychological Characteristics: Research Methods and Preliminary Results." *Religion and Health* 49: 18–31.

Xiao, Z., P. Mehrotra, and R. Zimmerman. 2011. "Sexual Revolution in China: Implications for Chinese Women and Society." *AIDS Care* 23(Supp. 1): 105–112.

Yalom, I. 2002. "Religion and Psychiatry." *American Journal of Psychotherapy* 56: 301–316.

Yip, K. 2004. "Taoism and Its Impact on Mental Health of the Chinese Communities." *International Journal of Social Psychiatry* 50: 25–42.

Zaccarinni, M. C. 2011. "Daoist Inspired Health in Daily Life." *Journal of Daoist Studies* 4: 80–103.

Ziaee, V., M. Razaei, Z. Ahmadinejad, H. Shaikh, R. Yousefi, L. Yarmohammadi, F. Bozorgi, and M. J. Behjati. 2006. "The Changes of Metabolic Profile and Weight during Ramadan Fasting." *Singapore Medical Journal* 47: 409–414.

CHAPTER SEVEN

Islamic Healing Approaches, Beliefs, and Health-Related Behaviors

Sujata R. Swaroop, Chanté D. DeLoach, and Fyeqa Sheikh

It is becoming clear that treating patients from a monocultural stance is grossly inadequate within the United States given the nation's composition of varied ethnicities, cultures, languages, and religions. Indeed, there is a growing movement for U.S. health professionals to build awareness of the multiple approaches to treatment present across cultures and develop an increased understanding of how providers' own cultural beliefs influence their work. Considering the cultural dimensions of health and mental health when treating patients of different backgrounds not only fosters culturally competent treatment, it also makes it more likely that non-dominant cultural groups access and are effectively treated within health care. Quan, Fong, De Coster, Wang, Musto, Noseworthy, and Ghali (2006) examined studies on racial and ethnic disparities in the use of health services and in health outcomes in the United States and reported that minorities are less likely to access health care and more likely to experience barriers than their White counterparts. These authors cite physicians' attitudes toward minority patients, patient unfamiliarity with the health care delivery system, and variables of language, poverty, transportation, education, health insurance coverage, and family support as central factors underlying ethnic disparities in health service usage. The insufficiency of universal application of Western forms of treatment can also be seen in health-seeking patterns of first and second generation immigrant communities, regardless of socioeconomic status (Watkins and Shulman 2008). Anecdotal evidence suggests that these communities predominantly seek services from traditional healers. The majority of these traditional healers are viewed as qualified and legitimate by these communities as their professional calling is seen as handed down through tribal law, religious custom, or cultural tradition (Inayat 2005).

Islamic populations comprise a growing segment of American society; yet, help-seeking attitudes and behaviors toward seeking formal health services as well as the experience of service utilization is largely understudied for American Muslims (Aloud 2004). Continued research on service utilization and the effectiveness of both formal and traditional treatments is necessary to better serve Muslim-American populations. Additionally, despite its long history in the United States, Americans understand relatively little about Islam or its followers (Altareb 1996). This chapter focuses on Muslim health-related beliefs and paradigms, offering valuable insight for interdisciplinary health professionals from a diversity of backgrounds.

Within this chapter, the terms "Muslim" and "Islamic populations" are used to refer to a community of people who recognize Islam as intrinsic to their worldview, in varying ways. Islamic populations living in the United States are ethnically, linguistically, and culturally diverse. In addition to these variables of diversity, Muslim populations also differ in religious beliefs and practices; further, individuals differ in the degree to which they identify with being Muslim in faith, function or culture. Thus, despite core commonalities, it should be clear there are no prototypical Muslim Americans (Ali, Abu-Ras, and Hamid 2009); health care professionals should be cautioned on developing stereotypic assumptions about beliefs and practices. In order to facilitate deeper understanding of the various ways Islamic populations living in the United States may experience, understand, and express concepts of health and wellness, this chapter will address the history and demography, beliefs and approaches to health and healing, and health care utilization and experiences of Islamic-Americans.

History and Demographics of Islamic-American Societies

It has been reported that there are over 1.5 billion Muslims in the world (Anwar 2008, Hasnain, Shaikh, and Shanawani 2008); yet, conflicting data exists regarding the size and demographic make-up of Islamic populations living in the United States. Estimates of the total population of this group range from 11 million to 1.6 million (Ali et al. 2009, Ali, Milstein, and Marzuk 2005, Pew 2007, Post and Sheffer 2007), with best estimates somewhere between 2.5 and 4.4 million (Ali et al. 2009, Nimer 2002). It is generally agreed that Muslims comprise one of the most rapidly growing minority groups in the United States (Ali et al. 2005, Hasnain et al. 2008, Husain 1998).

Immigrant Muslims living in the United States originally settled largely in metropolitan areas, such as New York City, Los Angeles, and Chicago. Over time, however, Islamic populations dispersed widely throughout the country. It is estimated that the majority of all Islamic populations living in the United States reside in California, Texas, New York, Washington, Illinois, Indiana, and Michigan (Anwar 2008, Hasnain, et al. 2008, Post and Sheffer 2007). It is also documented that Muslim populations tend to build regional communities along lines of ethnic ancestry; the Center for Immigration Studies (Camarota 2002) noted that Iranians have formed large ethnic communities in California, and South Asians have done so in Texas. Many Arabs and persons of African ancestry have formed large ethnic communities in the Midwest triangle. Muslims of East European descent, including Albanians, Bosnians, and Turks, have highly populated ethnic communities in Chicago, while Detroit is known to have the highest concentration of Muslims of Arab descent, including Lebanese, Iraqis, Palestinians, and Yemens. Muslim Somalis have formed large rural communities in Maine, New Hampshire, and Massachusetts. New York City, where the worldwide Muslim community is fully represented, is an exception to this generality (Ali et al. 2009).

Rough estimates indicate that two-thirds of all Muslims living in the United States are immigrants (Hasnain et al. 2008). Yet, American Muslims also represent a number of ethnonational diasporas; while some Islamic Americans are first- and second-generation immigrants, others can trace their origins to the colonization of the Americas (Ali et al. 2009). It is estimated that African-Americans, Arab-Americans, and South Asian-Americans evenly comprise 80 percent of American Muslims (Anwar 2008, Ali et al. 2009, Hasnain et al. 2008). Persons of African, East Asian, European, Caribbean, and Latino descent as well as American-born Whites of European descent comprise the remaining 20 percent of American practitioners of Islam (Ali et al. 2009, Anwar 2008, Hasnain et al. 2008).

The earliest Muslims to arrive in America in significant numbers were brought from West Africa as slaves between 1530 and 1831. It is noteworthy that Islam was brought to West and North Africa during the Arab invasion and therefore bears its own colonial history. This population comprised an estimated 14–20 percent of the hundreds of thousands of enslaved West Africans forcibly removed from their homelands (Ali et al. 2009, Anwar

2008). Due to discrimination against Muslims by slave-owners, many in this initial Islamic population were prohibited from practicing their religion and forced to convert to Christianity (Ali et al. 2009). Contextualizing this history promotes understanding that this same group of people were first introduced and/or forcibly converted to Islam during the Arab invasion of North and West Africa, then later enslaved in the Americas and forcibly converted to Christianity. Understanding the Arab colonial context and hegemonic history of Islam provides the historical and political landscape for which to understand the cultural demography of the religion as well as present day social and political relations.

In the late 19th and early 20th centuries, coinciding with the end of World War I and the decline of the Ottoman Empire, a second major wave of Muslims immigrated to the United States; this group sought economic opportunity and mainly originated from Syria, Lebanon, and other Arab nations (Ali et al. 2009, Anwar, 2008, Hasnain et al. 2008). Many immigrants in this group found work as manual laborers and factory workers. They also began to establish communities and mosques as their numbers grew (Anwar 2008, Hasnain et al. 2008).

In the 1930s, the Nation of Islam was founded in the United States by Wallace Fard Muhammad. This group considered itself different from the older Sunni and Shi'a denominations of Islam and was largely comprised of African-Americans (Hasnain et al. 2008). Forty years later, the Nation of Islam divided, and many of its followers, influenced by Malcolm X (also known as El Hajj Malik Shabazz), shifted to Sunni Islam (Hasnain et al. 2008).

A third wave of Islamic immigration began in the 1950s; immigrants in this group largely included professionals and university students seeking opportunities for advancement that they could not find in their countries of origin (Ali et al. 2009, Anwar 2008, Hasnain et al. 2008). This wave of immigrants tends to have larger incomes than their predecessors and lower levels of acculturation; it is estimated that 87 percent of the mosques in the United States were built following the immigration of this group (Hasnain et al. 2008).

In addition to this continuing third wave, groups of Muslims continue to arrive in the United States from areas affected by conflict. Human rights violations, poverty exacerbated by global economic decline, corrupt governments, and unequal distribution of power fueled the recent series of revolutionary demonstrations in Tunisia, Egypt, Yemen, Libya, Syria, and Bahrain, among other predominantly Muslim nations this past year; collectively, these revolts, civil wars, and protests have been referred to as the "Arab Spring." Iranians and Pakistanis have suffered similar economic, political, and military unrest, which has escalated in recent years. These alarming trends which span Arab, Persian, and Pashtun Islamic cultures in North Africa, the Middle East, and South Asia, make it likely that emigration trends for these populations will dramatically increase in coming years. These populations may be seeking escape from conditions such as underdevelopment, tyranny, persecution, lawlessness, poverty, civil strife, and war trauma (Hasnain et al. 2008). Immigrants in this group often held professional jobs with good incomes in their homeland, but have had to accept non-professional employment in the United States. Individuals in this group generally are less fluent in English, have lower incomes, and many lack benefits such as health insurance (Hasnain et al. 2008). The influx of this vulnerable group and the fact that they are seeking safety makes it only more urgent that clinicians, doctors, other health care professionals and the general public better understand the intersections between Islamic belief systems and Muslim health. Given the need for healthcare professionals to build awareness and maintain sensitivity regarding this client constituency's cultural, philosophical, moral, and spiritual-religious perspectives, the next section intends to assist healthcare providers in gaining familiarity with some of the basic concepts of Islam.

General Introduction to Islamic Beliefs

The dearth of research and culturally embedded Islamaphobia (particularly post 9/11) has contributed to the lack of knowledge about Islamic beliefs. Thus, a brief overview of core Islamic beliefs, practices, and differences across denominations pertinent to conceptualizations of health and health-related behaviors is necessary. The word "Islam" is derived from *Aslama,* an Arabic word which means to accept, surrender, or submit to God (Hasnain et al. 2008). Islam arose as a religion circa 610 C.E., when it is believed that the Prophet Muhammad[1] began receiving a series of revelations from God. These revelations now make up the Qur'an. Allah is an Arabic term for "The God," and Islam is considered to be one of the great monotheistic faiths. The many cultural variations among Muslims across the globe make it impossible to assert generalizations of a single Muslim culture or religion. However, common elements of belief and practice bind all followers of Islam.

---

[1] Peace be upon him (PBUH). When discussing the Prophet Muhammad, Muslim populations use the phrase *Peace be upon him* as a sign of reverence. Out of respect to Islamic beliefs, PBUH is inserted as an abbreviation throughout this chapter when referring to the Prophet Muhammad.

While several denominations exist within Islam, the Sunni and Shi'a groups are dominant within American Muslim populations (Hasnain et al. 2008, Husain 1998, Winter 2008). The division between these two groups can be traced to the decision on who would lead practitioners of Islam following the death of the Prophet Muhammad (PBUH) (Hasnain et al. 2008, Husain 1998, Winter 2008). Sunnis, or Sunnites, chose to accept Muhammad's (PBUH) close companion Abu Bakr as his successor and ideologically follow the *sunnah,* or custom of the Prophet (PBUH). Shi'ites chose to accept Ali, Muhammad's (PBUH) closest relative, as the successor and refer to themselves as followers of the family of the Prophet (PBUH). Estimates purport that Sunni Islam is comprised of 940 million attendants worldwide, while Shi'a Islam is comprised of 120 million attendants (Hasnain et al. 2008). Estimates of Sunnites and Shi'ites within the United States have been labeled unreliable (Hasnain et al. 2008); however, it is accepted that the majority of Muslims living in the United States identify as Sunnite though large communities of Shi'ites can also be found, particularly in southeast Michigan and northern California (Hasnain et al. 2008, Winter 2008). While the initial division between Sunnites and Shi'ites stemmed from differences in beliefs related to transmission of leadership, over time the Shi'a began to demonstrate preference for particular *hadith* and *sunnah* literature, particularly those credited to the Prophet's family and close associates. By contrast, Sunnites consider all *hadith* and *sunnah* equally valid. Such difference of emphasis resulted in different understandings of the laws and practices of Islam. Overall, the doctrinal and practical differences between Sunni and Shi'a are relatively slight, such as different schedules for prayer and the breaking of fasts (Hasnain et al. 2008, Winter 2008). For example, while all Muslims are required to pray five times daily, Shi'a practice permits combining some prayers into three daily prayer times. It should be noted that due to ethnic, cultural, and religious differences, Sunnites and Shi'ites can have as much intra-denominational diversity as they have inter-denominational diversity (Hasnain et al. 2008, Winter 2008).

Within the Islamic worldview, *tawhid,* or religious monotheism is fundamental (Altareb 1996, Husain 1998). According to Islamic belief, the universe was brought into being by Allah's command. Thus, the purpose of existence, as understood by this view, is to worship God. *Tawhid* enables followers of Islam to link total devotion and submission to God's will with lasting purity and peace (Altareb 1996, Husain 1998). While Allah is understood to be beyond all comprehension, He is also viewed as compassionate, merciful, and responsive to human distress (Ali 1975). Thus, for followers of Islam, every act carried out with the awareness of Allah, ranging from eating to child-rearing to conducting business, allows one to grow closer to Allah; this is connection between *tawhid* and *taqwa*, or God-consciousness. In mindfully striving towards embodying Islamic principles, Muslims demonstrate their belief in God (Altareb 1996).

According to Husain (1998), faith in Allah and carrying out righteous deeds are the springboard of the Qur'an. It is believed that Islamic holy texts were dictated by Allah through the prophets; the Arabic version of the Qur'an is believed to be God's final revelation (Ali 1975, Husain 1998). The Qur'an is comprised of 114 *suras,* or chapters, containing 6616 *ayahs,* or verses (Husain 1998). The Qur'an is the source from which followers of Islam derive not only their law and theology, but also their principles and institutions for public life; the central objective of the Qur'an is to influence and provide a framework for human conduct and Muslim spiritual life (Armstrong 2006, Husain 1998). Thus, the Qur'an is an essential element in understanding Muslim conceptualizations of all aspects of life, including health.

In addition to relying on Islamic texts for guidance, Muslims are expected to conduct their lives in accordance with model examples set by the prophets. The prophets of Islam are understood to have been chosen by Allah to serve as messengers (Armstrong 2006, Hasnain et al. 2008, Husain 1998). Muslims believe that the Prophet Muhammad (PBUH) was the last, not the only, prophet who exemplified God's message to mankind. Earlier prophets include Abraham, Ishmael, Isaac, David, Moses, and Jesus (Hasnain et al. 2008, Husain 1998). To this end, all followers of Islam are expected to emulate the example of the *sunnah*—which refers to the normative example of the Prophet Muhammad's (PBUH) life—including actions, conduct, and practical applications of the Qur'an—in their daily lives (Armstrong 2006, Hasnain et al. 2008, Husain 1998). Followers of Islam draw further religious teaching from the *hadith,* a collection of the sayings and actions of the Prophet Muhammad (PBUH). Transcending respect, love, and veneration for the Prophet is central for many followers of Islam; many Muslims thus utter the phrase *salla 'Llahu alayhi wa-sallam,* "Allah bless him and send him Peace," when using the prophet's name (Hasnain et al. 2008).

Finally, it is critical for health care professionals to understand the Five Pillars of Islam, which guide daily life for practicing Muslims. The Five Pillars of Islam are considered required practices for all believers and include *Al-shahadah,* or declaration of faith, which explicates the belief that there is only one God and that Muhammad is the last messenger of God; *Al-salah,* or daily prayers performed at the prescribed time and in particular manner; *Al-Zakah,* or almsgiving a proportionately fixed contribution of wealth to the needy; *Al-Sawm,* or fasting from dawn until sunset during Ramadan; and *Al-Hajj,* or pilgrimage to Mecca, at least once in one's lifetime (Altareb 1996, Husain 1998, Winter 2008). According to Altareb (1996), the Five Pillars of faith assist Muslims in integrating the material and spiritual worlds. Since in Islam it is believed that everything a person does or says with God in mind is an act of worship, the Five Pillars represent different forms of worship and relate to spiritual wholeness and development. In summary, an understanding of the major denominations of Islam, *tawhid,* and the guidance provided by the prophets, holy texts, and the Five Pillars of faith guide introduction to Islamic beliefs; familiarization with such concepts is necessary for American health care professionals given the growing population of American Muslims.

Islamic Approaches to Health and Healing

A basic understanding of these common principles of Islam allows this dialogue to shift to health-related beliefs and practices of Muslims living in the United States. Grounded in this context, we examine Islamic health-related paradigms, including cultural idioms of health and illness, approaches to spiritual healing, and Islamic understandings of mental health.

Muslim Health and Health-Related Paradigms

Western models of health typically present cultural and spiritual etiologies of health and idioms of distress in limiting ways that rarely warrant further investigation or inform the provision of health care (Greenwood et al. 2000). Yet, research on religious experience indicates that faith engages the body as much as it engages the mind (Mahmood 2001, Proudfoot 1985). As noted previously, Islamic teachings of health are holistic, connecting "knowledge, health, healing, the environment and the centrality of Allah" (Rajaram and Rashidi 2003, 87). This is in contrast to a Western allopathic perspective that maintains a dualistic separation of mind and body. Indeed within Islam, a person is comprised of four dynamic parts: the mind (*Aql*), body (*Jism*), self (*nafs*), and soul/spirit (*Ruh*) (Rajaram and Rashidi). The harmonious balance of all of these parts constitutes health in Islam whereas physical and mental disease is thought to occur when there is imbalance amongst these parts (Al-Zeera 2001, Ashy 1999, Rajaram and Rashidi 2003).

Thus, it is evident that Islam prioritizes health, as the body is viewed as being a gift from God. To this end, Islam requires a lifestyle of health promotion and encourages treatment to alleviate human suffering. Inhorn and Serour (2011) note that the Qur'an and *hadith* emphasize "early Islamic health prescriptions and injunctions . . . termed prophetic medicine"

(936). They quote the hadith that states, "for every disease there is a remedy" and therefore, "Muslims are encouraged to seek knowledge about their afflictions, and to pursue medical remedies administered by qualified healers" (ibid). Indeed, health care providers may be viewed as "human scientists under God's providence" or "undertaking God's handiwork" (937). Such a viewpoint aptly demonstrates the value and utility of allopathic medicine within Islam. Islamic medicine has a long history which helped develop the Islamic world community as well as contributed to Western science, including medicine (Ahmed 2000, Rajaram and Rashidi 2003).

Despite the high value placed upon allopathic medicine and health-seeking behaviors, there are some aspects of Islam that may conflict with the traditional practice of and advancements in medicine. Specifically, while there is widespread agreement on the use of biomedical technology that is life-saving and life-supporting (e.g. dialysis), there remain sectarian differences—primarily Shia and Sunni Muslims—in utilization of some types of health care such as reproductive assistance, stem cell therapies, and organ donation/transplantation (Inhorn and Serour 2011). Many Muslims may consult the *fatwas*, which refer to non-binding private or public statements issued by Muslim clerics or other Islamic authorities on moral issues, such as medical decision-making (Black 2009, Inhorn and Serour 2011). Yet, even the *fatwas* may vary around permissibility of scientifically complex phenomena that may blur the medical and moral, such as around reproductive assistance, third party donations, and human reproductive cloning. Such differences underscore the cultural pluralism within the Muslim community, even in understandings of health and the ethics of curative efforts. It also further illuminates the way in which religion may inform the health understandings of some Muslims, particularly in endorsing a "God-centric view of health and illness" (AlRawi et al. 2012, 492).

Some note that Muslims may have a fatalistic view as Allah is deemed the originator of all life and actions. In the Sufi tradition, which emphasizes mystical trends within Islam, illness may also be viewed as a gift that may be utilized to bring one closer to Allah. Chishti (1991) underscores this in quoting renowned Sufi Imam al-Ghazali: "Illness is one of the forms of experience by which humans arrive at the knowledge of God. . . . Illnesses are My servants which I attach to My chosen friends" (11). Thus, illness across Islamic traditions may also be viewed as a test of faith (*iman*) or punishment for sin (QHICQ 2010). Others also note that *nazr*, jealousy, ill intentions of others, and demonic possessions may contribute to physical illness (Abdussalam-Bali 2004). Evil *jinn* possession is theorized to contribute to multiple conditions including physical illness (e.g. chronic pain, epilepsy), psychological disorders, and relational problems (ibid). These beliefs illuminate the ways in which culture—including spiritual beliefs—can influence one's understanding of health and illness.

Traditional Healing

The confluence of religion and health may contribute to the high number of Muslims who seek assistance outside of allopathic medicine. It is estimated that 80–90 percent of people from the developing world utilize traditional healing for healthcare (WHO 2008). American Muslims engage traditional healing practices for a range of physical and mental ailments and typically include practices categorized as based upon Islamic religious texts Islamic worship practices, and folk healing practices (AlRawi et al. 2012). Similarly, Muslim immigrants may also seek traditional health practitioners when conditions are thought to have a spiritual etiology, when Western practitioners are perceived as lacking expertise with the particular condition, or if they have limited access to allopathic healthcare or health insurance (ibid). Within Islam, there is a lack of formal classification of traditional healers but available literature demonstrates that they may be male or female and may include:

> *al-fataha,* female fortune tellers; the *khatib* or *hajjab,* male healers providing amulets worn on the body for protection from negative energy; the *Dervish,* male or female healers using religious rituals and cultural traditions to treat mental illness; and *moalj belforan,* male healers using Islamic scripture for protection against negative energy and evil spirits (AlRawi et al. 2012, p.490).

From this range of types of healers, it becomes evident that there is diversity in the methodologies utilized by traditional healers as well. Given the high numbers of Muslims estimated to utilize traditional healing, a greater understanding of primary Islamic spiritual concepts thought to underlie or contribute to illness is pertinent.

Concepts of Islamic Spiritual Healing

According to Islamic understanding, the three essential elements of the human psyche, *ruh, nafs,* and *qalb,* reside within the human heart, an area commonly indicated to be the location of emotional pain (Inayat 2005, Sheikh and Gatrad 2000). Within the Muslim cultural system, both psychological and spiritual development is considered to take place in the *qalb.* Due to this shared location, problems of the psyche and soma are seen as interconnected. Distress is understood as the manifestation of an incongruent heart, which is lost or distant from Allah due to doubt or conflict (Sheikh and Gatrad 2000). Moreover, having a hard heart is understood to be a reflection of chronic ill feelings and ultimately a sign of Allah's displeasure. A person who suffers from a hard heart often describes symptoms of an aching heart, a trembling heart, or pressure in the heart. Thus psychological as well as most physical illnesses are understood as a reflection of illness of heart. In contrast, soundness of health is related to "well," true," "clear," or "guided" heart that is calm and in accordance with Islamic teachings (Husain 2006, Inayat 2005, Sheikh and Gatrad 2000).

As mental and physical distress in the practicing Muslim community is predominantly interpreted as the result of moral transgression or a consequence of Divine Will, primary intervention often involves spiritual healing. Islamic spiritual healing involves Islamic principles of the latent energy within the *ruh*, or soul, of an afflicted individual, as well as belief in the power contained in devotions, supplications, and meditations. For followers of Islam, spirituality is inseparable from awareness of Allah and daily living according to His will (Inayat 2005). Thus, spirituality and health—as an extension of one's spirituality—necessitates the principle of *tawhid*, or oneness, which Allah has revealed within the human soul. For followers of Islam, this means that Allah can treat *maradhun* (the sickness of the mind). Thus, faith is understood as the central factor in treatment (Husain 1998, Husain 2006, Inayat 2005, Sheikh and Gatrad 2000).

Spiritual approaches to healing within the context of Islam entail behavior modification regarding the relationship between the afflicted person and Allah, in which *iman* (faith) is central. According to Inayat (2005), *iman* is both a cognitive and an ethical construct. Because of this dual nature, *iman* pertains to both the belief in Allah's existence and the belief that service can remove *maradhun* (or sickness of the mind) from a person. Thus, healing involves purification of the body and soul through devotion. The essence of purification of the *ruh* (spirit or soul), *qalb* (essential heart), and *nafs* (ego or self) is to bring one's *nafs* under control (Inayat 2005).

Healing processes, then, commonly consist of *sawm* (fasting), *taubah* (repentance), and recitation of the Qur'an. For this reason, the majority of Islamic populations adhere to the Five Pillars that were previously discussed, in addition to obligatory practices related to diet, gender roles, dress, interpersonal relationships, and family values (Farooqi 2006). An essential aspect of devotion is that of prayer, defined as the process of communicating with the Divine or other spiritual forces, which can serve many functions, including healing (Eliade 1987, Javaheri 2006). Prayer healing in particular, "is classified as a spiritual category of alternative or complementary medicine" (Easthope 1998, 272 as cited in Javaheri 2006) and is a common practice in Muslim communities, such as Iran, yet is noted to have historical roots outside of Islam such as in ancient Zoroastrian tradition (AlRawi et al. 2012). Javaheri (2006) notes that prayer healing is prominent in Muslim theology across denominations and further describes how Qur'an scripture can be utilized for healing by both laypersons and faith healers alike. She quotes verse 82 of Chapter *Bani-Israel*: "We sent down the Qur'an which is a source of healing and mercy unto the believers, but it addeth not to the perdition" (172). This scripture demonstrates the enduring faith Muslims place not only in prayer but in the Qur'an as well.

In the Shiite tradition, it is common for followers to not only utilize scripture, but to flock to sacred places; health care providers may even bring patients to pray for healing by invoking the presence of holy leaders (Javaheri 2006). In the Sufi tradition, the healing of the sick is lauded as the most superior form of service to humanity and indeed, Allah. Accordingly, in Ajmer, India (home to Sufis), there is a free clinic that provides herbal-medicinal and spiritual assistance to an estimated sixty thousand people daily (Chishti 1991). Sufis, known for their mysticism and emphasis on faith healing, have healing methods that date back several hundred years (ibid). While scores of Muslims and non-Muslims alike seek the healing power of Allah through Sufi healers, it is noted that their methods are inexplicable by Western scientific inquiry.

As is evident, there is a clear relationship between Islamic philosophy and its healing practices. Inayat (2005) described the relationship between Islamic philosophy, *iman* (faith), and *din* (practice) as being understood within: *iman,* the belief in one God who is both "Creator" and "Cherisher" of the universe; *ihsan,* or right conduct and the process of perfecting character as set forth by the Qur'an; and *ibadat,* or religious duty as set forth by the *hadith* and *sunnah.* Essentially, Islamic spiritual healing recognizes that connection and intimacy with Allah enables a true understanding of the afflicted's situation; this understanding relieves distress, while promoting health and wellbeing.

Faith, service, and prayer underlie Islamic teachings of health. Yet, despite the global practice of prayer healing across religions—including Islam—prayer is not subject to empirical investigation; existing research on the impact of prayer healing is mixed (Javaheri 2006). While some speculate that its effects are placebo but may complement allopathic medicine, little is known about its effectiveness. As mentioned previously, Sufi healers are sought out because of their 'proven' effectiveness; the fact that such healing is not subject to traditional Western scientific inquiry only further contributes to its mysticism (Chisti 1991). A recent study of Muslim faith healing demonstrates that faith healers utilize a plurality of methods including blowing prayers onto patients, providing written prayers, utilizing hand movements, prescription of herbs and special diets (Javaheri 2006). Moreover, the author notes, "in comparison with mainstream medicine, prayer healing is associated with desirable, spiritual experiences for people" (179).

It is important to note that all faith healing in Islam is not deemed positive. Some spiritual healing categorized as magic, sorcery, or witchcraft is referred to as *sihr.* Sihr, whose etymology in Arabic, refers to witchcraft from the devil (Abdussalam-Bali 2004); caution is provided in seeking assistance from individuals who may utilize negative energy, such as female sorcerers.

In addition to traditional healers, there is little discussion of the role that imams and other Muslim leaders play in the health of this community. In a recent survey of community leaders, respondents identified four central roles for imams in healthcare: "(1) encouraging healthy behaviors through scripture-based messages in sermons; (2) performing religious rituals around life events and illnesses; (3) advocating for Muslim patients and delivering cultural sensitivity training in hospitals; and (4) assisting in healthcare decisions for Muslims" (Padela et al. 2011, 359). Clearly, there is a role for traditional healers, imams, and other Muslim leaders to promote health, facilitate healing, and possibly advocate for and facilitate more culturally informed healthcare for this population. Given the emphasis placed on the mind and soul, as well as healthy behaviors within Islam, it is pertinent to explore more specific Islamic understandings of psychology and how it relates to mental health.

Islamic Psychology

Islamic psychology is often defined by its contrast to Western philosophy, psychology, and psychotherapy. Critiques of Western models argue they are not equipped to fully explain or decrease mental health problems faced by Muslims (Alawi 1992). For example, the view of individuals as comprised mainly of urges and behaviors may present a highly reductionist and individualistic view in contrast to the general worldview of this population.

Differences in values-systems further illuminate how Western psychology may not serve as a good fit for Muslim populations. From an Islamic perspective, Western models tend to embody individualistic and competitive approaches, which emphasize self-interested and personal achievement goals (Jafari 1993). Additionally, it is viewed that Western psychotherapy focuses on worldly concerns and rationalizes guilt through positive regard and empathy (Jafari 1993). From this perspective, it is regarded that Western focus is also placed on freedom without limitations and boundaries (Jafari 1993) and these values are often reinforced in the therapeutic endeavors. Such a perspective may be viewed as in conflict with the teachings of Islam and guidelines of Muslim behaviors. In Islamic psychology, bounds and limits set by the Qur'an are utilized to help individuals determine how they can return to the straight path. For example, feelings of guilt may be viewed as indicators that one has offended Allah and may need to seek repentance, forgiveness, and realign one's thoughts and behaviors to be more consistent with Islam. This may be exemplified in the case of Samina below:

Case Example: Samina

Samina is a twenty-one year old Pakistani-American woman in her third year of college. Samina is the eldest of three sisters and her family is moderately religious. Samina currently lives with her parents in her home and commutes to college. Her mother is a pharmacist who immigrated to the United States in her mid-twenties and her father came to the United States two years after Samina was born. Samina considers herself well acculturated, while she considers her parents very traditional. Samina is currently single, though she experiences constant pressure from her parents to find an appropriate suitor and marry. Samina presents to a therapist at a college counseling center after attending a party and having a beer. She described feeling pressured to drink by her college friends. Samina disclosed to the therapist that she continues to experience great remorse after having engaged in drinking behavior. She shared, "I feel like I have greatly wronged Allah, my family, and myself." Samina also described feeling that she has strayed from her religious education and values, noting that after this incident, she has been afraid to pray and feels Allah is upset with her and will not want to listen to her prayers. Samina reported that she is also afraid to go to the mosque as other religious individuals may be able to sense her transgression. Samina has not been attending classes, indicating she has been experiencing headaches and an inability to get out of bed. She further reported that due to her failure to attend classes, her grades have been declining. Samina has not reported this incident to her parents, though they have indicated concern about her recent health status and behavior.

Discussion

Samina's experience illuminates internal conflict that may present when one's religious beliefs and traditions conflict with common practices in religiously dissimilar contexts. Clearly, this has been distressing for Samina. When practicing the principles of Islamic psychology, the counselor must take into account the larger socio-cultural context. In

Samina's case, the counselor should consider her family's Pakistani cultural roots and degree of religiosity and acculturation. As Samina feels more acculturated than her parents, she faces cultural dilemmas which cause conflict. Furthermore, Samina believes she has transgressed the bounds of religion, which is a motivating factor for mental health issues. In Islamic psychology, values are highly important in counseling (Jafari 1993); thus, it would be important for the counselor to examine Samina's values and how her actions may have transgressed her own boundaries. The counselor may seek to understand how Samina believes she has lost the pleasure of God and how she can return to a state of God-consciousness. The counselor may utilize methods such as *tawbah* (repentance) and exploring Samina's guilt while discussing her readiness to return to her methods of worship such as *salah* (prayer) (Jafari 1993). As it is common from her cultural and faith tradition to express mental health symptoms somatically (Inayat 2005), it would be essential to explore the mind-body connection and provide psychoeducation on how Samina's mental health symptoms may be impacting her physical state of being. Additional resources for Samina that may be therapeutic may include reading materials from Islamic scholars that speak to the diversity of experiences and beliefs within Islam. This may help her to critically reflect on her own faith as an adult and engage in the process of discernment, which may foster a deeper, more engaged, and informed faith system. Such materials may be helpful to integrate issues of faith and culture into the therapeutic encounter. In addition, it may be helpful to connect her with a Muslim student group (or other related cultural group where she is able to discuss issues with peers who may struggle with similar concerns) as well as an imam or another Muslim leader who can more directly speak to some of her religiously based questions.

Human Nature and Islamic Psychology

Islamic psychology posits that mental health issues result from three major sources, including imbalance between the needs of the *nafs* (physical self) and the *ruh* (spiritual self) (Khalili et al. 2002); experiencing religion as negative or restrictive (Murken and Shah 2002); and misusing freedom and choice. Tension related to any of these three sources leads to experiencing mental conflict (Alawi 1992). By contrast, mental health is defined by the inner heart directing intellect, while both of these aspects direct the *nafs ammara* (Skinner 2010). Diagnosis is evaluated by identifying from which level of the self the experience of discomfort is arising; thus, psychological treatment can be targeted at the physical, spiritual, or psychological level (Skinner 2010). An example of this holistic view of mental health is provided by Skinner (2010), who posits that anxiety can result from either physical (excess caffeine), psychological (suppressing drives), or spiritual (straying from the divine path) sources as well as by combination of these factors.

As stated earlier in this chapter, the self is referred to as *nafs*, also known as the ego and material part of the self. The *nafs* possesses three dimensions: *nafs ammara*, or the soul, which commands man to evil and is egotistic, *nafs lawwama*, the soul aware of one's own imperfections, and *nafs mutmainna*, the soul at peace (Husain 2006). These features of the self are theorized to be in conflict and must be balanced in order to achieve a well-adjusted sense of self. Non-material aspects of the self include the *qalb* (heart), *ruh* (soul), and *aql* (intellect). The *ruh* is responsible for meeting all spiritual and emotional needs; thus from a psychological perspective, it is the driving force of behavior. The *nafs*, which is again the "I," or personhood, can exist independently of the body and has egocentric tendencies (Husain 2006).

The goal in Islamic psychology then, is to overcome these egocentric tendencies and to align towards the path prescribed by Allah. The *nafs* is encompassed in the *ruh* and comprises the non-material self. The *qalb* is the main source of spiritual and moral disease, and is also associated with *aql*. *Qalb* can refer to the physical heart or the divine entity that possesses the qualities of knowledge and perception. These concepts are described in more detail in the preceding section and can also be seen in the case of Samina, given her struggles with some of the material challenges of college life. An Islamic psychological perspective may encourage Samina to consider her egocentric tendencies that may impede her alignment with Allah. Thus, the heart and soul are essential to psychological health and healing in Islam.

The Qur'an mentions diseases of the heart such as *nifaq* (hypocrisy) or *'Ama* (blindness), which is critical, as it is stated if the heart is blocked, the senses serve no purpose (Husain 2006). The *qalb* is the emotional center and is tied to the physical body. Both *aql* and *qalb* combine to form decisions regarding human behavior. Thus, behavior is motivated by the *nafs* and is moderated by the *qalb* and *aql*. In other words, in Islamic psychology, the heart and soul are primary and outweigh what is defined as the self in Western psychology. Clearly, this perspective is counter to traditional Western models of psychology and has implications for behavioral change and clinical interventions.

In the Islamic model of behavior, four mental states precede action (Safi 1998). The first of these is *Al-khatir* (impression), which refers to an image through thought. Secondly, *Al-mayl* refers to disposition, in which an impression becomes an urge. *Hukum* refers to judgment, at which stage an individual evaluates his or her own behavior according to his or her own values. Finally, *Al-ham,* volition, indicates behavior is only hindered by external conditions (Safi 1998). *Iradah* refers to the possibility of *tazkiyah* (sublimation), which indicates the transformation of personality or character. In Islamic psychotherapy, the goal is to reconcile with weakness to achieve transcendence rather than focusing on symptom reduction, which can be seen as motivational in nature (Safi 1998).

Guilt, shame, and anxiety serve as acknowledgement that one has committed sin (Murken and Shah 2002) and this is explored in therapy. In the Islamic perspective, *tawbah* (repentance) is utilized to correct or modify behavior (Jafari 1993). Repentance is promised to all individuals who seek it. In Islam, the entire body, including the organs, follows the path of Allah. Complete submission to Allah's will, thus, brings peace, and prevents conflicts in personality (Alawi 1992). In the Islamic view, man is regulated by a divine course but also possesses free will. Mental unrest occurs when the heart is incongruent and the soul is unstable (Inayat 2005). *Fitrah* refers to human nature and signifies intrinsic goodness (Khalili et. al. 2002). Values are highly important in shaping whether one adheres to or strays from *Fitrah* (Khalili et al 2002). Man must achieve balance between his worldly and spiritual needs (Khalili et al. 2002). Overpowering the *nafs al ammara* and stopping pathological behavior through the *nafs al-lawwamah* is critical to achieving overall health (Jafari 1993, Husain 2006). The target is *nafs al mutma'innah* or contentment. The well-balanced Islamic personality is appropriately integrated and receives all the pleasure of God (Jafari 1993, Inayat 2005).

Islamic Psychotherapy

An Islamic approach to psychotherapy emphasizes the cognitive, psychological, biological, and spiritual aspects of the individual (Khalili et al. 2002). The cognitive element refers to the individual being capable of learning about his or her own environment while the psychic refers to feelings and emotions such as desire or anger. The biological refers to the actualization of desires, while the spiritual refers to human knowledge and choice (Safi 1998). The individual achieves balance through thought and action while also caring for the collective welfare of the society (Jafari 1993). While individual concerns are taken into account, the collective responsibility, importance of brotherhood, and achieving social peace are of utmost importance (Jafari 1993). This is exemplified by the *hadith,* "Every one of you is a shepherd and each one of you is responsible for his flock" (al Bukhari, n.d. in Jafari 1993). In this view, psychological problems result from confusion about social and religious values, and thus are solved in accordance with social and religious guidelines (Khalili et al. 2002). The clinician reflects the client's values rather than imposing his or her own values (Khalili et al. 2002). Khalili and colleagues (2002) advise the clinician to maintain a stance which is empathic and active. Counseling through this perspective also values selflessness, altruism, perfecting oneself, and wishing the best for others (Jafari 1993). Islamic psychotherapy is directive, reflective, and critically supportive while focusing on the present problem; one's past is utilized as a learning tool (Khalili et al. 2002). For example, thoughts and actions which are not in accordance with Islamic tradition are analyzed. Moreover, society and interpersonal relationships are very important and also analyzed (Khalili et al. 2002). The client is urged to give up materialistic needs and understand his or her own weaknesses (Khalili et al. 2002). The goal for therapy is to attain holistic growth in both physical and spiritual domains (Jafari 1993).

The following case of Murad may help illuminate how symptoms may be associated with issues of spirit and religion. This case may provide insight into how health care professionals may more fully incorporate understanding of Islamic healing approaches, beliefs, and health-related behaviors into effective and ethical practice with Islamic populations living in the United States.

Case Example: Murad

Murad is a forty-five year old Palestinian male. Murad is married to his wife of eighteen years, Layla, and they have three children. Murad works as a cardiac surgeon and spends very long hours in the hospital. Murad's wife is a teacher and has been a homemaker for many years. Murad's eldest son, Zahir, is currently fifteen years-old and attends a public high school. Murad's daughter, Zehra, is ten years-old and attends public elementary school. The youngest daughter, Marwa, is eight years-old and attends a private Muslim school. Murad presents to an outpatient clinic with concerns that his children, particularly his eldest son Zahir, are straying from the path of Islam. Additionally, Murad described feelings of regret that he often misses his prayers while working long hours in surgery. He also regrets not being able to provide his children with the religious education his parents provided to him. Murad described feeling concerned for his family after his friends from the mosque informed him they believe Zahir has a girlfriend due to his postings on the social networking website, Facebook. Zahir also has many non-Muslim friends, of whom Murad does not approve. Murad informed the counselor that he is worried that it may be too late to steer Zahir in the path of Islam and that his younger children may follow the same direction. Murad also shared that he does not agree with Layla working outside of the home; he asserted that if one parent were home, the children would have a religious educator to guide them. Murad reported to the counselor that his wife is unaware that he is attending counseling and he is only doing so because the Imam (religious leader) at the mosque suggested this as a course of action.

Discussion

In the case of Murad, it is evident that Islam is central for him: he experiences distress from his impaired practice of Islam, including daily prayers. Thus, the health care professional may consider it important to examine the patient's feelings of guilt and regret. The health care provider must understand how Murad's feelings of regret and concern for his son may be stemming from his confusion about his own actions in addition to feelings of shame regarding his children's actions (Khalili et al. 2002). The provider should also consider how the family system is implicated in this case and understand how to intervene on a systemic level. The provider may assist Murad in processing his own guilt regarding straying from his own Islamic beliefs, and help him acknowledge how he can find balance between his physical worldly needs (his occupation) and his spiritual needs (prayer) (Khalili et al. 2002). Indeed, it may be imperative to explore what a re-alignment spiritually may mean for him and his family. It is important to bring awareness to Murad that this is a family issue and encourage him to involve his family in the process. Exploring Murad's values, as well as the family's values, is essential in guiding the family towards the course they believe is best for them. The health care professional must refrain from imposing his or her own values (Khalili et al. 2002); thus, before suggesting a course of action, it is essential to explore the value placed on religious beliefs by the entire family, while demonstrating respect for familial structure. It is important also for Murad to understand he can guide his children towards "the right path," but cannot control their actions. Understanding the role of freedom of choice and own volition is highly essential for Murad to better comprehend his children's actions.

While health care professionals in the United States may not typically provide spiritually-centered treatment, clearly issues of faith are central to Murad's sense of well-being. Accordingly, it may be particularly therapeutic to discuss with Murad ways in which he may want to work on his practice of Islam and his spiritual development in general. Murad may want or need guidance around questions of repentance, for example. Accordingly, it may be helpful to assess if he has a relationship with an imam, or other spiritual leader. Such an assessment may further illuminate the ways in which Murad conceptualizes his own health and healing, in addition to working through the family related concerns. This approach is more aligned with an Islamic conceptualization of health, which more readily connects the mind, body, and spirit and therefore may feel more culturally consistent for Murad.

Help-Seeking Patterns of Islamic American Communities

The diversity of America's Muslim population adds to the complexity of understanding Islamic health care service utilization in the United States. To provide appropriate and effective health services, health providers must recognize that this population represents varied complex histories influenced by an array of sociopolitical, socioeconomic, cultural, and religious factors. Islamic tradition promotes the idea that every disease has a cure. Due to this cultural belief, Muslims generally maintain positive health-related help-seeking attitudes (Ali, Abu-Ras, and Hamid 2009). However, the inflexibility of Western treatment paradigms appears to hinder service utilization. The fact that Islam plays a major role in the Muslim understanding, experience, and expression of distress is well documented (Ansari 1992, Badri 2000, Hussain 1999). Islamic populations generally consider supportive treatment as involving religious and spiritual interventions as well as efforts to facilitate a sense of community (Ali, Abu-Ras, and Hamid 2009). Kelly and colleagues (1996) found that Muslims in the United States tend to view professional health interventions with skepticism, as applicability of Western treatments are regarded to be limited to problems in Western culture. In fact, their research indicated that among Muslim individuals who do access helping professionals within the United States, preference is often given to those with an understanding of Islam. Additional research has indicated that the use of traditional healers and resources, lack of knowledge and familiarity with local Western services, and perceived social stigma may deter use of professional health services by Muslim-Americans. Socio-political concerns, including immigration status and fear of discrimination, detention, or deportation further impede access to and utilization of health care services for many in this population (Ali, Abu-Ras, and Hamid 2009, Aloud 2004).

Health Care Utilization and Experiences

While spiritual origins of illness are part of some Muslims understanding of health, Islam also places a high value on the use of allopathic medicine. The early history of medicine in Islam is noted to have contributed to the global Islam community as well as Western science and medicine (Ahmed 2000). Despite the fact that of the 800,000 physicians in the United States, more than 60,000 are Muslim (Hanley 2009), there is limited empirical research on culturally specified healthcare delivery for Muslims (Padela et al. 2011). Available research on Muslims and healthcare delivery models indicates latent cultural biases and mixed findings. An ethnographic content analysis of Medline abstracts from 1966 to 2005 revealed the following themes: 1) that being an observant Muslim poses health risks; 2) Muslims are negatively affected by tradition, and should adopt modernity; 3) that "Islam" is a problem for biomedical healthcare delivery; and 4) a contrasting theme that being Muslim may promote positive health outcomes (Laird, de Marrais, and Barnes 2009). These biases in the research likely parallel experiences with healthcare delivery and patient experiences.

The diversity within the Muslim population may also contribute to healthcare experiences. In a study of African American, South Asian, and Arab Muslims in the Detroit area, participants reported being discriminated against within the healthcare system (Padela et al. 2011). Interestingly, in a study of Muslim physicians in Saudi Arabia, the overwhelming majority (91 percent) stated that religion had a positive influence on health, yet 62.2 percent reported that religion could hinder patient treatment compliance (Al-Yousefi 2012). Over half of respondents did not ask about patients' religious backgrounds despite their own religious identification; such findings underscore the lack of medical attention in this area.

Treating Muslim Patients in the United States

Given the ongoing exponential growth in Islamic populations living in the United States, it is quite likely that health care professionals will encounter Muslim patients in their practice. As seen from this chapter, Islamic perspectives offer methodologies towards resolving physical, spiritual, and mental health-related problems. Thus, increased familiarity with and understanding of the Islamic worldview, including healing or health-related beliefs and practices, enables health care providers to become more sensitive to the diversity of needs which exist within the American Muslim community (Altareb 1996, Kelly et al. 1996).

By now, it should be understood that Islam is a religion, philosophy, moral or ethical code, culture, and a sociopolitical system; thus, assessment should explore the Muslim patient's religiosity, cultural heritage, and meaning-making beliefs concerning Islam. Whether Islam is an integral aspect of a Muslim patient's presenting concern depends on both the individual and the issue. In assessing culture, it is important to note that indigenous American Muslims are likely to have been impacted by different social, economic, and political conditions than immigrant Muslims (Altareb 1996). Additionally, dialogue related to gender roles and relationships, forbidden practices, and the role of the family are likely essential to understanding an individual from an Islamic context. Providing a framework for therapy can be helpful for Muslim clients to orient them to the process (Hasnain et al. 2008). It may be important to integrate religious, spiritual, and cultural values into solutions to the patient's presenting concern. Accordingly, the provider may ask the patient for information about his presenting concern from an Islamic perspective or consult with imams when forming a treatment plan.

Health care providers should also be aware of their own perceptions, stereotypes, and beliefs about Islam and Muslims as preconceived notions may lead health care professionals to assume they understand a cultural or spiritual belief when they do not. Additionally, given the current post 9–11 political climate, some Muslim clients may assume that health care professionals assume pathologizing stances towards deeply meaningful religious and cultural beliefs; thus, the patient may be reticent to articulate his worldview unless genuine openness, respect, and acceptance are conveyed (Garzon 2005). Further, health care providers may find it helpful to assure patients who strongly identify as Muslim that they will attempt to understand the patient's perspective and not change it (Kelly et al. 1996). Health care providers should be aware that Muslim patients may object to treatment plans which prevent them from observing their religious duties, such as prayer or adherence to medications that may be inconsistent with dietary restrictions. Understanding the patient's apprehensions may help health care professionals develop alternative treatment plans while conveying respect for the patient's traditions.

Conclusion

Within Islamic models of health, the mind, body, self, and soul or spirit are considered interconnected, and wellness is achieved when these components are harmoniously in balance. Further, the centrality of Allah and additional cultural and religious knowledge are formative to Islamic understandings and experiences of health and wellness. Illness is believed to occur when one is distant from Allah or the Islamic community or when the four dynamic parts of the person are imbalanced (Al-Zeera 2001, Ashy 1999, Rajaram and Rashidi 2003). Resulting Islamic health seeking patterns and healing conventions may therefore not align with prototypical systems and approaches maintained by all Western health care providers.

It is also notable that in a post 9–11 milieu, increased American xenophobia towards Islamic populations interferes with health care providers' ability to learn about and better understand how Islamic teachings and traditions may impact health and wellness for American Muslims. Such shortcomings are becoming increasingly deleterious given the continuing increase of immigrants from Muslim countries. The diversity within Islamic populations cannot be over-stressed, and health care providers should remain cognizant that Muslims living in the United States differ among variables of ethnicity, language, cultural and religious practices and beliefs, and degree of identification with Islam. Given that Muslim immigrants who have come to the United States seeking refuge since 2011's Arab Spring may lack health insurance, have limited economic resources, and face additional barriers to accessing health services, there is a distinct and growing need for health care providers to develop increasing competence in culturally centered models of health care delivery, including mental health. Such models would suitably support the clear connection between spiritual, physical, and mental health which is central for many Muslims. Additionally, health literacy is a primary component of health care utilization and treatment compliance, yet little is known about the health literacy of the Muslim population. Haq and colleagues (2011) advocate for demarketing strategies for the self-management of common illnesses (e.g. hypertension) and to increase health literacy and the promotion of overall healthy lifestyles.

As seen throughout this chapter, cultural competency in health care professionals is a first necessary step towards providing optimal services and outcomes for American Muslim populations. It is clear that treatment efficacy depends not only on the ability of a health care professional to properly identify and treat a given condition, but also on the patient's access to, belief in, and collaborative participation in the treatment process. Overall, empathic understanding of the Muslim patient's worldview can enhance the provider-patient alliance, increase the validity of assessment, and allow for valuable religious and cultural coping resources to be used effectively in treatment. As health care providers, we should strive to learn from patients who pursue transforming healing encounters (Garzon 2005).

References

Abdussalam-Bali. W. 2004. *Sword against Black Magic and Evil Magicians.* India: Al-Firdous Books.

Achoui, M. "Human Nature from a Comparative Psychological Perspective." *The American Journal of Islamic Social Sciences* 15(4): 71–95.

Ahmed, A. A. 2000. "Health and Disease: An Islamic Framework." In *Caring for Muslim Patients, 2nd* Ed., edited by A. Sheikh and A. R. Gatrad, 35–43. Radcliffe Publishing: New York, NY.

Alawi, A. H. 1992. "The Quranic Concept of Mental Health." In *Quranic Concepts of Human Psyche,* edited by Z. Ansari, 87–97. Lahore, Pakistan: Islamic Research Institute.

Ali, A.Y. 1975. *The Holy Quran: Text, Translation and Commentary.* Leicester, UK: Islamic Foundation.

Ali, O.M., W. Abu-Ras, and H. Hamid. 2009. "Cultural Profile of Muslim Americans." NKI Center of Excellence in Culturally Competent Mental Health. http://ssrdqst .rfmh.org/cecc/

Ali, O.M., G. Milstein, and P. M. Marzuk. 2005. "The Imam's Role in Meeting the Counseling Needs of Muslim Communities in the United States." *Psychiatry Services* 56(2): 202–205.

Aloud, N. 2004. "Factors Affecting Attitudes toward Seeking and Using Formal Mental Health and Psychological Services among Arab-Muslim Populations." Retrieved from Proquest Digital Dissertations.

Alrawi, S., M. D. Fetters, A. Killawi, A. Hammad, and A. Padela. 2012. "Traditional Healing Practices among American Muslims: Perceptions of Community Leaders in Southeast Michigan." *Journal of Immigrant and Minority Health* 14: 489–496.

Altareb, B.Y. 1996. "Islamic Spirituality in America: A Middle Path to Unity." *Counseling and Values* 41(1): 29–37.

Al-Yousefi, N.A. 2012. "Observations of Muslim Physicians Regarding the Influence of Religion on Health and Their Clinical Approach." *Journal of Religion and Health* 51: 269–280.

Al-Zeera, Z. 2001. *Wholeness and Holiness in Education: An Islamic Perspective.* Herndon, VA: International Institute of Islamic Thought.

Ansari, Z. 1992. *Quranic Concepts of Human Psyche.* Lahore, Pakistan: Islamic Research Institute.

Anwar, M. 2008. "Muslims in the West: Demographic and Socio-Economic Position." In: *Caring for Muslim Patients,* edited by A. Sheikh, and A. R. Gatrad. New York: Radcliffe Publishing.

Armstrong, K. 2006. *Muhammad: A Prophet for Our Time.* New York: Harper Collins.

Ashy, M. A. 1999. "Health and Illness from an Islamic Perspective." *Journal of Religion and Health* 38: 241–257.

Badri, M. 2000. *Contemplation: An Islamic Psychospiritual Study.* Kuala Lumpur, Malaysia: Medina Books.

Black, A. 2009. "Fatwas and Surgery: How and Why a Fatwa May Inform a Muslim Patient's Surgical Options." *ANZ Journal of Surgery* 79(12): 866–871.

Camarota, S. A. 2002. "Immigrants in the United States—2002: A Snapshot of America's Foreign-Born Population." Center for Immigration Studies. http://www.cis.org/articles/2002/back1302.pdf

Chishti, S. H. M. 1991. *The Book of Sufi Healing.* Rochester, Vermont. Inner Traditions International.

Coker, N. 2001. *Racism in Medicine: An Agenda for Change.* King's Fund: London.

De Jong, J. T., and R. Reis. 2010. "Kiyang-Yang, a West-African Postwar Idiom of Distress." *Culture, Medicine, and Psychiatry* 34(2): 301–21.

Eliade, M. 1987. *The Encyclopedia of Religion,* Vol. 11, New York: Library of Congress Cataloging in Publication Data.

Farooqi, Y. N. 2006. "Traditional Healing Practices Sought by Muslim Psychiatric Patients in Lahore, Pakistan." *International Journal of Disability, Development, and Education* 53: 401–415.

Faruqi, I. R. 1995. *Islamization of Knowledge: General Principles and Work Plan.* Herndon, VA: International Institute of Islamic Thought.

Garzon, F. L. 2005. "Inner Healing Prayer in 'Spirit-Filled' Christianity." In *Integrating Traditional Healing Practices into Counseling and Psychotherapy,* edited by R. Moodley and W. West, 159–169. London, UK: Sage Publications.

Greenwood, N., F. Hussain, T. Burns, and F. Raphael. 2000. "Asian In-Patient and Career Views of Mental Health Care. Asian Views of Mental Health Care." *Journal of Mental Health* 9(4): 397–408.

Hanley, D. C. 2009. "Muslim American Leaders, Physicians Join Effort to Reform Health Care." *Washington Report on Middle East Affairs* 28(8): 44–45.

Haque, A. 1998. "Psychology and Religion: Their Relationship and Integration from an Islamic Perspective." *The American Journal of Islamic Social Sciences* 15(4): 97–116.

Haq, F., A. Medhekar, and T. Fardous. 2011. "Health Literacy for Muslim Consumers: A Strategic Demarketing Approach." *Journal of Global Intelligence and Policy* 4(4): 54–66.

Haque, A. and K. A. Masuan. 2002. "Religious Psychology in Malaysia." *The International Journal for the Psychology of Religion* 12(4): 277–289.

Hasnain, R., L. C. Shaikh, and H. Shanawani. 2008. "Disability and the Muslim Perspective: An Introduction for Rehabilitation and Health Care Providers." *Center for International Rehabilitation Research Information and Exchange CIRRIE* Database. http://cirrie.buffalo.edu/culture/monographs/muslim/#s1b

Husain, A. 2006. *Islamic Psychology: Emergence of a New Field.* Daryaganj, New Delhi: Global Vision Publishing House.

Husain, S. A. 1998. "Religion and Mental Health from the Muslim Perspective." In *Handbook of Religion and Mental Health.* H.G. Koenig New York: Academic Press.

Hussain, J. 1999. *Islamic Law and Society.* Leichardt: Federation Press.

Inayat, Q. 2005. "Islam, Divinity, and Spiritual Healing." In *Integrating Traditional Healing Practices into Counseling and Psychotherapy,* edited by R. Moodley and W. West, 159–169. London, UK: Sage Publications.

Inhorn, M., and G. Serour, G. 2011. "Islam, Medicine, and Arab-Muslim Refugee Health in America after 9/11." *The Lancet* 378: 935–943.

Jafari, M. F. 1993. "Counseling Values and Objectives: A Comparison of Western and Islamic Perspectives." *The American Journal of Islamic Social Sciences* 10(3): 326–339.

Javaheri, F. 2006. "Prayer Healing: An Experiential Description of Iranian Prayer Healing." *Journal of Religion and Health* 45(2): 171–181.

Kelly, E. W., A. Aridi, and L. Bakhtiar. 1996. "Muslims in the United States: An Exploratory Study of Universal and Mental Health Values." *Counseling and Values* 40(3): 206–218.

Khalili, S., S. Murken, K. H. Reich, A. A. Shah, and A. Vahabzadeh. 2002. "Religion and Mental Health in Cultural Perspective: Observations and Reflections after the First International Congress on Religion and Mental Health, Tehran, 16–19 April 2001." *The International Journal for the Psychology of Religion* 12(4): 217–237.

Koenig, H. G. 1999. Religion and Medicine. *Lancet* 353: 1803.

Koenig, H. G., M. E. McCollough, and D. B. Larson. 2001. *Handbook of Religion and Health.* OUP: Oxford.

Laird, L. D., J. de Marrais, and L. L. Barnes. 2007. *Social Science and Medicine* 65(12): 2425–2439.

Mahmood, S. 2001. "Feminist Theory, Embodiment, and the Docile Agent: Some Reflections on the Egyptian Islamic Revival." *Cultural Anthropology* 162: 202–236.

Murken, S. and A. A. Shah. 2002. "Naturalistic and Islamic Approaches to Psychology, Psychotherapy, and Religion: Metaphysical Assumptions and Methodology—A discussion." *The International Journal for the Psychology of Religion* 12(4): 239–254.

Nichter. 1981. "Idioms of Distress: Alternatives in the Expression of Psychological Distress." *Culture, Medicine, and Psychiatry* 5: 379–408.

Nimer, M. 2002. *The North American Muslim Resource Guide: Muslim Community Life in the United States and Canada.* New York: Routledge.

Padela, A., A. Killawi, M. Heisler, S. Demonner, and M. D. Fetters. 2011. "The Role of Imams in American Muslim Health: Perspectives of Muslim Community Leaders in Southeast Michigan." *Journal of Religion and Health* 50(2): 359–73.

Parkin, D. 1999. "Suffer Many Healers." In *Religion, Health, and Suffering,* edited by J. R. Hinnells and R. Porter Kegan. Paul: London.

Pew Research Center. 2007. "Muslim Americans: Middle Class and Mostly Mainstream." http://pewresearch.org/assets/pdf/muslim-americans.pdf

Post, J. M. and G. Sheffer. 2007. "The Risk of Radicalization and Terrorism in U.S. Muslim Communities." *The Brown Journal of World Affairs* 13(2): 101–112.

Proudfoot, W. 1985. *Religious Experience.* Berkeley, CA: University of California Press.

Quan, H., A. Fong, C. De Coster, J. Wang, R. Musto, T. Noseworthy, and W. Ghali. 2006. "Variation in Health Services Utilization among Ethnic Populations." *Canadian Medical Association Journal* 174(6): 787–791.

Queensland Health and Islamic Council of Queensland QHICQ. 2010. *Health Care Providers' Handbook on Muslim Patients.* 2nd ed. Division of the Chief Health Officer, Queensland Health, Brisbane.

Rahman, F. 1989. *Major Themes of the Qur'an.* Kuala Lumpur, Malaysia: Islamic Book Trust.

Rajaram, S. S. and A. Rashidi. 2003. "African American Muslim Women and Health Care." *Women and Health* 37(3): 81–95.

Richards, P. and A. Bergin. 1997. *A Spiritual Strategy for Counseling and Psychotherapy.* Washington D.C.: American Psychological Association.

Safi, L. M. 1998. "Islamicization of Psychology: From Adaption to Sublimation." *The American Journal of Islamic Social Sciences* 15(4): 117–125.

Sheikh, A. and A. R. Gatrad. 2000. *Caring for Muslim Patients.* London: Radcliffe Medical Press.

Sheikh, A. and A. R. Gatrad, 2008. "Conclusions: Breaking Barriers, Building Bridges." In *Caring for Muslim Patients*, edited by A. Sheikh and A. R. Gatrad. New York: Radcliffe Publishing.

Skinner, R. 2010. "An Islamic Approach to Psychology and Mental Health." *Mental Health, Religion, and Culture* 113(6): 547–551. doi: 10.1080/13674676 .2010.488441.

Sloan, R. P., P. Bagiella, and T. Powell. 1999. "Religion, Spirituality, and Medicine." *Lancet* 353: 664–667.

Watkins, M. and H. Shulman. 2008. *Towards Psychologies of Liberation.* New York: Palgrave Macmillan.

Winter, T. J. 2008. "The Muslim Grand Narrative." In *Caring for Muslim Patients*, edited by A. Sheikh and A.R. Gatrad. New York: Radcliffe Publishing.

World Health Organization. 2008. Traditional Medicine Fact Sheet. http://www .who.int/mediacentre/factsheets/fs134/en/

CHAPTER EIGHT

The Health and Wellness of Sexual and Gender Minorities

David W. Pantalone, John E. Pachankis, Brian A. Rood, and Sarah M. Bankoff

Sexual and gender minority individuals have appeared throughout history and across cultures. In the United States, having a minority sexual orientation was labeled as a mental disorder in the American Psychiatric Association's *Diagnostic and Statistical Manual of Mental (DSM) Disorders* until it was removed by a consensus vote of the APA's leadership in a landmark 1973 meeting. Having a transgender gender identity continues to be codified in the current DSM under the diagnostic label of gender dysphoria (GD) (APA 2013). Many scholars argue that, eventually, GD will be removed from the DSM in the same way that homosexuality was removed earlier: because of activism, and within a context of changing social norms.

Until then, however, individuals who possess an identity, either related to their sexuality or gender, that is "different" from that of the mainstream heterosexual majority will often face discrimination—and, based on empirical research, it has been suggested that stress associated with discrimination and stigma is often associated with negative health. Thus, in this chapter, we aim to review

1. the role of stigma and discrimination in the health of sexual and gender minority individuals
2. the extant literature on the mental and physical health disparities facing these populations; and

3. information regarding the treatment of sexual and gender minority individuals that could potentially be helpful for counselors or other healthcare workers interacting with members of these populations.

To understand how gender and sexuality fit together, it is essential first to understand how sex and gender are related. In its use as an adjective, *sex* refers to the biological aspects of being a man or woman (e.g., chromosomes, genitalia). *Sex* is commonly understood as a binary—colloquially we talk about men and women being "the opposite sex"—and it is a common practice, for example, to ask new parents whether their baby is "a boy or a girl" when those are not the only options. Indeed, there are people who do not fit into the rigid categories of male or female, termed *intersex*. These are individuals who, either because of chromosomal, morphologic, genital, or gonadal atypicalities, exemplify the notion that even biological sex is multi-dimensional.

Gender is the enacted correlate of sex; a socially constructed notion of masculinity and femininity that describes the overt behaviors and behavioral tendencies of all people. Gender identity, also, is typically understood to exist on a binary but is, in practice, more fluid. When we speak of gender, we are often really speaking about gendered behaviors or gender performance—that is, the behaviors that we consider feminine are those more typical of biological females, and the behaviors that we consider masculine are those more typical of biological males. However, gender, like sex, is deceptively complex. Many men, for example, frequently engage in typical masculine behaviors (e.g., fixing cars or completing home renovations) and also frequently engage in typical feminine behaviors (e.g., crying when upset). Having a male gender identity, then, does not or should not preclude a man from engaging in behaviors that are typically associated with the female sex or with a female gender identity.

Although the intricacies of sex and gender are unfamiliar to many, acknowledging differences in sexual orientation is more commonplace. Because of heterosexual individuals' numeric majority, non-heterosexual individuals are sometimes termed *sexual minority individuals* or said to have a minority sexual orientation. Sexual minority individuals include any people who do not identify as exclusively heterosexual. Typically this term is used as a superordinate category that includes gay men, lesbian women, bisexual individuals of any sex, and people who wish to express their sexual orientation as *queer*. The term queer, formerly understood to be derogatory and oppressive, was reclaimed by some sexual minority individuals in the 1980s and 1990s, especially the youth of those and more contemporary eras, as an umbrella term and synonym for sexual minority.

Sexual orientation is the most widely accepted term for referring to the way in which an individual defines his or her sexual identity. Examples of sexual orientation are "opposite sex" or "heterosexual," and "same sex" or "lesbian," "gay," or "bisexual." Sexual orientation is typically viewed more favorably than terms such as "homosexual," or referring to one's "sexual preference" or "lifestyle," which are seen as pathologizing, invalidating, or trivializing an individual's sexual identity. It is also important to note that sexual identity and sexual behavior are not synonymous. Behavior is what people *do*, whereas identity is how people view themselves and how they represent themselves to the world. For example, a woman may engage in same-sex sexual behaviors but not identify as lesbian, or may self-identify as lesbian without engaging in same-sex sexual behaviors. Researchers and clinicians who inevitably work with sexual and gender minority individuals would do well to understand these nuances. For further reading, we suggest *The Fenway Guide to Lesbian, Gay, Bisexual, and Transgender Health* (Makadon et al. 2008) or *The Health of Sexual Minorities: Public Health Perspectives on Lesbian, Gay, Bisexual and Transgender Populations* (Meyer and Northridge 2007). A recent journal article (Mayer et al. 2012) summarizes some of the relevant content, as well.

The Role of Stigma in the Health of Sexual and Gender Minority Individuals

There are many, varied factors, both proximal and distal, that impact the health of all people—the case is not different for sexual and gender minority individuals. However, for any group that is a numeric minority, and especially when holding that identity violates some or all societal mores, there is the potential for stigma and associated discrimination to impact the lived experience of group members. Individuals can be stigmatized by anyone in society, including people close to them as well as strangers, and including members of helping professions like medical or mental health providers (Eliason and Schope 2001, Neville and Henrickson 2006). Increasingly strong empirical evidence suggests that stigma plays a key role in threatening the mental and physical health of sexual and gender minority individuals. Sexual orientation related stigma exerts possible health-depleting effects on sexual minority individuals across structural, interpersonal, and internalized sources. Numerous studies have shown that self-reports of perceived and objective sexual orientation stigma are associated with negative mental health, including mood, anxiety, and substance use disorders (McLaughlin, Hatzenbuehler, and Keyes 2010). This association between discrimination and health among gay and bisexual men also extends to physical health markers, including physician visits, nonprescription medication use, and HIV risk behavior (Huebner and Davis 2007, Lelutiu-Weinberger et al. 2012, Mays and Cochran 2001). Similarly, stigma and discrimination specific to transgender individuals have also been shown to be associated with HIV risk behaviors and decreased utilization of healthcare services (Clements et al. 1999, Clements-Nolle et al. 2001, Sugano, Nemoto, and Operario 2006).

Recent studies have operationalized sexual orientation stigma at a societal level as

1. state laws and policies affecting sexual minority individuals (e.g., same-sex marriage prohibition, the relative absence of anti-bullying school policies recognizing sexual minority individuals) (Hatzenbuehler et al. 2010);
2. the proportion of adherents to religions that are hostile to sexual minority individuals in a given locale (Hatzenbuehler, Pachankis, and Wolff 2012);
3. the number of supportive resources available to sexual minority youth in a county (e.g., school-based gay-straight alliances) (Hatzenbuehler 2011); and
4. the presence of LGBT-supportive resources on college campuses (Eisenberg 2002, Eisenberg and Wechsler 2003).

These objective indicators of stigma have been shown to be associated with indicators of poor mental health, such as the presence of mental disorders, substance use, suicidality, and, among gay and bisexual men, lack of condom usage (Eisenberg 2002, Eisenberg, and Wechsler 2003, Hatzenbuehler et al. 2010, Hatzenbuehler 2011, Hatzenbuehler et al. 2012). There appear to be even fewer supportive laws and policies specific to transgender individuals. For example, the recent repeal of the "Don't Ask Don't Tell" policy in the military does not apply to transgender persons, who continue to be banned from military service (Kerrigan 2012). Even the recent emergence of school policies designed to better protect LGB individuals often do not provide protections based on gender identity or expression (McGuire et al. 2010).

In the ensuing sections, we will present a review of the published literature to date examining sexual orientation related health disparities for sexual minority men, sexual minority women, and transgender individuals. We use those categories not because we believe they are especially meaningful (as the former two reify the gender binary of "women and men") but simply because our task is to chronicle and critique from an existing literature—and those are the groupings typically employed. Further, there is a varied literature about health disparities and, for the sake of brevity, we report for each group only on the health disparities that appear most consistently in the literature. For other work that reports more broadly on sexual orientation health disparities, we encourage readers to consult a recent consensus report published by the Institute of Medicine

(Institute of Medicine [IOM], Committee on Lesbian, Gay, Bisexual, and Transgender Health Issues and Research Gaps and Opportunities 2011).

Sexual Minority Men's Health Disparities

Significant sexual orientation disparities in men's health exist for mental health, substance use problems, and HIV infection. Although most sexual minority men do not contend with poor health, across epidemiological samples and across age cohorts, gay and bisexual men are twice as likely to report lifetime experiences with major depression and anxiety disorders than heterosexual men (Meyer 2003). Further, several well-designed studies demonstrate alcohol use disparities for men (Drabble, Midanik, and Trocki 2005, McCabe et al. 2009) and, across studies, sexual orientation disparities clearly exist for men's tobacco, marijuana, and illicit drug use (McCabe et al. 2005, McCabe et al., 2009, Trocki, Drabble, and Midanik 2009). Further, HIV infection represents the most significant physical health disparity faced by sexual minority men in terms of the number of HIV-infected men, the chronic course of the disease, and its associated mortality (Centers for Disease Control and Prevention [CDC] 2008, 2010).

In addition to disparities in mental health, substance abuse, and HIV infection, gay and bisexual men also report significant exposure to various forms of social stigma and discrimination—which serve as important risk factors for mental and physical health problems (Hatzenbuehler, Nolen-Hoeksema, and Erickson 2008, Rosario et al. 2006, Rotheram-Borus et al. 1995). These risk factors combine with disparities in mental health, substance use, and HIV infection to produce a synergistic conglomeration of health risks, known as a "syndemic" (Stall et al. 2003). A syndemic occurs when a marginalized population faces multiple, co-occurring psychosocial threats to health and wellbeing that interact synergistically to increase the risk of disease in this population (e.g., Singer and Clair 2003).

Sexual Minority Men—Mental Health

Gay and bisexual men are significantly more likely than heterosexual men to report depression and anxiety symptoms and diagnoses. Aggregating across studies containing both sexual minority and heterosexual participants, Meyer (2003) found that lifetime rates of any mood or anxiety disorder diagnosis were more than twice as high among gay and bisexual, compared to heterosexual, men. For example, Cochran, Mays, and Sullivan (2003) found prevalence estimates of Major Depression to be at 31 percent for gay and bisexual men, in comparison to 10 percent for heterosexual men. In another study, Sandfort and colleagues (2001) found prevalence estimates of Social Anxiety Disorder to be at 14.6 percent for sexual minority men, again in comparison to only 5.5 percent for heterosexual men. Therefore, it appears crucial that health providers remain mindful of possible mental health disparities present among sexual minority men in comparison to heterosexual men.

The impact of stigma likely underlies the noted health disparities specific to gay and bisexual men. For example, sexual orientation stigma may increase vulnerability to depression and anxiety through the efforts required to cope with them (Meyer 2003). Efforts to avoid being the target of stigma may include concealing or downplaying one's sexual orientation on a daily basis. Although concealment may represent a functional adaptation to a hostile social climate (Pachankis and Goldfried 2006), it is also associated with symptoms of depression and anxiety among gay and bisexual men (Beals, Peplau, and Gable 2009, Frost, Parsons, and Nanin 2007, Pachankis and Bernstein 2012). Similarly, early experiences of being rejected because of one's sexual orientation by important others, such as one's parents, may instill chronic anxious expectations of interpersonal rejection (Pachankis, Goldfried, and Ramrattan 2008), which has been shown to be associated with symptoms of depression and social anxiety disorder among gay and bisexual men (Feinstein, Goldfried, and Davila 2012).

Further, sexual orientation stigma is also associated with elevations in depression and anxiety through psychological processes such as social isolation, hopelessness, maladaptive self-schemas, and rumination (Hatzenbuehler 2009). One prospective study showed that sexual minority individuals who experienced a stigmatizing event reported increased rumination and social isolation immediately following the event, and these elevations fully accounted for the relation between experiencing the event and symptoms of depression and anxiety (Hatzenbuehler et al. 2009). Low self-esteem (Hershberger and D'Augelli 1995) and hopelessness (Safren and Heimberg 1999) have similarly been shown to mediate the association between sexual orientation stigma and depression and anxiety.

Although many sexual minority men do not have substance use problems, some national studies have shown gay and bisexual men to be at increased odds of substance use problems compared to heterosexual men (e.g., Cochran et al. 2004, McCabe et al. 2005). These disparities seem to be strongest for marijuana and illicit drugs (e.g., sedatives, stimulants, inhalants) (McCabe et al. 2009), although recent evidence shows a decrease in sexual minority men's use of many substances over the past several years (Pantalone et al. 2010). In this study, which examines a series of cross-sectional data points from 2002–2007, 14.6 percent to 23.5 percent of the men sampled reported any club drug use in the 90 days prior to assessment, and 4.6 percent to 12.1 percent reported polydrug use—with HIV-positive men consistently more likely to report use across years (Pantalone et al. 2010). Studies also indicate that sexual minority men, compared to their heterosexual peers, are at increased risk of alcohol dependence (McCabe et al. 2009) are less likely to abstain from alcohol (Drabble et al. 2005), and are more likely to endorse being smokers *(Greenwood et al. 2007)*. Young gay and bisexual men who report more investing effort to appear masculine are especially likely to be smokers (Pachankis, Westmaas, and Dougherty 2011).

Explanations for disparities in men's substance use, similar to anxiety and depression, have focused on stressors such as stigma related to sexual orientation. Having experienced sexual orientation-related discrimination in the past year is associated with nearly twice the odds of having a substance use disorder that year (McCabe et al. 2010). Internalized homophobia also consistently demonstrates positive associations with substance use problems across studies (Brubaker, Garrett, and Dew 2009). However, whereas concealing one's sexual orientation is associated with depression and anxiety as reviewed above, the stress of being open about one's sexual orientation has been shown to increase risk of using at least some illicit substances (e.g., *Ecstasy*) (Kipke et al. 2007, Klitzman et al. 2002). Although sexual orientation disclosure ostensibly makes one a more visible target of stigma (Green and Feinstein 2012), greater openness with one's orientation could also be associated with greater exposure to more permissive substance use norms embedded in the gay community (Hatzenbuehler, Corbin, and Fromme 2008). In fact, greater affiliation with the gay community has consistently been associated with elevated rates of substance use (e.g., Halkitis and Parsons 2002, Kipke et al. 2007).

Sexual Minority Men—Physical Health

Gay, bisexual, and other men who have sex with men (MSM) represent the population most severely affected by HIV in the United States and one of the only risk groups for which new HIV infections continue to rise (CDC 2008, 2010, Jaffe, Valdiserri, and DeCock 2007). MSM account for 53 percent of all new HIV infections, and one in five MSM in major U.S. cities is infected with HIV. MSM are 44 to 86 times more likely to be diagnosed with HIV compared to heterosexual men (CDC 2010). Because unprotected anal intercourse represents a primary route of HIV transmission, sexual minority men have been disproportionately impacted by this chronic disease, since the beginning of the HIV epidemic in 1981.

Advances in biomedical approaches have significantly improved treatment of HIV, especially since the advent of highly active antiretroviral medications in the mid-1990s (called antiretroviral therapies or ARVs) began significantly increasing the lifespan and quality of life of people living with HIV. More recently, ARVs have been shown to be effective in preventing the spread of HIV when taken regularly (Golub, Operario, and Gorbach 2010) or when taken after a high-risk exposure (CDC 2005). These advances ultimately rely on individuals' behavioral patterns, especially medication adherence, a behavior closely associated with psychosocial factors among sexual minority men, including depression and anxiety (Pantalone, Hessler, and Simoni 2010), HIV stigma (Mahajan et al. 2008), and substance use (Hendershot et al. 2009).

Among gay and bisexual men, anxiety and depression, often in combination with substance abuse, have been shown to be significantly associated with unprotected sex and increased health risk behaviors (Hart and Heimberg 2005, Hutton et al. 2004, Kashdan, Collins, and Elhai 2006, Mustanski et al. 2007, Perdue et al., 2003, Reisner et al. 2009, Rosario et al. 2006, Stall et al. 2003). Further, depression and anxiety appear to co-occur with sexual orientation-related stress, which may synergistically propel sexual minority men's HIV risk behavior. In one recent study, sexual orientation stigma predicted gay and bisexual men's unprotected anal intercourse in the previous 30 days; perceived stigma predicted anxiety that fully mediated the association between stigma and HIV risk behavior (Lelutiu-Weinberger et al. 2012). Numerous other studies have shown that sexual orientation-related stressors, in combination with mental health disorders, predict sexual minority men's HIV risk behaviors, such as high numbers of sexual partners, unprotected anal intercourse, and sex under the influence of substances (Hatzenbuehler et al. 2008, Rosario et al. 2006, Rotheram-Borus et al. 1995).

Sexual Minority Men—Healthcare Access and Utilization

The U.S. Department of Health and Human Services (2013) document, "Healthy People 2020," highlights some of the major areas of improvement for the U.S. healthcare system and, among them, are recommendations related to the health of sexual minority individuals. Given the increased risk of certain health problems among sexual minority men, specifically, providers need to be skilled at assessing sexual orientation, assessing for and intervening to decrease sexual risk behaviors (that could lead to STIs) and alcohol and substance use. However, there is a lack of training in sexual minority cultural competence in many healthcare training programs (Sanchez et al. 2006). Some sexual minority men report experiencing overt discrimination in health care settings (Kaiser Family Foundation 2001) while others note more subtle forms of disapproval. While there is a range of potentially stigmatizing behaviors—from non-verbal gestures to disparaging remarks or outright ridicule—the consequences appear similar: sexual minority men are less likely to openly discuss their sexual identity with their providers and may be less likely to provide accurate sexual histories in the context of stigma (Scott, Pringle, and Lumsdaine 2004). Experiences of discrimination may be especially likely with sexual minority men who are living with HIV (Mimiaga et al. 2007, Schuster et al. 2005), given their multiple minority identities. The cumulative impact of the aforementioned stressors, then, likely impacts the extent to which sexual minority men access and utilize healthcare services.

Sexual Minority Women's Health Disparities

The research literature suggests that, compared to heterosexual women, sexual minority women may be at increased risk of worse mental and physical health, as well as insufficient access to healthcare (e.g., Bowen, Balsam, and Ender 2008, Brown and Tracy 2008, Diamant et al. 2000, Gilman et al. 2001). In terms of mental health, evidence points to increased rates of anxiety and depression (Gilman et al. 2001) and increased risk of substance use and abuse (Hughes et al. 2010), including alcohol, tobacco, marijuana, and cocaine, among sexual minority compared to heterosexual women. Regarding physical health, sexual minority women appear to have higher rates of obesity, resulting in increased risk to cardiovascular health (e.g., Boehmer, Bowen, and Bauer 2007), as well as higher rates of certain cancer diagnoses (Brandenburg et al. 2007, Matthews et al. 2004). Finally, sexual minority women seem to be less likely than heterosexual women to access healthcare, including routine care and screenings (Diamant et al. 2000, Matthews et al. 2004).

In examining the impact of minority stress on sexual minority women's health, researchers have found minority stressors, such as violence, victimization, internalized homophobia, and sexual orientation concealment, as well as one's social-psychological resources, to significantly impact anxiety and depressive symptoms among sexual minority women (Lehavot and Simoni 2011). Gender expression is another factor that appears to underlie the experience of minority stress. For example, Levitt and Horne (2005) found that sexual minority women who present with a more masculine gender expression are more likely to experience discrimination and prejudice, which can then impact health outcomes. Other studies have demonstrated that sexual minority women who are gender-nonconforming are at risk for drug and alcohol use and smoking (e.g., Rosario, Schrimshaw, and Hunter 2008). Overall, increased mental health symptoms and substance use will likely impact sexual minority women's physical health, and their ability to access healthcare services.

Sexual Minority Women—Mental Health

Compared to heterosexual women, sexual minority women appear to be at an increased risk for indicators of poor mental health (e.g., Gilman et al. 2001). Specifically, evidence points to sexual minority women exhibiting higher rates of anxiety and depressive symptoms, including suicidal ideation (Austin and Irwin 2010, Diamant and Wold 2003, Koh and Ross 2006), with women reporting same-sex sexual partners being significantly more likely than women reporting only opposite-sex partners to endorse any anxiety disorder (40 percent vs. 22 percent) or mood disorder (35 percent vs. 14 percent) diagnosis (Gilman et al. 2001). Among women diagnosed with a depressive disorder, lesbian women also seem to be more likely than heterosexual women to report taking an antidepressant medication (Diamant and Wold 2003), which suggests that, to warrant use of a pharmacological treatment, depression may be more severe among lesbian women, or alternatively, lesbian women may be more willing to seek psychopharmacologic treatment. In a study considering disclosure of one's sexual orientation, "not out" lesbian and "out" bisexual women were more likely to have experienced suicidal ideation in the past 12 months, while "out" lesbian and "not out" bisexual women were more likely to have made a suicide attempt (Koh and Ross 2006). These authors suggest that one's degree of "outness" could affect bisexual and lesbian women differently, as bisexual women may feel isolated from both the heterosexual and lesbian communities, and bisexual women presumed to be heterosexual before coming out may experience greater stigmatization after disclosure, due to societal prejudice against sexual minority individuals. In addition to higher rates of recent and current mental health problems compared to heterosexual women, bisexual and lesbian women also report having experienced more emotional stress as teenagers, potentially due to struggles to understand, accept, and disclose their non-heterosexual sexual orientation (Koh and Ross 2006).

Disparities in substance use and abuse between heterosexual and sexual minority women are also well documented in the research literature. Past-year prevalence of any substance use disorder has been found to be nearly five times greater among lesbian (25.8 percent) and bisexual (24.3 percent) women compared to heterosexual women (5.8 percent) (McCabe et al. 2010). Sexual minority women appear to be more likely than exclusively heterosexual women to report hazardous drinking, including heavy drinking, binge drinking, intoxication, adverse consequences from drinking, and potential signs of alcohol dependence (Hughes et al. 2010). Findings from this study suggest that increased rates of lifetime sexual victimization and revictimization, when compared to heterosexual women, may explain in part the higher rates of hazardous drinking among sexual minority women (Hughes et al. 2010).

Research also points to discrimination as a factor explaining the increased prevalence of substance use disorders among sexual minority women. In one study, LGB adults who reported having experienced three types of discrimination (i.e., sexual orientation, gender, and race discrimination) in their lifetime were four times more likely to have been diagnosed with a substance use disorder in the past year (McCabe et al 2010).

Smoking has also been identified as a substance use behavior in which sexual minority women engage at increased rates. In a statewide household-based study, sexual minority women were more likely to report daily or nondaily smoking, compared to approximately 12 percent of the general population of women in California who reported smoking, with approximately 29 percent of lesbian women, 27 percent of bisexual women, and 44 percent of women reporting having sex with women (WSW) also endorsing being smokers (Gruskin et al. 2007). Results from a population-based study conducted in Washington and Oregon confirmed higher rates of current and lifetime smoking among lesbian and bisexual, compared to heterosexual, women, in spite of similar attitudes and behaviors regarding secondhand smoke (Pizacani et al. 2009).

Sexual Minority Women—Physical Health

Given these disproportionate rates of substance use and abuse among sexual minority versus heterosexual women—including drinking alcohol and smoking cigarettes—it is unsurprising that some physical health disparities also exist between these groups. Two of the most prominent physical health issues affecting sexual minority women that are discussed in the research literature are obesity and cancer. Regarding weight, studies have found increased prevalence of body weight in the overweight or obese range among lesbian women, specifically (Boehmer et al. 2007), and sexual minority women, in general (Boehmer and Bowen 2009, Jun et al. 2012). In a national population-based study, lesbian women, specifically, were twice as likely to report a body mass index (BMI) categorized as overweight or obese compared to heterosexual women (Boehmer et al. 2007). These results are supported by a recent literature review that examined obesity and related issues among sexual minority women compared to heterosexual women (Brown and Tracy 2008). Of 19 studies reviewed, nine found higher weight or obesity rates among lesbian than heterosexual or control participants (ranging from 1–5 pounds), five found no differences, and four did not report comparisons (Brown and Tracy 2008). Although lesbian and bisexual women appear to be more likely than heterosexual women to exhibit adverse weight gain trajectories over the course of adulthood (Jun et al. 2012), these patterns may begin during adolescence. Binge eating behaviors have been found to be more prevalent among girls between the ages of 12 and 23 years who identify a minority sexual orientation as compared to heterosexual girls (Austin et al. 2009). Researchers have speculated that both minority stress and gender socialization and norms may account in part for the increased rates of binge eating behaviors and, subsequently, overweight and obesity among sexual minority girls and women.

Additionally, and possibly related to the likelihood of increased body weight among sexual minority women, results of a recent literature review reveal that disparities in cancer risk have been understudied in sexual minority women (Brown and Tracy 2008). A majority of related studies conducted over the past three decades have focused on breast and cervical cancer screenings. A dearth of information is available in the literature examining sexual minority women's experiences with ovarian, lung, and colorectal cancers (Brown and Tracy 2008). However, sexual minority women demonstrate higher prevalence estimates of several risk factors for each of these types of cancer, including alcohol use, smoking, and overweight/obesity, as discussed above. Evidence also suggests that sexual minority women are less likely to participate in some routine cancer screenings, such as Pap tests (Matthews et al. 2004). Although tailored risk counseling efforts have effectively increased rates of breast and gynecological cancer screening among lesbian women, sexual minority women remain at higher risk of breast (Brandenburg et al. 2007) and cervical (Matthews et al. 2004) cancers, among others, given the aforementioned elevated risk factors. As such, additional research is needed to explore all aspects of these disparities in cancer risk among sexual minority women.

Sexual Minority Women—Healthcare Access and Utilization

Given these mental and physical health issues disproportionately affecting sexual minority women, the importance of access to and utilization of prevention and treatment services is clear. Unfortunately, research evidence also suggests that sexual minority women face barriers in access to healthcare and tend to underutilize available services. In a population-based sample, lesbian and bisexual women were less likely to have health insurance and more likely to report difficulty accessing necessary medical care due to barriers, including financial reasons (Diamant et al. 2000). More specifically, findings also suggest that lesbian women are less likely to access gynecologic care, including Pap testing (Matthews et al. 2004), and also to report a recent clinical breast exam (Diamant et al. 2000). Identified barriers to healthcare access among sexual minority women, including both personal barriers and structural barriers, can be traced to stigma—enacted stigma, felt stigma, and internalized stigma (IOM 2011). Thus, it is imperative that healthcare providers possess high levels of cultural competency to work with sexual minority women.

Transgender Health Disparities

Transgender (not "transgendered") is an umbrella term that describes gender-variant identities and expressions. It is commonly used to note when one's biological sex (anatomical male, anatomical female, or intersex) does not match one's gender identity (culturally defined characteristics specific to men and women) (Mallon 1999). Although some transgender individuals choose to identify themselves based on a more traditional gender binary system (i.e., transitioning from male-to-female [MTF] or female-to-male [FTM]), others may choose to identify as bigender (to identify as both male and female), gender queer (an example of the rejection of the binary system), or as any number of culturally transcendent categories of gender (IOM 2011). However, after individuals fully transition to their gender of choice (e.g., by undergoing sex reassignment surgery), some may cease from identifying as transgender at all and, rather, identify solely as the newly realized gender category. Gender identity and sexual orientation are conceptually distinct; therefore, a current or formerly transgender individual may have sexual or romantic feelings towards women, men, both women and men, other transgender individuals, or some combination thereof (IOM 2011). Although prevalence estimates vary, it is estimated that transgender individuals comprise 0.3 percent of the total population in the United States (Gates 2011). Transgender individuals can be found in all geographical regions, and represent the full range of sociodemographic characteristics, including race, ethnicity, education level, religious affiliation, and marital status (e.g., Rosser et al. 2007).

Transgender individuals may be assigned the *DSM-IV* diagnosis of gender dysphoria (GD, APA 2000). Criteria include a strong desire for cross-gender identification, and persistent discomfort in and preoccupation with one's biological sex—both primary and secondary sex characteristics—to the extent that these disturbances lead to significant distress and impairment in day-to-day functioning. This diagnosis remains highly controversial, however, as many clinicians argue that it reinforces gender stereotypes, devalues social nonconformity, and may lead to emotional and psychological distress in the individual (Lev 2005). GD is further complicated when considered in the context of gender nonconforming children, who are becoming increasingly visible (Pleak 2009). Mental disorders are believed to originate from within the individual (APA 2000), yet the stress that gender nonconforming children experience is typically associated with social condemnation and rejection, and is therefore largely extrinsic (e.g., Bartlett, Vasey, and Bukowski 2000; Wester et al. 2010). Thus, GD remains unclear as a diagnosis and as a representation of psychological distress. Regardless, transgender individuals may choose to utilize psychotherapy as a way to address transgender-related distress and stigmatization, to find support and affirmation, and sometimes, as a way to begin the process of transitioning from one gender to another. This process can involve hormone treatment, vocal conditioning (raising or lowering the pitch of the voice), dressing and living day-to-day in the gender of choice, silicone injections, and, although less common, surgical procedures.

Sex reassignment surgery (SRS) is a procedure through which individuals can surgically alter biologically assigned sex characteristics to match those of the opposite sex. Although SRS is a goal for some transgender individuals, an acceptance of one's gender identity and gender role can be achieved with or without surgery and/or hormone treatment (Bockting 2008). Thus, there is no definitive standard for how and to what extent a given individual will transition or affirm their gender. Yet, in order to undergo SRS, an individual will need a letter of recommendation from two trained, mental health professionals (i.e., the client's psychotherapist and an outside consultant on the case). Decisions are made based on a rather rigorous evaluation that includes psychotherapy and requires that the individual live full time in the identified gender role prior to authorization (Meyer et al. 2001). One can imagine, then, that having one's therapist be a potential facilitator or barrier to SRS complicates the therapeutic alliance, to be sure.

Currently, there are limited data available regarding the health of transgender individuals. Compared to sexual minority individuals, transgender individuals appear to be less visible, and even from within sexual minority communities, transgender individuals can remain highly marginalized. From the available data, however, it appears that transgender individuals are disproportionately impacted by several mental and physical health concerns—specifically, depression and suicidality, HIV, and substance abuse. It has been documented that transgender individuals are at an increased risk for experiencing stigma and discrimination compared to the general population—and even compared to sexual minority individuals. Researchers and clinicians are only now beginning to conceptualize theoretical frameworks that may accurately capture the mechanisms through which poor mental and physical health indicators may develop among transgender individuals. For example, emerging data suggest that Meyer's minority stress model (Meyer 2003) can be adapted and applied to transgender health—that the experience of gender-related victimization and discrimination may be associated with internalized transphobia, expectations of future rejection, and psychological distress (Hendricks and Testa 2012).

Transgender Individuals—Mental Health

There are relatively few transgender-inclusive studies that have examined mental health, and those that have been conducted typically have not involved representative samples—so we must be highly cautious against drawing conclusions that are assumed to be reliable over time and across geographic locations. The majority of these studies identify depression (or depressive symptoms) as an area of particular salience. Estimates of depression among transgender individuals are often higher than those in the general population (e.g., 36.2 percent vs. 6.8 percent) (Pitts et al. 2009). Further, depressive symptomology is present across multiple studies (e.g., Bith-Melander et al. 2010, Clements-Nolle et al. 2001, Garofalo et al. 2007, Haas et al. 2011, Pitts et al. 2009, Shipherd, Green, and Abramovitz 2010). Thus, depression appears to be a specific area of concern in the lives of transgender individuals—which is especially meaningful, given the association of psychosocial concerns with depression (e.g., substance abuse and sexual risk taking behaviors).

In addition to depression, suicidality is identified as a psychological factor relevant to this population (Haas et al. 2011). In one study of 67 MTF persons, 16 percent reported suicidal ideation in the last 30 days, and lifetime prevalence was 60 percent (Risser et al. 2005). In another study that included 392 MTF and 123 FTM individuals, 32 percent of each population had attempted suicide (Clements-Nolle et al. 2001). General psychological distress—to what severity remains questionable—appears to be common among transgender individuals. This likely extends from the prejudicial and discriminatory social environments in which transgender individuals live (e.g., Clements-Nolle, Marx, and Katz 2006).

Transgender Individuals—Physical Health

The most common physical health concern noted for transgender individuals in the scientific literature is HIV/AIDS acquisition. HIV prevalence has been shown to be particularly high among this group, and especially in comparison to the general population. HIV prevalence estimates have been shown to range from 13.5 percent to 27 percent (Garofalo et al. 2006, Guadamuz et al. 2011, Prabawanti et al. 2011, Risser et al. 2005, Wilson et al. 2009). It is important to note these rates are based on studies that include only MTF participants—which reflects the limited number of studies available. Rates of sexually transmitted infections (STIs) are also varied; however, STI infections are believed to be common, especially among those who engage in high-risk sexual activities, including inconsistent condom use and sex with anonymous partners (Prabawanti et al.

2011, Reisner, Perkovich, and Mimiaga 2010, Risser et al. 2005, Stephens, Bernstein, and Philip 2011). Currently, there are no definitive statistics regarding STIs and it remains unclear if these numbers generalize to all transgender individuals.

In addition to HIV risk, substance abuse has been identified as a salient concern for this population. Compared to the general population, transgender individuals face a number of unique psychosocial issues (e.g., disclosing or concealing one's gender identity), and substance use may be used as a way to cope (e.g., Phillips and Patsdaughter 2010). Drug and alcohol use is commonly cited by transgender individuals across several studies, and is often associated with transgender-related stressors (Bith-Melander et al. 2010, Garofalo et al. 2007, Wilson et al. 2009, 2010). For example, Clements-Nolle and colleagues (2006) found that among a sample of 515 transgender individuals, 28 percent had been in a substance abuse treatment program at some point in the past. Further, injection silicone and hormone use may impact a certain portion of this population—which has implications for HIV risk if needles are shared (Garofalo et al. 2006, Guadamuz et al. 2011). Given that transgender individuals may have difficulty accessing medical services (e.g., due to provider mistrust, prior negative experiences with the healthcare system, lack of health insurance), there is the possibility that they will seek out hormones from non-medical environments, and from persons unfamiliar with possible medical concerns. Thus, lack of provider cultural competence may place transgender individuals at an increased risk for negative health outcomes.

Although commercial/transactional sex work and unprotected sex are commonly cited as behavioral risks present in the transgender population (e.g., Barrington et al. 2012, Bith-Melander et al. 2010, Garofalo et al. 2007, Guadamuz et al. 2011, Phillips and Patsdaughter 2010, Prabawanti et al. 2011, Reisner et al. 2010, Risser et al. 2005, Wilson et al. 2009), researchers and clinicians should use caution when generalizing this information to the larger transgender community, which is incredibly vast and diverse. Sex work should be understood as a means to gain resources for those who may not be able to access these otherwise—largely due to the result of discrimination, stigma, and marginalization (e.g., Clements-Nolle et al. 2006). Thus, "survival sex work" is a more accurate descriptor for transgender individuals who engage in these behaviors as a way to meet basic needs.

Transgender Individuals—Healthcare Access and Utilization

Even with the overrepresentation of adverse health outcomes present in the transgender population, there appears to be a lack of accessible resources and services. Many transgender individuals report difficulties accessing and utilizing services due to a number of factors: provider incompetence; lack of provider acceptance regarding gender variance; lack of sensitive and inclusive language in health-related questions; general discrimination and stigma; and unwelcoming medical environments (Alegria 2011, Boyce et al. 2012, De Santis, Martin, and Lester 2010, Ryan et al. 2010, Shipherd et al. 2010, Vanderleest and Galper 2009). Yet, studies have shown that transgender individuals who receive services from health clinics and know their HIV status engage in healthier behaviors than those who do not receive services (Melendez and Pinto 2009, Prabawanti et al. 2011, Sanchez, Sanchez, and Danoff 2009, Thornhill and Klein 2010).

Provider Recommendations

The extant literature on the health and wellness of sexual and gender minority individuals clearly documents disproportionate experience with physical and mental health problems among members of these groups. Providers working with LBGT individuals, thus, should take special care to provide culturally competent services to members of these communities. Empirical work on sexual and gender minority cultural competence (e.g., Riggs and Fell 2010, Wilkerson et al. 2011) is lacking. For example, it is notable that there are no published reports that investigate, for example, the differences in outcome between LGBT culturally competent treatments and standard care. Thus, any recommendations for providing this type of care must be understood within that context. Work that investigates such differences is sorely needed.

Despite limited empirical evidence on this point, here we provide recommendations for working clinically with members of sexual and gender minority communities. There is some evidence that many health-care providers espouse "neutral" views about working with sexual minority individuals (Willging, Salvador, and Kano 2006), that is, that they aim to treat all clients/patients "the same." However, such a stance fails to take into account some of the unique aspects of the lived experience of LGBT individuals which, it seems clear, influence their psychosocial status, health behaviors, and physical health. We argue, then, that the competent clinical care of sexual and gender minority individuals does require some modifications from a "standard" treatment, and here we indicate some suggestions for those modifications. What we have listed below are two major, overarching recommendations based upon our own collective research and clinical experiences, as well as extrapolations from the published literature on LGBT physical and mental health more generally.

Recommendation 1: Providers should engage in honest self-assessment and information gathering.

Clinicians who work with people who are different from themselves in any way, including but not limited to sexual and gender minority individuals, must make an honest appraisal of their own biases. It is naïve to believe that anyone is completely without bias. Even when our biases are not ill-intentioned, we can still make errors. Without living within the culture of a particular client, it is easy to make assumptions that are based on stereotypes, and to remain unaware of the ways that such assumptions bias our decision-making processes. Thus, culturally competent clinicians must make *a lifelong commitment* to understanding the breadth of differences across people, and to engaging in introspection to recognize where their own cultural experiences blind them to the experiences of others.

From the mental health literature, there are a variety of self-assessment questions that a provider could ponder, or could discuss in a consultation group. These questions include assumptions of morality that are tied up in sexual behavior (e.g., Do I believe that people who engage in same-sex sexual behavior are bad or wrong?), increasing awareness of reactions to people who are different (e.g., Do I become anxious when I interact with a person who doesn't conform strongly to traditional gender norms, for example, when I interact with a masculine woman or a feminine man?), and noting the ways in which one's behavior may be shaped by implicit biases (e.g., more likely to "see" psychpathology in LGB clients, or more likely to "see" Axis II personality disorders in trans clients). Space constraints preclude a more thorough description of these questions, however, interested readers should consult Martell and colleagues (2004) for self-questions about working with LGB clients, and Pantalone and colleagues (2009) who noted a list of additional self-assessment questions that aim to identify biases and "blind spots" related to work with a member of any group that is different from oneself.

Further, it is necessary to become knowledgeable about the sociocultural groups of which clients are members. Such education should come from a combination of reading books, articles in professional journals, the popular press, courses, travel, and cultural events or informal discussions with friends or peers. Remember to use the information gleaned as a guide, rather than to treat it as a rigid absolute. Within-group differences can be significant, and it will be most helpful to use any newly discovered knowledge to help generate hypotheses or to demonstrate interest in, and connection with, the client. General information about a sociocultural group cannot substitute for thorough assessment of an individual client's unique experience of the world.

Recommendation 2: In healthcare interactions, providers should approach rather than avoid, and assess rather than make assumptions.

In our experience, one problem with current healthcare delivery practices is that providers may suspect but not assess, or infer without confirming, information about an individual's sexual orientation, gender identity, or sexual behavior. Many providers may believe that such information is not necessary. However, it seems clear from the information summarized in this chapter that there are systematic differences in the physical and mental health status of sexual and gender minority individuals and, thus, that information is absolutely necessary to understand the sociocultural context of the clients we serve. The most generous assumption about this assessment omission is that providers do not want to offend or upset clients who may already be maligned by society by asking, or by using outmoded language that inadvertently offends. We applaud that kindness and caring and, thus, suggest that providers can use open-ended questions to gather important information about sexuality and gender, and ask clients what terminology they prefer to use for sensitive aspects of their identity.

Open-ended questions are those which cannot be answered with a simple "yes" or "no" and, instead, require a qualitative (vs. quantitative) response. In this arena, examples would be "How do you identify your sexual orientation?" or "Tell me about your recent sexual partners." Questions like, "Do you have sex with men, women, or both?" can be useful for some patients, however, questions like that also reify the gender binary (i.e., the only possible genders of their sexual partners are "male" and "female") and imply that there is congruence between a sex partner's biological sex and gender identity. There is increasing evidence (e.g., Kuper, Nussbaum, and Mustanski 2012, Levy and Johnson 2012) that today's younger individuals are more likely than older individuals to eschew traditional labels for sexual orientation (gay, lesbian, bisexual) in favor of more contemporary choices (queer, pansexual) without implications for a narrow construal of gender.

To that end, we suggest that providers ask clients directly what terminology they prefer for their sexual orientation (e.g., "How do you identify your sexual orientation?") and gender identity (e.g., "What label do you prefer for your gender identity?"). We have found that asking clients to give us information about how they think about, and how they most prefer to talk about, those intimate aspects of their identity is the best way to minimize the likelihood of using biased or incorrect language. It also seems that addressing issues of sexuality and gender directly communicates to clients that the healthcare setting is a safe and accepting space no matter what their response, and gives the message that providers understand the importance of sexual orientation and gender identity to the client's health.

Finally, it is important—in addition to not making assumptions about other areas—that providers not make assumptions about aspects of an individual's relationship simply because some information is provided. For example, it is important to always take a thorough sexual history regardless of the client's partner/marital status. Many gay men, for example, have negotiated open relationships in which they engage in extra-dyadic sexual behavior. Further, even clients who identify as heterosexual may occasionally engage in same-sex sexual behavior.

Conclusions

Sexual and gender minority individuals, although often grouped under the "LGBT umbrella," are incredibly diverse and varied with regard to their identities, beliefs, practices, and unique health needs. Compared to heterosexual or non-transgender individuals, LGB-identified and transgender-identified individuals are at a greater risk for experiencing discrimination and prejudice, as well as internalizing those experiences as stigma, which have been shown to be associated with indicators of poorer mental and physical health. Although sexual and gender minority individuals are often resilient in employing strategies to cope with their psychosocial stress, health providers can offer clinical support and care in an effort to further minimize health disparities and strengthen health-promoting practices. To provide an optimal level of care for patients/clients, providers must first engage in the practice of cultural humility—specifically, the acknowledgment that we all carry personal biases, assumptions, and beliefs. With this awareness, and by engaging with LGBT individuals in an open and honest manner, a more informed and effective level of care will emerge which, we hope, will translate into improvements in the health and wellness of all LGBT people.

References

Alegria, C. 2011. "Transgender Identity and Health Care: Implications for Psychosocial and Physical Evaluation." *Journal of the American Academy of Nurse Practitioners* 23(4): 175–182.

American Psychiatric Association. 2013. *Diagnostic and Statistical Manual of Mental Disorders* (5th ed.). Arlington, VA: American Psychiatric Publishing.

Austin, E. L. and J. A. Irwin. 2010. "Health Behaviors and Health Care Utilization of Southern Lesbians." *Women's Health Issues* 20(3): 178–184.

Austin, S. B., N. J. Ziyadeh, H. L. Corliss, M. Rosario, D. Wypij, J. Haines, and A. E. Field. 2009. "Sexual Orientation Disparities in Purging and Binge Eating from Early to Late Adolescence." *Journal of Adolescent Health* 45(3): 238–245.

Barrington, C., C. Wejnert, M. Guardado, A. Nieto, and G. Bailey. 2012. "Social Network Characteristics and HIV Vulnerability among Transgender Persons in San Salvador: Identifying Opportunities for HIV Prevention Strategies." *AIDS and Behavior* 16(1): 214–224.

Bartlett, N., P. Vasey, and W. Bukowski. 2000. "Is Gender Identity Disorder in Children a Mental Disorder?" *Sex Roles* 43: 753–785.

Beals, K. P., L. A. Peplau, and S. L. Gable. 2009. "Stigma Management and Wellbeing: The Role of Perceived Social Support, Emotional Processing, and Suppression." *Personality and Social Psychology Bulletin* 35: 867–879.

Bith-Melander, P., B. Sheoran, L. Sheth, C. Bermudez, J. Drone, W. Wood, and K. Schroeder. 2010. "Understanding Sociocultural and Psychological Factors Affecting Transgender People of Color in San Francisco." *Journal of the Association of Nurses in AIDS Care* 21(3): 207–220.

Bockting, W. O. 2008. "Psychotherapy and the Real-Life Experience: From Gender Dichotomy to Gender Diversity." *Sexologies* 17(4): 211–224.

Boehmer, U., and D. J. Bowen. 2009. "Examining Factors Linked to Overweight and Obesity in Women of Different Sexual Orientations." *Preventive Medicine* 48(4): 357–361.

Boehmer, U., D. J. Bowen, and G. R. Bauer. 2007. "Overweight and Obesity in Sexual-Minority Women: Evidence from Population-Based Data." *American Journal of Public Health* 97(6): 1134–1140.

Bowen, D. J., K. F. Balsam, and S. R. Ender. 2008. "A Review of Obesity Issues in Sexual Minority Women." *Obesity* 16(2): 221–228.

Boyce, S., C. Barrington, H. Bolaños, C. Arandi, and G. Paz-Bailey. 2012. "Facilitating Access to Sexual Health Services for Men Who Have Sex with Men and Male-to-Female Transgender Persons in Guatemala City." *Culture, Health and Sexuality* 14(3): 313–327.

Brandenburg, D. L., A. K. Matthews, T. P. Johnson, and T. L. Hughes. 2007. "Breast Cancer Risk and Screening: A Comparison of Lesbian and Heterosexual Women." *Women and Health* 45(4): 109–130.

Brown, J. P. and J. Tracy. 2008. "Lesbians and Cancer: An Overlooked Health Disparity." *Cancer Causes and Control* 19(10): 1009–1020.

Brubaker, M., M. Garrett, and B. Dew. 2009. "Examining the Relationship between Internalized Heterosexism and Substance Abuse among Lesbian, Gay, and Bisexual Individuals: A Critical Review." *Journal of LGBT Issues in Counseling* 3: 62–89.

Centers for Disease Control and Prevention. 2005. "Antiretroviral Postexposure Prophylaxis after Sexual, Injection-Drug Use, or Other Non-Occupational Exposure to HIV in the United States: Recommendations from the U.S. Department of Health and Human Services." *MMWR. Recommendations and Reports: Morbidity and Mortality Weekly Report. Recommendations and Reports / Centers for Disease Control*, 54(RR-2): 1–16.

Centers for Disease Control and Prevention 2008. *HIV/AIDS Surveillance Report, 2008.* Atlanta, GA: Author.

Centers for Disease Control and Prevention. 2010. *HIV among Gay, Bisexual and Other Men Who Have Sex with Men (MSM).* Atlanta, GA: Author.

Clements, K., W. Willy, K. Kitano, and R. Marx. 1999. "HIV Prevention and Health Service Needs of the Transgender Community in San Francisco." *International Journal of Transgenderism* 3(1).

Clements-Nolle, K., R. Marx, R. Guzman, and M. Katz. 2001. "HIV Prevalence, Risk Behaviors, Health Care Use, and Mental Health Status of Transgender Persons: Implications for Public Health Intervention." *American Journal of Public Health* 91(6): 915–921.

Clements-Nolle, K., R. Marx, and M. Katz. 2006. "Attempted Suicide among Transgender Persons: The Influence of Gender-Based Discrimination and Victimization." *Journal of Homosexuality* 51: 53–69.

Cochran, S. D., D. Ackerman, V. M. Mays, and M. W. Ross. 2004. "Prevalence of Non-Medical Drug Use and Dependence among Homosexually Active Men and Women in the U.S. Population." *Addiction* 99: 989–998.

Cochran, S., V. Mays, and J. Sullivan. 2003. "Prevalence of Mental Disorders, Psychological Distress, and Mental Health Services Use among Lesbian, Gay, and Bisexual Adults in the United States." *Journal of Consulting and Clinical Psychology* 71(1): 53–61.

De Santis, J. P., C. W. Martin, and A. Lester. 2010. "An Educational Program on HIV Prevention for Male-to-Female Transgender Women in South Miami Beach, Florida." *Journal of the Association of Nurses in AIDS Care* 21(3): 265–271.

Diamant, A. L. and C. Wold. 2003. "Sexual Orientation and Variation in Physical and Mental Health Status among Women." *Journal of Women's Health* 12(1): 41–49.

Diamant, A., C. Wold, K. Spritzer, and L. Gelberg. 2000. "Health Behaviors, Health Status, and Access to and Use of Health Care: A Population-Based Study of Lesbian, Bisexual, and Heterosexual Women." *Archives of Family Medicine* 9(10): 1043–1051.

Drabble, L., L. T. Midanik, and K. Trocki. 2005. "Reports of Alcohol Consumption and Alcohol-Related Problems among Homosexual, Bisexual and Heterosexual Respondents: Results from the 2000 National Alcohol Survey." *Journal of Studies on Alcohol* 66: 111–120.

Eisenberg, M. E. 2002. "The Association of Campus Resources for Gay, Lesbian, and Bisexual Students with College Students' Condom Use." *Journal of American College Health* 51: 109–116.

Eisenberg, M. E. and H. Wechsler. 2003. "Social Influences on Substance-Use Behaviors of College Students with Same-Sex Experience: Findings from a National Study." *Social Science and eMedicine* 57: 1913–1923.

Eliason, M. J. and R. Schope. 2001. "Does 'Don't Ask Don't Tell' Apply to Health Care? Lesbian, Gay, and Bisexual People's Disclosure to Health Care Providers." *Journal of the Gay and Lesbian Medical Association* 5(4): 125–134.

Feinstein, B. A., M. R. Goldfried, and J. Davila. 2012. "The Relationship between Experiences of Discrimination and Mental Health among Lesbians and Gay Men: An Examination of Internalized Homonegativity and Rejection Sensitivity as Potential Mechanisms." *Journal of Consulting and Clinical Psychology* 80(5): 917–927.

Frost, D. M., J. T. Parsons, and J. E. Nanín. 2007. "Stigma, Concealment, and Symptoms of Depression as Explanations for Sexually Transmitted Infections among Gay Men." *Journal of Health Psychology* 12(4): 636–640.

Garofalo, R., J. Deleon, E. Osmer, M. Doll, and G. W. Harper. 2006. "Overlooked, Misunderstood and At-Risk: Exploring the Lives and HIV Risk of Ethnic Minority Male-to-Female Transgender Youth." *Journal of Adolescent Health* 38(3): 230–236.

Garofalo, R., E. Osmer, C. Sullivan, M. Doll, and G. Harper. 2007. "Environmental, Psychosocial, and Individual Correlates of HIV Risk in Ethnic Minority Male-to-Female Transgender Youth." *Journal of HIV/AIDS Prevention in Children and Youth* 7(2): 89–104.

Gates, G. 2011. *How Many People Are Lesbian, Gay, Bisexual, and Transgender?* The Williams Institute, University of California, Los Angeles. http://williamsinstitute .law.ucla.edu/research/census-lgbt-demographics-studies/how-many -people-are-lesbian-gay-bisexual-and-transgender/

Gilman, S. E., S. D. Cochran, V. M. Mays, M. Hughes, D. Ostrow, and R. C. Kessler. 2001. "Risk of Psychiatric Disorders among Individuals Reporting Same-Sex Sexual Partners in the National Comorbidity Survey." *American Journal of Public Health* 91(6): 933–939.

Golub, S. A., D. Operario, and P. M. Gorbach. 2010. "Pre-Exposure Prophylaxis State of the Science: Empirical Analogies for Research and Implementation." *Current HIV/AIDS Reports* 7(4): 201–209.

Green, K. E. and B. A. Feinstein. 2012. "Substance Use in Lesbian, Gay, and Bisexual Populations: An Update on Empirical Research and Implications for Treatment." *Psychology of Addictive Behaviors* 26: 265.

Gruskin, E. P., G. L. Greenwood, M. Matevia, L. M. Pollack, and L. L. Bye. 2007. "Disparities in Smoking between the Lesbian, Gay, and Bisexual Population and the General Population in California." *American Journal of Public Health* 97(8): 1496–1502.

Guadamuz, T., W. Wimonsate, A. Varangrat, P. Phanuphak, R. Jommaroeng, J. McNicholl, and F. van Griensven. 2011. "HIV Prevalence, Risk Behavior, Hormone Use and Surgical History among Transgender Persons in Thailand." *AIDS and Behavior* 15(3): 650–658.

Haas, A. P., M. Eliason, V. M. Mays, R. M. Mathy, S. D. Cochran, A. R. D'Augelli, and G. K. Brown. 2011. "Suicide and Suicide Risk in Lesbian, Gay, Bisexual, and Transgender Populations: Review and Recommendations." *Journal of Homosexuality* 58(1): 10–51.

Halkitis, P. N. and J. T. Parsons. 2002. "Recreational Drug Use and HIV-Risk Sexual Behavior among Men Frequenting Gay Social Venues." *Journal of Gay and Lesbian Social Services* 14: 19–39.

Hart, T. A. and R. G. Heimberg. 2005. "Social Anxiety as a Risk Factor for Unprotected Intercourse among Gay and Bisexual Male Youth." *AIDS and Behavior 9*: 505–512.

Hatzenbuehler, M. L. 2009. "How Does Sexual Minority Stigma 'Get Under the Skin'? A Psychological Mediation Framework." *Psychological Bulletin 135*(5): 707.

Hatzenbuehler, M. L. 2011. "The Social Environment and Suicide Attempts in a Population-Based Sample of LGB Youth." *Pediatrics 127*: 896–903.

Hatzenbuehler, M. L., W. R. Corbin, and K. Fromme. 2008. "Trajectories and Determinants of Alcohol Use among LGB Young Adults and Their Heterosexual Peers: Results from a Prospective Study." *Developmental Psychology 44*: 81.

Hatzenbuehler, M. L., K. A. McLaughlin, K. M. Keyes, and D. S. Hasin. 2010. "The Impact of Institutional Discrimination on Psychiatric Disorders in Lesbian, Gay, and Bisexual Populations: A Prospective Study." *American Journal of Public Health 100*: 452–459.

Hatzenbuehler, M., S. Nolen-Hoeksema, and J. Dovidio. 2009. "How Does Stigma 'Get under the Skin'?: The Mediating Role of Emotion Regulation." *Psychological Science 10*: 1282–1289.

Hatzenbuehler, M. L., S. Nolen-Hoeksema, and S. J. Erickson. 2008. "Minority Stress Predictors of HIV Risk Behavior, Substance Use, and Depressive Symptoms: Results from a Prospective Study of Bereaved Gay Men." *Health Psychology 27*: 455.

Hatzenbuehler, M. L., J. Pachankis, and J. Wolff. 2012. "Religious Climate and Health-Risk Behaviors in Sexual Minority Youth: A Population-Based Study." *American Journal of Public Health 102*: 657–663.

Hendershot, C. S., S. A. Stoner, D. W. Pantalone, and J. M. Simoni. 2009. "Alcohol Use and Antiretroviral Adherence: Review and Meta-Analysis." *Journal of Acquired Immune Deficiency Syndromes 52*(2): 180–202.

Hendricks, M. L., and R. J. Testa. 2012. "A Conceptual Framework for Clinical Work with Transgender and Gender Nonconforming Clients: An Adaptation of the Minority Stress Model." *Professional Psychology: Research and Practice 43*(5): 460–467.

Hershberger, S. L., and A. R. D'Augelli. 1995. "The Impact of Victimization on the Mental Health and Suicidality of Lesbian, Gay, and Bisexual Youths." *Developmental Psychology 31*(1): 65–74.

Huebner, D. M., and M. C. Davis. 2007. "Perceived Antigay Discrimination and Physical Health Outcomes." *Health Psychology 26*: 627–634.

Hughes, T. L., L. A. Szalacha, T. P. Johnson, K. E. Kinnison, S. C. Wilsnack, and Y. Cho. 2010. "Sexual Victimization and Hazardous Drinking among Heterosexual and Sexual Minority Women." *Addictive Behaviors 35*(12): 1152–1156.

Hutton, H. E., C. G. Lyketsos, J. M. Zenilman, R. E. Thompson, and E. J. Erbelding. 2004. "Depression and HIV Risk Behaviors among Patients in a Sexually Transmitted Disease Clinic." *American Journal of Psychiatry 161*: 912–914.

Institute of Medicine, Committee on Lesbian, Gay, Bisexual, and Transgender Health Issues and Research Gaps and Opportunities. 2011. *The Health of Lesbian, Gay,*

Bisexual, and Transgender (LGBT) People: Building a Foundation for Better Understanding.* Washington, DC: National Academies Press.

Jaffe, H. W., R. O. Valdiserri, and K. M. De Cock. 2007. "The Reemerging HIV/AIDS Epidemic in Men Who Have Sex with Men." *Journal of the American Medical Association* 298: 2412–2414.

Jun, H. J., H. L. Corliss, L. P. Nichols, M. J. Pazaris, D. Spiegelman, and S. B. Austin. 2012. "Adult Body Mass Index Trajectories and Sexual Orientation: The Nurses' Health Study II." *American Journal of Preventive Medicine* 42(4): 348–354.

Kaiser Family Foundation. 2001. "Inside-OUT: A Report on the Experiences of Lesbians, Gays and Bisexuals in America and the Public's Views on Issues and Policies Related to Sexual Orientation." http://www.kff.org/kaiserpolls/loader.cfm?url=/commonspot/security/getfile.cfmandpageid=13875

Kashdan, T. B., R. L. Collins, and J. D. Elhai. 2006. "Social Anxiety and Positive Outcome Expectancies on Risk-Taking Behaviors." *Cognitive Therapy and Research* 30(6): 749–761.

Kerrigan, M. F. 2012. "Transgender Discrimination in the Military: The New Don't Ask, Don't Tell." *Psychology, Public Policy, and Law* 18(3): 500–518.

Kipke, M. D., G. Weiss, M. Ramirez, F. Dorey, A. Ritt-Olson, E. Iverson, and W. Ford. 2007. "Club Drug Use in Los Angeles among Young Men Who Have Sex with Men." *Substance Use and Misuse* 42: 1723–1743.

Klitzman, R. L., J. D. Greenberg, L. M. Pollack, and C. Dolezal. 2002. "MDMA ('Ecstasy') Use, and Its Association with High Risk Behaviors, Mental Health, and Other Factors among Gay/Bisexual Men in New York City." *Drug and Alcohol Dependence* 66: 115–126.

Koh, A. S. and L. K. Ross. 2006. "Mental Health Issues: A Comparison of Lesbian, Bisexual and Heterosexual Women." *Journal of Homosexuality* 51(1): 33–57.

Kuper, L. E., R. Nussbaum, and B. Mustanski. 2012. "Exploring the Diversity of Gender and Sexual Orientation Identities in an Online Sample of Transgender Individuals." *Journal of Sex Research* 49(2/3): 244–254.

Lehavot, K. and J. M. Simoni. 2011. "The Impact of Minority Stress on Mental Health and Substance Use among Sexual Minority Women." *Journal of Consulting and Clinical Psychology* 79(2): 159–170.

Lelutiu-Weinberger, C., J. E. Pachankis, S. Golub, J. J. Walker, A. J. Bamonte, and J. Parsons. 2012. "Differential Association of Psychosocial Factors and HIV Risk Behavior for Younger and Older Sexual Minority Men." *AIDS and Behavior* 17(1): 340–349.

Lev, A. I. 2005. "Disordering Gender Identity: Gender Identity Disorder in the DSM-IV-TR." *Journal of Psychology and Human Sexuality* 17: 35–69.

Levitt, H. M., and S. G. Horne. 2005. "She Looked Like a Dyke: The Relation between Homophobic Discrimination and Gender Expression." Research on Non-Heterosexual Women's Experiences: Informing Future Psychological Work, moderated by H. Levitt. Symposium session held at the meeting of the Association for Women in Psychology, Tampa, FL.

Levy, D. L., and C. W. Johnson. 2012. "What Does the Q Mean? Including Queer Voices in Qualitative Research." *Qualitative Social Work* 11(2): 130–140.

Mahajan, A. P., J. N. Sayles, V. A. Patel, R. H. Remien, D. Ortiz, G. Szekeres, and T. J. Coates. 2008. "Stigma in the HIV/AIDS Epidemic: A Review of the Literature and Recommendations for the Way Forward." *AIDS* 22(Suppl 2): S67-S79.

Makadon, H. J., K. H. Mayer, J. Potter, and H. Goldhammer, eds. 2008. *The Fenway Guide to Lesbian, Gay, Bisexual, and Transgender Health*. Philadelphia, PA: American College of Physicians.

Mallon, G. P. 1999. "Appendix: A Glossary of Transgendered Definitions." *Journal of Gay and Lesbian Social Services* 10(3/4): 143–145.

Martell, C. R., S. A. Safren, and S. E. Prince. 2004. *Cognitive-Behavioral Therapies with Lesbian, Gay, and Bisexual Clients*. New York, NY: Guilford Press.

Matthews, A. K., D. L. Brandenburg, T. P. Johnson, and T. L. Hughes. 2004. "Correlates of Underutilization of Gynecological Cancer Screening among Lesbian and Heterosexual Women." *Preventative Medicine* 38(1): 105–113.

Mayer, K., L. Bekker, R. Stall, A. Grulich, G. Colfax, and J. Lama. 2012. "Comprehensive Clinical Care for Men Who Have Sex with Men: An Integrated Approach." *Lancet* 380(9839): 378–387.

Mays, V. M., and S. D. Cochran. 2001. "Mental Health Correlates of Perceived Discrimination among Lesbian, Gay, and Bisexual Adults in the United States." *American Journal of Public Health* 91(11): 1869–1876.

McCabe, S., W. B. Bostwick, T. L. Hughes, B. T. West, and C. J. Boyd. 2010. "The Relationship between Discrimination and Substance Use Disorders among Lesbian, Gay, and Bisexual Adults in the United States." *American Journal of Public Health* 100(10): 1946–1952.

McCabe, S. E., T. L. Hughes, W. Bostwick, and C. J. Boyd. 2005. "Assessment of Difference in Dimensions of Sexual Orientation: Implications for Substance Use Research in a College-Age Population." *Journal of Studies on Alcohol* 66(5): 620–629.

McCabe, S. E., T. L. Hughes, W. B. Bostwick, B. T. West, and C. J. Boyd. 2009. "Sexual Orientation, Substance Use Behaviors and Substance Dependence in the United States." *Addiction* 104(8): 1333–1345.

McGuire, J. K., C. R. Anderson, R. B. Toomey, and S. T. Russell. 2010. "School Climate for Transgender Youth: A Mixed Method Investigation of Student Experiences and School Responses." *Journal of Youth and Adolescence* 39(10): 1175–1188.

McLaughlin, K. A., M. L. Hatzenbuehler, and K. M. Keyes. 2010. "Responses to Discrimination and Psychiatric Disorders among Black, Hispanic, Female, and Lesbian, Gay, and Bisexual Individuals." *American Journal of Public Health* 100(8): 1477–1484.

Melendez, R. M., and R. M. Pinto. 2009. "HIV Prevention and Primary Care for Transgender Women in a Community-Based Clinic." *Journal of the Association of Nurses in AIDS Care* 20(5): 387–397.

Meyer, I. H. 2003. "Prejudice, Social Stress, and Mental Health in Lesbian, Gay, and Bisexual Populations: Conceptual Issues and Research Evidence." *Psychological Bulletin* 129: 674–697.

Meyer, I. H., M. E. Northridge, eds. 2007. *The Health of Sexual Minorities: Public Health Perspectives on Lesbian, Gay, Bisexual and Transgender Populations.* New York, NY: Springer.

Meyer, W., W. O. Bockting, P. Cohen-Kettenis, E. Coleman, D. DiCeglie, H. Devor, and C. Wheeler. 2001. "The Harry Benjamin International Gender Dysphoria Association's Standards of Care for Gender Identity Disorders, Sixth Version." *Journal of Psychology and Human Sexuality* 13(1): 1.

Mimiaga, M., H. Goldhammer, C. Belanoff, A. Tetu, and K. Mayer. 2007. "Men Who Have Sex with Men: Perceptions about Sexual Risk, HIV and Sexually Transmitted Disease Testing, and Provider Communication." *Sexually Transmitted Diseases* 34(2): 113–119.

Mustanski, B., R. Garofalo, A. Herrick, and G. Donenberg. 2007. "Psychosocial Health Problems Increase Risk for HIV among Urban Young Men Who Have Sex with Men: Preliminary Evidence of a Syndemic in Need of Attention." *Annals of Behavioral Medicine* 34: 37–45.

Neville, S., and M. Henrickson. 2006. "Perceptions of Lesbian, Gay and Bisexual People of Primary Healthcare Services." *Journal of Advanced Nursing* 55(4): 407–415.

Pachankis, J. E., and L. Bernstein. 2012. "An Etiological Model of Anxiety in Young Gay Men: From Early Stress to Public Self-Consciousness." *Psychology of Men and Masculinity* 13: 107–122.

Pachankis, J. E., and M. R. Goldfried. 2006. "Social Anxiety in Young Gay Men." *Journal of Anxiety Disorders* 20: 996–1015.

Pachankis, J. E., M. R. Goldfried, and M. Ramrattan. 2008. "Extension of the Rejection Sensitivity Construct to the Interpersonal Functioning of Gay Men." *Journal of Consulting and Clinical Psychology* 76: 306–317.

Pachankis, J. E. and J. L. Westmaas, and L. R. Dougherty. 2011. "The Influence of Sexual Orientation and Masculinity on Young Men's Tobacco Smoking." *Journal of Consulting and Clinical Psychology* 79: 142–152.

Pantalone, D. W., D. S. Bimbi, C. A. Holder, S. A. Golub, and J. T. Parsons. 2010. "Consistency and Change in Club Drug Use by Sexual Minority Men in New York City, 2002 to 2007." *American Journal of Public Health* 100(10): 1892–1895.

Pantalone, D. W., D. M. Hessler, and J. M. Simoni. 2010. "Mental Health Pathways from Interpersonal Violence to Health-Related Outcomes in HIV-Positive Sexual Minority Men." *Journal of Consulting and Clinical Psychology* 78: 387–397.

Pantalone, D. W., G. Y. Iwamasa, and C. R. Martell. 2009. "Adapting Cognitive-Behavioral Therapies to Diverse Populations." *Handbook of Cognitive-Behavioral Therapies* (3rd ed.), edited by K. S. Dobson, 445–464. New York, NY: Guilford Press.

Perdue, T., H. Hagan, H. Thiede, and L. Valleroy. 2003. "Depression and HIV Risk Behavior among Seattle-Area Injection Drug Users and Young Men Who Have Sex with Men." *AIDS Education and Prevention* 15: 81–92.

Phillips, J. and C. Patsdaughter. 2010. "Toward a Healthier Tomorrow: Competent Health and HIV Care for Transgender Persons." *Journal of the Association of Nurses in AIDS Care* 21(3): 183–185.

Pitts, M. K., M. Couch, H. Mulcare, S. Croy, and A. Mitchell. 2009. "Transgender People in Australia and New Zealand: Health, Wellbeing and Access to Health Services." *Feminism and Psychology* 19(4): 475–495.

Pizacani, B. A., K. Rohde, C. Bushore, M. J. Stark, J. E. Maher, J. A. Dilley, and M. J. Boysun. 2009. "Smoking-Related Knowledge, Attitudes and Behaviors in the Lesbian, Gay and Bisexual Community: A Population-Based Study from the U.S. Pacific Northwest." *Preventive Medicine* 48(6): 555–561.

Pleak, R. R. 2009. "Formation of Transgender Identities in Adolescence." *Journal of Gay and Lesbian Mental Health* 13(4): 282–291.

Prabawanti, C., L. Bollen, R. Palupy, G. Morineau, P. Girault, D. Mustikawati, and R. Magnani. 2011. "HIV, Sexually Transmitted Infections, and Sexual Risk Behavior among Transgenders in Indonesia." *AIDS and Behavior* 15(3): 663–673.

Reisner, S. L., M. J. Mimiaga, S. A. Safren, and K. H. Mayer. 2009. "Stressful or Traumatic Life Events, Post-Traumatic Stress Disorder (PTSD) Symptoms, and HIV Sexual Risk Taking among Men Who Have Sex with Men." *AIDS Care* 21: 1481–1489.

Reisner, S. L., B. Perkovich, and M. J. Mimiaga. 2010. "Mixed Methods Study of the Sexual Health Needs of New England Transmen Who Have Sex with Non-transgender Men." *AIDS Patient Care and STDs* 24(8): 501–513.

Riggs, D. W. and G. R. Fell. 2010. "Teaching Cultural Competency for Working with Lesbian, Gay, Bisexual, and Trans Clients." *Psychology Learning and Teaching* 9(1): 30–38.

Risser, J. H., A. Shelton, S. McCurdy, P. Padgett, J. Atkinson, B. Useche, and M.Williams. 2005. "Sex, Drugs, Violence, and HIV Status among Male-to-Female Transgender Persons in Houston, Texas." *International Journal of Transgenderism* 8(2/3): 67–74.

Rosario, M., E. W. Schrimshaw, and J. Hunter. 2008. "Butch/Femme Differences in Substance Use and Abuse among Young Lesbian and Bisexual Women: Examination and Potential Explanations." *Substance Use and Misuse* 43: 1002–1015.

Rosario, M., E. W. Schrimshaw, J. Hunter, and L. Braun. 2006. "Sexual Identity Development among Lesbian, Gay, and Bisexual Youths: Consistency and Change over Time." *Journal of Sex Research* 43: 46–58.

Rosser, B., J. Oakes, W. O. Bockting, and M. Miner. 2007. "Capturing the Social Demographics of Hidden Sexual Minorities: An Internet Study of the Transgender Population in the United States." *Sexuality Research and Social Policy* 4(2): 50–64.

Rotheram-Borus, M. J., M. Rosario, H. Reid, and C. Koopman. 1995. "Predicting Patterns of Sexual Acts among Homosexual and Bisexual Youths." *The American Journal of Psychiatry* 152: 588–595.

Ryan, C., S. T. Russell, D. Huebner, R. Diaz, and J. Sanchez. 2010. "Family Acceptance in Adolescence and the Health of LGBT Young Adults." *Journal of Child and Adolescent Psychiatric Nursing* 23(4): 205–213.

Safren, S. A. and R. G. Heimberg. 1999. "Depression, Hopelessness, Suicidality, and Related Factors in Sexual Minority and Heterosexual Adolescents." *Journal of Consulting and Clinical Psychology* 67(6): 859–866.

Sanchez, N., J. Rabatin, J. Sanchez, S. Hubbard, and A. Kalet. 2006. "Medical Students' Ability to Care for Lesbian, Gay, Bisexual, and Transgendered Patients." *Family Medicine* 38(1): 21–27.

Sanchez, N. F., J. P. Sanchez, and A. Danoff. 2009. "Health Care Utilization, Barriers to Care, and Hormone Usage among Male-to-Female Transgender Persons in New York City." *American Journal of Public Health* 99(4): 713–719.

Sandfort, T. G., R. de Graaf, R. V. Bijl, and P. Schnabel. 2001. "Same-Sex Sexual Behavior and Psychiatric Disorders: Findings from the Netherlands Mental Health Survey and Incidence Study (NEMESIS)." *Archives of General Psychiatry* 58: 85–91.

Schuster, M., R. Collins, W. Cunningham, S. Morton, S. Zierler, M. Wong, and D. Kanouse. 2005. "Perceived Discrimination in Clinical Care in a Nationally Representative Sample of HIV-Infected Adults Receiving Health Care." *Journal of General Internal Medicine* 20(9): 807–813.

Scott, S. D., A. Pringle, and C. Lumsdaine. 2004. *Sexual Exclusion—Homophobia and Health Inequalities: A Review of Health Inequalities and Social Exclusion Experienced by Lesbian, Gay, and Bisexual People.* http://www.glhv.org.au/files/gmhn_report.pdf

Shipherd, J. C., K. E. Green, and S. Abramovitz. 2010. "Transgender Clients: Identifying and Minimizing Barriers to Mental Health Treatment." *Journal of Gay and Lesbian Mental Health* 14(2): 94–108.

Singer, M. and S. Clair. 2003. "Syndemics and Public Health: Reconceptualizing Disease in Biosocial Context." *Medical Anthropology Quarterly* 17(4): 423–441.

Stall, R., T. C. Mills, J. Williamson, T. Hart, G. Greenwood, J. Paul, and J. A. Catania. 2003. "Association of Co-Occurring Psychosocial Health Problems and Increased Vulnerability to HIV/AIDS among Urban Men Who Have Sex with Men." *American Journal of Public Health* 93: 939–942.

Stephens, S. C., K. T. Bernstein, and S. S. Philip. 2011. "Male to Female and Female to Male Transgender Persons Have Different Sexual Risk Behaviors Yet Similar Rates of STDs and HIV." *AIDS and Behavior* 15(3): 683–686.

Sugano, E., T. Nemoto, and D. Operario. 2006. "The Impact of Exposure to Transphobia on HIV Risk Behavior in a Sample of Transgendered Women of Color in San Francisco." *AIDS and Behavior* 10(2): 217–224.

Thornhill, L. and P. Klein, P. 2010. "Creating Environments of Care with Transgender Communities." *Journal of the Association of Nurses in AIDS Care* 21(3): 230–239.

Trocki, K. F., L. A. Drabble, and L. T. Midanik. 2009. "Tobacco, Marijuana, and Sensation Seeking: Comparisons across Gay, Lesbian, Bisexual, and Heterosexual Groups." *Psychology of Addictive Behaviors* 23: 620–631.

U.S. Department of Health and Human Services, Office of Disease Prevention and Health Promotion. 2013. *Healthy People 2020.* http://www.healthypeople.gov/2020/topicsobjectives2020/overview.aspx?topicId=25

Vanderleest, J. G., and C. Q. Galper. 2009. "Improving the Health of Transgender People: Transgender Medical Education in Arizona." *Journal of the Association of Nurses in AIDS Care* 20(5): 411–416.

Wester, S. R., T. A. McDonough, M. White, D. L. Vogel, and L. Taylor. 2010. "Using Gender Role Conflict Theory in Counseling Male-to-Female Transgender Individuals." *Journal of Counseling and Development* 88: 214–219.

Wilkerson, J., S. Rybicki, C. A. Barber, and D. J. Smolenski. 2011. "Creating a Culturally Competent Clinical Environment for LGBT Patients." *Journal of Gay and Lesbian Social Services: The Quarterly Journal of Community and Clinical Practice* 23(3): 376–394.

Willging, C., M. Salvador, and M. Kano. 2006. "Brief Reports: Unequal Treatment: Mental Health Care for Sexual and Gender Minority Groups in a Rural State." *Psychiatric Services* 57(6): 867–870.

Wilson, E. C., R. Garofalo, D. Harris, and M. Belzer. 2010. "Sexual Risk Taking among Transgender Male-to-Female Youths with Different Partner Types." *American Journal of Public Health* 100(8): 1500–1505.

Wilson, E., R. Garofalo, R. Harris, A. Herrick, M. Martinez, J. Martinez, and M. Belzer. 2009. "Transgender Female Youth and Sex Work: HIV Risk and a Comparison of Life Factors Related to Engagement in Sex Work." *AIDS and Behavior* 13(5): 902–913.

CHAPTER NINE

Childhood Obesity and Cultural Influences

Jacqueline Woods, Stephen K. Trapp, and Marilyn Stern

Rates of obesity in children and adults have reached levels that call for public health alarm. More concerning is that these rates have increased across all race, ethnic, gender, and age groups. Minority individuals face a greater risk for overweight and obesity than their Caucasian counterparts (Franko and George 2009). As obesity has a strong correlation with lifelong health, health care providers are often seen as a "first line of defense" in dealing with obese individuals. In the same manner that providers must consider multicultural nuances (e.g., cultural health, beliefs, and practices) in treatments for other disorders, health care providers must also operate within a culturally valid framework when treating childhood obesity. Despite the good intentions of a health care provider, providing recommendations that contradict the cultural beliefs of patients may impede adherence to the recommended health-related behaviors and practices for overweight children and their caregivers. Increasing an understanding of cultural differences and maintaining a commitment to lifelong learning about the intersection of culture and health can aid health care professionals in tailoring treatment plans that respect the beliefs of their patients, foster effective patient-provider communication, and ultimately improve child health outcomes.

This chapter examines childhood obesity within the intersection of several sociocultural contexts. The relationship between each of these identities and health behaviors is not orthogonal; meaning, it is not useful to examine the effect of class, race, gender, religion, and culture separately on health behaviors because such an analysis would obscure the combined effect of each of those identities. Instead, we examine how these identities work in combination to better understand minority patients' health beliefs and behaviors. Using an intersectionality framework is appropriate for studying childhood obesity in minority communities because it examines the ways in which several socially constructed identities act in concert to drive systematic social and health disparities (Collins 2000). The purpose of examining obesity prevalence rates across minority groups is not to contradict the significance of obesity in Caucasian adults and children (Franko and George 2009), but rather to bring attention to systemic sociocultural factors that may be driving differential rates among ethnic and racial groups. Critical examinations of obesity must consider culture as a proximal variable because culture shapes many obesogenic factors such as food preferences, food preparation, attitudes toward diet and exercise, and body image (Kumanyika 2008).

In this chapter, we provide an overview of the prevalence of obesity within the United States, as well as the effects of obesity on physical and psychological health. We also review the ways in which cultural beliefs and sociocultural factors affect eating behaviors, physical activity, and body image within several ethnic minority groups. While the focus of this chapter is to provide education on multicultural implications regarding childhood obesity, we also discuss cultural beliefs among minority adults as these messages are likely transmitted to children by caregivers and adults in the larger community. Moreover, we take the perspective that understanding cultural health beliefs will facilitate effective communication between healthcare providers and caregivers of obese children. We therefore review and examine these health messages to provide health care professionals with culturally relevant tools to integrate into their treatment and prevention of obesity in minority children.

Prevalence of Obesity in the United States

Obesity is classified by Body Mass Index (BMI), which is computed based on height and weight. For children and adolescents obesity is defined as having a BMI above the 95th percentile for one's age and gender (Daniels 2009, Flegal et al. 2012). Data from the 2010 National Health Examination Survey (NHANES) indicate that the prevalence of overweight and obesity among U.S. adult men is 35.5 percent and 36.3 percent for adult women (Flegal et al. 2012). Among American children and adolescents, the prevalence of being overweight and obesity has tripled since 1980 (Ogden et al. 2010). Data from the 2010 NHANES indicate that 16.9 percent of children aged 2–19 had body mass index levels within the obese range (Flegal et al. 2012), an increase from 11.9 percent of the children surveyed in the 2008 NHANES study (Ogden et al. 2010).

While the focus of this chapter is on obesity in minority children, it is important to consider obesity trends among adults. Prevalence rates suggest that adult obesity is common in minority communities, and it is likely that obese children may have obese parents or other family members. Parental weight is associated with child weight status (Strauss and Knight 1999) and child weight loss (Hunter, Steele, and Steele 2008), and is therefore important to consider when discussing the treatment and prevention of childhood obesity. Data from the 2010 NHANES research indicate that minority individuals had the highest rates of obesity: 49.6 percent of African American adults and 37.9 percent of Hispanic adults surveyed had BMI scores within the obese range. The obesity prevalence rate among Caucasian adults was 34.9 percent. Considering race and gender together, African American women face the highest risk for obesity at 58.6 percent (Flegal et al. 2012). However, compared to African American and Hispanic adults, Asian/Pacific Islander and American Indian adults have relatively higher rates of obesity. Data collected from the Racial and Ethnic Approaches to Community Health 2010 Risk Factor survey indicate that approximately 42.2 percent of American Indian men and 36.7 percent of American Indian women are obese. Additionally, 30.5 percent of Asian and Pacific Islander men and 3.3 percent of Asian and Pacific Islander women are obese (CDC 2004). Considering these results together, obesity is prevalent among adults in minority communities.

Similar to trends seen in adults, significant differences in the prevalence of obesity have been found as a function of race and ethnicity among African American, Hispanic, and Caucasian children. Data from the 2010 NHANES research estimate that Hispanic and African American children are more likely to be obese than their Caucasian peers (Flegal et al. 2012). Almost one fourth (24.3 percent) of African American children were obese, compared to 21.2 percent of Hispanic and 14 percent of Caucasian children. Gender differences in the prevalence of obesity are also seen in children. Among all racial and ethnic groups surveyed, 18.6 percent of male children had BMI percentiles within the obese range compared to 15.8 percent of female children. Examining race and gender together, both male and female African American children and Hispanic males have the highest rates of obesity, at 24.3 percent. Prevalence rates are lowest among Caucasian female children and are found to be 11.7 percent of the population

(Flegal et al. 2012). Data from U.S. adolescents enrolled in the National Longitudinal Study of Adolescent Health Add Health Survey indicate 22.8 percent of Asian males and 10.3 percent of Asian females were obese (Gordon-Larsen, Adair, and Popkin 2003). Considering that 26.5 percent of Caucasian, 25.5 percent of African American, and 27.7 percent of Hispanic boys and 22.2 percent of Caucasian, 38 percent of African American, and 29.6 percent of Hispanic girls were overweight, prevalence rates among Asian American adolescents in the Add Health sample is relatively low compared to their peers (Gordon-Larsen et al. 2003).

Data on obesity prevalence rates within Asian American samples should be interpreted with caution in light of research indicating that in many Asian populations individuals have higher percentage body fat than Caucasians at the same BMI (Consultation 2004). Such findings indicate that the relation between BMI and percentage body fat varies across ethnic groups; the World Health Organization encourages using lower BMI cut off points for determining obesity with Asian individuals (Consultation 2004). Finally, within the literature, research on the prevalence of obesity in American-Indian children is sparse because many national surveys (such as the NHANES and Add Health surveys reviewed above) exclude this population due to small sample size (Story, Sherwood, Himes, Davis, Jacobs, Cartwright, and Rochon 2003). One study of over 13,000 school aged American Indian children living on or near reservations in the Midwest found that obesity prevalence rates were high: 39.1 percent and 38 percent for males and female respectively (Zephier, Himes, and Story 1999). In summary, childhood obesity is prevalent among minority American youth, and no gender or ethnic community seems to be "free" from this health issue.

Obesity and Health

The childhood obesity epidemic warrants serious attention due to significant physical risks associated with pediatric obesity in childhood and into adulthood. Compared to their healthy-weight peers, overweight and obese individuals have an increased risk of developing type 2 diabetes, asthma, and sleep apnea (CDC 2009). Obese children also have a greater likelihood of remaining obese into adulthood (CDC 2009). Further, overweight and obese children are also more likely to have elevated blood pressure, insulin, and cholesterol levels, putting them at risk for developing premature cardiovascular disease (Deckelbaum and Williams, 2001, Freedman, Dietz, Srinivasan, and Berenson, 1999). Developing these health problems in childhood puts obese children and adolescents at greater risk for major health problems and chronic diseases as they age (Franko and George 2009).

Additionally, obese children are likely to remain obese into adulthood (Reilly et al. 2003). One study tracking the weight status of obese children into young adulthood found that 69 percent of obese 6 to 9 year olds, 85 percent of obese 10 to 14 year olds, and 77 percent of obese 15–17 year olds remained obese into adulthood (Whitaker et al. 1997). Childhood obesity warrants attention from health care providers in order to mitigate the immediate health impacts, and also to prevent the long term health consequences associated with obesity.

Pediatric obesity is also associated with detrimental effects to the child's psychosocial well-being. Compared to their healthy weight peers, obese children exhibit lower self-esteem and other indicators of quality of life, usually associated with social stigmatization and teasing. Additionally, experiencing weight-related teasing is a significant predictor of the quality of life of obese children (Stern et al. 2006). Eisenberg and colleagues (2003) well as others (Porter et al. in press) have found that adolescents who experienced weight-based teasing from peers and family members were likely to endorse low body satisfaction, low-self-esteem, and depressive symptoms, including suicidal ideation.

Obesity is associated with poor physical and psychological health outcomes in childhood and adulthood. While working with caregivers to treat obese children, it is important that health professionals provide culturally relevant treatments to their patients. One way for health providers to foster culturally relevant dialogue is to recognize that minority parents may encourage different developmental outcomes than those espoused by mainstream culture (Ogbu 1985). Minority caregivers may be operating from different cultural imperatives, which may value different ethno-theories (e.g., cultural models that provide frameworks for social behaviors, such as parenting (Keller et al. 2006)) and competencies than the dominant culture (Ogbu 1985). Remaining aware of these cultural differences in health behaviors can help health care professionals improve patient-provider communication and child health outcomes.

Patient-Provider Communication

Patients' perception of how they may be treated by health care providers shape weight management health behaviors, and may exacerbate the poor health outcomes associated with obesity. The stigma associated with overweight in our society (Puhl and Brownell 2001) may impede obese individuals from seeking services from medical providers, making it more difficult for obese individuals to manage their weight in healthy ways (O'Dea 2005). For overweight and obese adults, fears about negative interactions, shaming, and weight prejudice from health care professionals may make some less likely to visit doctors for preventive screenings and routine care (O'Dea 2005). Research on patient-physician communication has validated some of obese patients' fears; one study found that health providers were likely to hold negative attitudes toward obese patients, viewing them as lazy or possessing little self-control (Price et al. 1987). Additionally, doctors' self-report of respect held toward obese patients has been found to be negatively associated with patient BMI (Huizinga et al. 2009). It is likely that obese children may internalize similar attitudes, learning to dread and avoid interactions with doctors for fear of being lectured about their weight, and continuing the cycle of neglecting preventive care across generations. To facilitate effective communication between obese pediatric patients and their caregivers, health care professionals should be sensitive to feelings of shame, guilt, or trepidation obese patients may experience.

Framing rising obesity rates as a "social problem" and an "epidemic" may also encourage obese children and adults to adopt drastic, quick fix behaviors in order to control their weight (Schwartz and Henderson 2009). O'Dea (2005) cautions that even well intentioned messages from concerned health care providers may be misunderstood and misconstrued, leading to the development of disordered weight control behaviors such as vomiting, laxative abuse, and cigarette smoking to control weight. Shifting the focus of lifestyle interventions from weight to overall health and fitness can help facilitate health behavior change without shaming obese patients (Bean et al. 2011, Wickham et al. 2009). Ultimately, being aware of cultural beliefs and attitudes that shape patients' health behaviors will foster effective patient-provider communication by ensuring that the patient feels the health professional respects his or her cultural beliefs. For this reason, we present a review of cultural correlates of physical inactivity, dietary patterns, and body image in minority cultures to give health care providers tools for engaging in culturally relevant conversations with obese pediatric patients and their caregivers.

Physical Inactivity

Physical inactivity has been repeatedly cited as a significant predictor of poor long-term health, including obesity in children (Blair 2009, Cecchini et al. 2010, Hallal et al. 2006). In general, it has been found that children in the United States are not meeting the criteria for optimal levels of physical activity (Gordon-Larsen, Nelson, and Popkin 2004, Nelson et al. 2006) and compared to non-Hispanic Caucasians, high rates of inactivity and excessive sedentary behaviors are greater among ethnic minorities (Eaton et al. 2008, Whitt-Glover et al. 2009). Specifically, a recent review article noted that Mexican Americans, followed by American Indian/Alaskan Natives, and African Americans had the highest rates of physical inactivity during leisure-time (Kurian and Cardarelli 2007). Considering these high rates of inactivity, as well as the noted disparity in obesity prevalence rates, it is imperative that greater examination of the cross-cultural trends of physical inactivity and the construction of culturally valid behavioral weight-management interventions are undertaken (Evans al. 2009).

Conceptualizing the etiology for the high rates of physical inactivity in children include a variety of interacting factors, including ecological considerations (Sallis and Kerr 2006) and social cognitive variables, such as self-regulation, social support, and cultural beliefs (Anderson et al. 2006, Caperchione, Kolt, and Mummery 2009). Ecological models offer explanations regarding how elements in the environment either promote or hinder physical activity (Sallis and Glanz 2009). Specifically, four environmental settings have been proposed to account for the variance of increased or decreased physical activity: occupational, recreational, transportation, and household environments. For example, it was found that the way a recreational environment is set up, such as the design of a public park, can influence an individual's level of physical exertion. Floyd and colleagues (2008) noted that greater physical exertion occurred in parks featuring tennis and basketball courts, while parks featuring picnic shelters and baseball/softball fields were associated with lower physical exertion. Other environmental considerations include occupational-related physical activity, such as school environments that demand a great amount of desk time (e.g., schools with limited physical education and recess). These environmental characteristics provide insight into an individual's normative level of activity and highlight ecological variables that may be creating barriers to healthy physical activity. Conversely, this understanding also allows for opportunities to increase physical activity in daily behaviors, such as choosing to play at a park that contains high exertion activity spaces. Opportunities for physical activity range in settings that include the home, neighborhood, school, and other places that the child frequents. It is appropriate to consider the ecological differences experienced by ethnic minority patients, as they likely play a role in their level of physical activity.

Although physical environment may account for some of the variance accounting for the rise in sedentary behaviors, social cognitive variables have also been found to help explain an individual's reasons to engage (or not engage) in physical activity (Eyler al. 2003, Schwarzer et al. 2008). Specifically, cultural beliefs and attitudes have been found to relate to levels of physical activity, willingness to exercise, and level of health literacy (Caperchione et al. 2009, Crespo et al. 2000, D'Alonzo and Fischetti 2008, Kafatos et al., 1999). Attitudes regarding a concern about perspiration, disheveled hair, and disturbed make-up were found as main reasons for not exercising in a qualitative study of middle school African American and Latino girls (Stern et al. 2006, Taylor et al. 2000).

Cultural messages, such as exercise beliefs and health beliefs, may reinforce these "reasons" for sedentary behavior and are therefore important to integrate into children's clinical care. Beliefs and attitudes associated with cultural and ethnic identity have also been examined as barriers to physical activity (Harrison, Lee, and Belcher 1999). Specifically, culturally derived preferences regarding physical activities (e.g., walking, team sports), appearance (e.g., hair, body shape), and weight control practices (e.g., dieting, eating habits) have been cited as identity-based factors for physical activity in ethnic minority girls (Airhihenbuwa et al. 1995). Consequently some activities may be more congruent with a child's ethnic identity, such as a valued community activity or sport, and therefore be considered more appropriate to engage in as a means for physical activity. This can both increase and decrease physical activity depending on the culturally-valued activity. For example, it is found that Latino boys receive culturally transmitted messages encouraging playing soccer, while Latino girls tend to be discouraged from engaging in soccer (Evenson et al. 2002). Work has been done for a number of years examining trends, preferences of and participation in physical activities according to variables such as ethnicity, gender, and socioeconomic status (Greendorfer and Ewing 1981). Culturally-based identity values associated with physical activity, or inactivity, have been identified. For example, greater time is spent by Asian Americans on home-based educational practices, such as taking extra time on studying and homework, while greater time is spent in faith-based activities by African Americans, and greater time is spent on home-based family activities, such as eating and chores, in Latino homes (Hofferth and Sandberg 2001). As there is wide variability of behaviors that are congruent with a patient's cultural and ethnic identity, querying a patient for activities most salient to his or her cultural identity and providing education about related activities can increase the effectiveness of patient-provider communication.

Social class has also been associated with physical inactivity in both adults and children (Allison 1996, Epstein et al. 1996, Winkleby et al. 1998, 1999). Because of the high prevalence of ethnic minorities that share a lower socioeconomic status (SES), some research has indicated that it may be more common to encounter SES-related constraints on physical activity in ethnic minority groups (Goran, Reynolds, and Lindquist 1999,

Kington and Smith 1997, National Heart, Lung, and Blood and Institute 1995). However, varying reasons for the role of SES and physical inactivity in ethnic minority groups have been found. In one study, SES has been found to moderate the association between race/ethnicity and inactivity, in which education level, family income, and marital status qualified the relationship (Marshall et al. 2007). Other research casts doubt upon whether current indicators of SES adequately explain low rates of physical activity in ethnic minorities (Crespo et al. 2000). Specifically, co-varying constructs, such as acculturation and ecological variables related to SES, are often left unaccounted for in traditional SES studies. For example, in a sample of Latino and Asian-American adolescents, acculturation was related to lower frequency of physical activity and other unhealthy behaviors (Unger et al. 2004). The authors offered explanations that ranged from wanting to play like an "American," by engaging in sedentary activities (e.g., video games, watching television), as well as some ecological variables, namely unsafe neighborhoods and environments lacking resources that promote physical activity. Sedentary activity among obese minority children can be explained in part by social cognitive and ecological factors. Remaining aware of these sociocultural determinants of physical inactivity can help health care providers working with obese minority patients and their caregivers to encourage physical activity in culturally valid ways.

Eating Behaviors

Nutrition and Cultural Eating Behaviors

In addition to regular physical activity, a healthy diet, consisting of portion controlled nutritious meals, is considered a primary factor in preventing childhood obesity (Krebs and Jacobson 2003). Unfortunately, poor nutrition and unhealthy eating behaviors have been cited as a primary factor in childhood obesity rates in ethnic minority groups (Kumanyika and Grier 2006). Culture has been considered a primary factor informing individuals' eating behaviors (Axelson 1986, Mintz and Du Bois 2002, Murcott 1988). Cultural eating is defined as the eating beliefs, values, and customs related to the multiple, and interacting, components of one's identified culture. Cultural eating can be considered the traditional foods and eating behaviors found to commonly occur within a specified culture. In light of the prominent role of culture in the healthy nutritional choices made by ethnic minority groups, understanding the role of dietary acculturation as well as the traditional cultural norms of minority groups is critical.

As non-Western individuals immigrate to Western countries, dietary acculturation, or the acceptance of the host country's food practices is common. Dietary acculturation is considered to occur in a non-linear path in which an immigrant group, characterized and influenced by a variety of socioeconomic, demographic, and cultural factors, become immersed in a host culture (Satia-Abouta et al. 2002). Once imbedded in the host culture, the immigrant group experiences changes in psychosocial factors (e.g., changes in dietary values, changes in nutritional knowledge), as well as changes in environmentally based food options. The intersection of traditional food values and the host culture's values alter overall food attitudes and behaviors.

Unfortunately, acculturation into the United States has been cited as a predictive factor of poorer diet choices associated with higher levels of acculturation (Ayala, Baquero, and Klinger 2008, Lin, Bermudez, and Tucker 2003, Satia-Abouta et al. 2002). In a systematic review of the literature pertaining to Latino immigrants, it was found that less acculturated individuals ate more culturally-traditional and healthier foods (e.g., fruit, grains, legumes), as well as fewer foods and beverages based on a high sugar content than individuals who reported greater levels of acculturation (Ayala et al. 2008). Furthermore, there is evidence to show that second generation Latino immigrants have higher intakes of monosaturated fat than the previous, often less acculturated generations (Monroe et al. 2003). In a Chinese-American immigrant sample, it was found that acculturated food behaviors were mainly influenced by cost and convenience (Satia et al. 2000). In other words, unhealthy, host culture food choices were based less on interest in the food, but chosen for practical reasons. Although much of these acculturated food behaviors are based on parent involvement with diet (i.e. primary grocery shopping, food preparation), food behaviors as a function of the level of acculturation of ethnic minority children have yielded similar results. In samples of Latino, African immigrant, Thai/Laos-born Hmong-American children, it was found that higher levels of acculturation predicted poor dietary choices, and consequently a greater likelihood of obesity and other food-related health problems (e.g., heart disease, diabetes) (Buscemi, Beech, and Relyea 2011, Mulasi-Pokhriyal et al. 2012). These findings may help guide the development of interventions that focus on the benefits of culture-of-origin food practices and provide education about the many unhealthy food practices associated with acculturated diets.

Unhealthy food choices have also been found in ethnic minorities who have been settled in the United States for multiple generations. For example, research has demonstrated that African American diets tend to be high in fat intake, and characterized by an underconsumption of vegetables and fruits (James 2009). Additionally, increased rates of consumption of beverages containing a high sugar content, such as corn syrup-based juices and other commercial products, has been linked to obesity in African American children (Lim et al. 2009). Reasons for unhealthy eating vary from contextual limitations to cultural practices. A study that included a large cohort of African Americans noted fewer opportunities for fresh vegetables and fruits in grocery stores located near the African American communities (Morland, Wing, and Roux 2002). Cultural behaviors, such as the symbolic importance of feeding family and friends, has also been cited as barriers to good nutrition (Bramble, Cornelius, and Simpson 2009). Understanding the contextual limitations and cultural behaviors may inform culturally and ecologically appropriate solutions, such as using family feeding as an opportunity to share nutritious meals.

Eating Disorders

Eating disorders are defined as a cluster of eating disturbances influenced by a distorted body image and often based on the intent to control weight (DSM-IV-TR 2000). These disorders include anorexia nervosa, bulimia nervosa, and binge eating disorder. The World Health Organization (WHO 2005) reported eating disorders to be the third leading chronic illness among adolescent girls in the United States. For some time, eating disorders were considered to be relegated to middle-upper class, Caucasian females (Bruch 1979), but epidemiological findings have begun to demonstrate cross-ethnic incidences at higher rates than once believed (Bisaga et al. 2005, Crago, Shisslak, and Estes 1996, Smolak and Striegel-Moore 2001). As cultural components, such as culturally-valued body shapes and sizes are considered meaningful factors in the etiology of eating disorders, scholars have asserted that acculturation and disordered eating can be attributed to the spread of western values (Rieger et al. 2001, Weiss 1995). More specifically, as non-Western based people integrate Western values into their cultural milieu, disordered eating has been found to increase. In a naturalistic experimental design, researchers exposed a sample of naïve Fijian schoolgirls to prolonged television exposure (Becker et al. 2002). Results demonstrated higher rates of disordered eating attitudes and behaviors post exposure, thus indicating that exposure to culturally endorsed images of beauty were shown to be a predictive factor in alterations of eating behavior.

Although the prevalence of anorexia nervosa and bulimia among ethnic minority groups is still relatively small, there is evidence for equal and higher rates of binge eating disorder among ethnic minorities compared to that of Caucasian Americans (Azarbad et al. 2010, Marques et al. 2011, Mazzeo, Saunders, and Mitchell 2005, Shaw et al. 2004). Binge eating is characterized by a lack of controlled eating, but unlike bulimia nervosa there are no associated weight limiting behaviors, such as purging or fasting

(NIMH 2012). Not unexpectedly, binge eating is highly comorbid with obesity (Blaine 2009). A recent study found lifetime prevalence rates for binge eating in a nationally representative sample of adolescents (N=10,123) to range from 2.4 percent for Hispanics, 1.5 percent for Non-Hispanic African Americans, 1.3 percent for other ethnic minorities, 0.7 percent for Caucasians (Swanson et al. 2011). These rates are only slightly lower than what is found in adult samples (Marques et al. 2011). Furthermore, it was found that the median age of onset for sub-threshold binge-eating disorder and diagnosable binge eating disorder occurred at 12.6 years of age with dramatic increases until early adulthood. These rates indicate that a critical prevention time point may occur before middle childhood and adolescence when the disorder begins to manifest.

Compared with other ethnic groups, binge eating has been found to be relatively common in African American children and Latino females compared to that of Caucasian and Asian American children (Croll et al. 2002, Johnson, Rohan, and Kirk 2002). Common disturbed eating behaviors related to binge eating include: inhibited eating, secretive eating, and overeating (Stice, Agras, and Hammer 1999). Inhibited eating is characterized by highly controlled and attentive eating; this often leads to later hunger and uncontrolled eating. Secretive eating is characterized by private eating, oftentimes done in bedrooms or late at night. It is not uncommon for secretive eaters to hide food in their rooms in order to eat unnoticed by others. Overly enjoying and excessively consuming a type of food, as well as loss of control while eating characterizes overeating. Vomiting post binge is not uncommon due to over eating. This can be mistaken for purging, but is behaviorally different, as overeating induces the vomiting—not a desire to control weight. Predictors of childhood binge eating include obesity, hunger, body dissatisfaction, maternal eating disinhibition, and paternal obesity. A meta-analysis also found similar predictors that included obesity, depression, body dissatisfaction, modeled disturbed eating behaviors, low self-esteem, low social support, and overvaluation of appearance (Stice 2002). These predictors may aid in the identification of patients that may be vulnerable to binge eating. However, clearly, a greater understanding of the multiple and interactive biopsychosocial factors involved is needed (Marcus and Kalarchian 2003).

Body Image

Body image refers to an individual's perception and appraisal of his or her body shape and size (Franko and George 2009). A related, but different construct, body dissatisfaction, refers to the discrepancy between one's perceived body weight, shape, or size and one's ideal body (Grabe and Hyde 2006). Body image can be shaped by a variety of factors including family, peers, and media images. Similar to physical activity and dietary patterns, body image satisfaction and dissatisfaction are strongly influenced by cultural norms. The dominate message in mainstream American culture is that being thin is ideal and beautiful for women and that muscular builds are desired for men; however, minority children may espouse different body ideals informed by their own cultural beliefs. Body image concerns affect all ethnic groups; environmental and cultural factors may protect some and put others at risk for developing eating pathology (Franko and George 2009).

There are conflicting findings in the literature about body satisfaction in African American women. Many assert that African American girls and women are more likely to endorse satisfaction at higher body weight than Caucasian women and girls and are less likely to endorse body dissatisfaction compared to women of other ethnic groups (Kelly, Bulik, and Mazzeo 2011, Ruiz, Pepper, and Wilfley 2004). In a sample of obese adolescent African American girls seeking weight management treatment, body satisfaction was found to partially mediate the association between teasing and self-esteem, and teasing and depression (Porter, in press). These data suggest that body satisfaction is relevant to the well-being of obese African American adolescents. However, overweight and obese African American women are less likely than other overweight women to correctly identify their weight status (Chandler-Laney et al. 2009), making it less likely that they will engage in healthy weight management behaviors. Compared to their Caucasian peers, African American male school-aged children (Thompson, Corwin, and Sargent 1997) and adolescents (Thompson, Sargent, and Kemper 1996) have been found to prefer larger body silhouettes. Differences in endorsement rates of body dissatisfaction between Caucasian and African American individuals may be influenced by the fact that beauty norms within the African American community may emphasize other factors besides weight, such as skin color, hair texture, or personality (Dawson-Andoh et al. 2011).

Similar to the literature on African American body image, research on body image within Hispanic cultures focuses mainly on comparisons to Caucasian norms (Grabe and Hyde 2006). Findings within the literature vary: some studies conclude that Hispanic women endorse lower levels of body dissatisfaction than Caucasian women (Franko and Herrera 1997) while others assert that Hispanic women and girls endorse body dissatisfaction at the same frequency as their Caucasian counterparts (Shaw et al. 2004). One study comparing body dissatisfaction among middle school aged girls found that Hispanic girls endorsed the highest rates of body dissatisfaction compared to their Caucasian and Asian peers (Robinson et al. 1996). Among Hispanic youth, studies have found no differences in the levels of body satisfaction endorsed between boys and girls (Mirza et al. 2011). While there is some discrepancy in the literature, the findings indicate that body image dissatisfaction is prevalent among Hispanic youth. This information is important for health care providers to assess because body image dissatisfaction has been associated with low self-esteem (Erickson, Hahn-Smith, and Smith 2009) and increased rates of disordered eating (Croll et al. 2002) among Hispanic youth.

The limited body of research on body satisfaction among Asian Americans is characterized by contradictory findings (Nouri, Hill, and Orrell-Valente 2011). Some research suggests that Asian Americans endorse body dissatisfaction at rates similar to Caucasian Americans (Nicdao, Hong, and Takeuchi 2007), whereas, other studies have reported that Asian Americans report lower levels of body dissatisfaction than their Caucasian counterparts (Gluck and Geliebter 2002). One study of over 900 middle school aged girls found that among those in the lowest weight quartile in the sample, Asian girls endorsed higher levels of body dissatisfaction compared to Caucasian and Hispanic peers (Robinson et al. 1996). In a study of over 4000 adolescents, Neumark-Stzainer and colleagues (2002) found that Asian American boys endorsed the lowest levels of body satisfaction and were the most likely to endorse chronic dieting compared to boys from other ethnic groups even though Asian Americans had the lowest prevalence rate of obesity in the sample. Overall, these findings suggest that body image dissatisfaction is common among Asian American youth and is important for health providers to consider when assessing risk for eating pathology and unhealthy weight management in obese patients.

Within the obesity and body image literature, the research on Native Americans is sparse. One study of over 2,000 school-aged Caucasian, Native American, and Hispanic children found that Native American boys endorsed the highest levels of body satisfaction compared to male peers. Female Native American children, however, endorsed wanting to be smaller than they currently perceived themselves to be at rates equivalent to those of Caucasian girls (Lynch et al. 2007). However, a study of school aged, urban Native American youth found that both girls and boys endorsed body dissatisfaction and a desire to be thinner; obese girls endorsed the highest levels of body dissatisfaction (Rinderknecht and Smith 2002). The experience of Native Americans is largely missing from the obesity literature (Story et al. 2003), and more research with this population in general is needed. Based on the existing research, body image dissatisfaction is common among Native American youth and is likely associated with their physical and psychological well-being. In light of this research, body image dissatisfaction, and its related problems of unhealthy weight management behaviors, are prevalent across ethic groups and warrant attention from health care providers.

Gender

One weakness of the obesity and body image literature is that the majority of research focuses on the experience of girls and women (Schwartz and Brownell 2004). One study of obese Asian and Latino youth found that the relationship between self-esteem and body dissatisfaction was stronger among girls compared to their male peers (Xie et al. 2010). In their meta-analysis of the literature, Cohane and Pope (2001) found that body image dissatisfaction was common among boys across ethnic backgrounds and was related to low self-esteem. In contrast to the findings with obese girls, the majority of obese boys' body dissatisfaction focused on a desire to be bigger, stronger, and more muscular, rather than being thin. The absence of research on the experience of obese men of color may reflect perceived cultural norms that lead some men to view overweight as evidence of masculinity and strength, rather than a health problem (Cash and Hicks 1990). Understanding the cultural context of size and weight as a perception of masculinity may provide an opportunity to counter these unhealthy beliefs by educating patients about the health risks of being overweight and obese.

Religion

Religion plays an important role in shaping body image. Some religious sects and denominations may downplay the importance of weight and encourage believers to focus on spiritual matters. However, other religious teachings emphasize that physical and spiritual health are intertwined, and encourage worshippers to make health and fitness a priority (Cline and Ferraro 2006). As is true for the obesity literature in general, research on the intersection of body image, obesity, religion, and other constructs related to one's cultural identity has primarily focused on the experience of women. One study of Muslim women found that women who wore veils and primarily non-Western clothing were less likely to endorse body dissatisfaction and more likely to endorse preference for larger body sizes than their peers who preferred to wear Western clothing. These authors suggested that religion and cultural dress customs served as protective factors against the internalization of the Western thin ideal (Dunkel, Davidson, and Qurashi 2010). Although relatively little research is available that examines these relations, religion has been identified as serving as a protective factor against the development of unhealthy weight control eating behavior for Christian women (Kim, Schulz, and Carver 2007) and as a significant influence on body image for African American Muslim women (Odoms-Young 2008) and Jewish women (Gluck and Geliebter 2002). Integrating the patient's spiritual values into treatment is one way health care providers can provide culturally relevant care to obese patients.

Acculturation

Level of acculturation has been found to be related to body image satisfaction. As noted above, acculturation is a nonlinear, multidimensional process that results when individuals from different cultures come into contact with each other. Over time, individuals internalize various aspects of mainstream culture and integrate the mainstream worldview with that of their own culture (Berry 1997). Considering the level of acculturation of obese minority patients may provide insight into the degree to which patients have internalized the Western thin ideal as well as suggest important information about their body image. Some researchers hypothesize that the loss of cultural heritage orientation, as subsequent generations acculturate to mainstream U.S. norms, may be associated with overweight and obesity; for example, increased acculturation is associated with increased sedentary activity (Wang et al. 2011). In a study of Hispanic and Asian youth, acculturation was found to mediate the relation between obesity and depressive symptoms for girls but not boys; girls with higher levels of acculturation were more likely to endorse body dissatisfaction and depressive symptoms (Xie et al. 2010). Additionally, difficulty learning to reconcile conflicting messages from the thin ideal of mainstream American culture and the body image ideals of specific minority cultures may lead some minority youth to develop body dissatisfaction, eating pathology (Franko and George 2009), and depression (Xie et al. 2010).

Examining body image satisfaction and dissatisfaction supplements medical knowledge of obesity by illuminating the psychosocial effects of obesity on children (Schwartz and Brownell 2004). Body dissatisfaction increases as weight increases, a trend true for those at the higher end of the BMI spectrum regardless of race. It is important for health care providers to remain aware of likely body image concerns among obese children because body dissatisfaction has been associated with poor health outcomes and behaviors, such as disordered eating behaviors to control weight. Culturally competent health care providers counseling minority patients about weight or eating behaviors should be mindful of the various sociocultural forces, such as race, gender, religion, and acculturation, informing patient body image in order to present health care recommendations to patients in a culturally relevant way.

Obesity Interventions

As childhood obesity has been deemed a critical public health concern in the United States, it is not surprising that researchers have begun constructing and testing interventions to attend to this problem (Daniels et al. 2009). With the etiology and maintenance of childhood obesity being multifactorial (e.g., diet, physical activity), identifying which components to address in interventions can be challenging. A recent meta-analysis of obesity interventions directed towards ethnic minority children revealed that the most effective interventions included approaching the patient with at least three components (Seo and Sa 2010). Efficacious components were found to include parental involvement, changes directed at overall lifestyle, culturally-tailored approaches, and use of new technology, such as computer and internet-based programming. Programs that emphasized parent involvement included teaching methods to provide optimal social support for the children, healthy food selection, and participation in the intervention sessions with the child (Sothern et al. 2002, Wilfley et al. 2007). Culturally-tailored programs included the use of same-race interventionists, and community faith-based approaches (Resnicow et al. 2005, Story et al. 2003). Programs that utilized new technology (e.g., internet applications, interactive computer programs) included online goal setting, nutrition monitoring, and lifestyle changes (Goran and Reynolds 2005, Williamson et al. 2005, 2006). A second systematic review of obesity prevention studies for children and adolescents found that programs characterized by time-limited treatment (i.e., no more than one year), held in school-based settings and emphasizing topics regarding diet and exercise, were most efficacious in preventing obesity. Specifically, 41 percent of the studies reviewed demonstrated a positive program effect (Flodmark, Marcus, and Britton 2006). Although the review was unable to conduct a formal meta-analysis, the trends indicate that children can benefit from prevention programs targeting obesity-related health behaviors. While the implementation of these programs can be challenging due to the resources necessary to initiate and sustain them, when properly constructed, programs targeting obese ethnic-minority children can be effective methods to attend to this public health crisis. Even at the individual level, health care providers armed with culturally relevant knowledge can serve as an effective "first line of defense" in treating and preventing childhood obesity.

References

Airhihenbuwa, C. O., S. Kumanyika, T. D. Agurs, and A. Lowe. 1995. "Perceptions and Beliefs about Exercise, Rest, and Health among African-Americans." *American Journal of Health Promotion* 9(6): 426–429.

Alegria, M., M. Woo, Z. Cao, M. Torres, X. Meng, and R. Striegel-Moore. 2007. "Prevalence and Correlates of Eating Disorders in Latinos in the United States." *International Journal of Eating Disorders* 40(S3): S15–S21.

Allison, K. 1996. "Predictors of Inactivity: An Analysis of the Ontario Health Survey." *Canadian Journal of Public Health. Revue Canadienne de Sant Publique* 87(5): 354–358.

American Psychiatric Association. 2000. *Diagnostic and Statistical Manual of Mental Disorders* (4th ed., text rev.). Washington, DC: Author.

Anderson, E. S., J. R. Wojcik, R. A. Winett, and D. M. Williams. 2006. "Social-Cognitive Determinants of Physical Activity: The Influence of Social Support, Self-Efficacy, Outcome Expectations, and Self-Regulation among Participants in a Church-Based Health Promotion Study." *Health Psychology* 25(4): 510–520.

Axelson, M. 1986. "The Impact of Culture on Food-Related Behavior." *Annual Review of Nutrition* 6(1): 345–363.

Ayala, G. X., B. Baquero, and S. Klinger. 2008. "A Systematic Review of the Relationship between Acculturation and Diet among Latinos in the United States: Implications for Future Research." *Journal of the American Dietetic Association* 108(8): 1330–1344.

Azarbad, L., J. Corsica, B. Hall, and M. Hood. 2010. "Psychosocial Correlates of Binge Eating in Hispanic, African American, and Caucasian Women Presenting for Bariatric Surgery." *Eating Behaviors* 11(2): 79–84.

Bean, M. K., S. E. Mazzeo, M. Stern, R. K. Evans, D. Bryan, Y. Ning, and J. Laver. 2011. "Six-Month Dietary Changes in Ethnically Diverse, Obese Adolescents Participating in a Multidisciplinary Weight Management Program." *Clinical Pediatrics* 50(5): 408–416.

Becker, A. E., R. A. Burwell, D. B. Herzog, P. Hamburg, and S. E. Gilman. 2002. "Eating Behaviours and Attitudes Following Prolonged Exposure to Television among Ethnic Fijian Adolescent Girls." *The British Journal of Psychiatry* 180(6): 509–514.

Berry, J. W. 1997. "Immigration, Acculturation, and Adaptation." *Applied Psychology* 46(1): 5–34.

Bisaga, K., A. Whitaker, M. Davies, S. Chuang, J. Feldman, and B. T. Walsh. 2005. "Eating Disorder and Depressive Symptoms in Urban High School Girls from Different Ethnic Backgrounds." *Journal of Developmental and Behavioral Pediatrics* 26(4): 257–266.

Blaine, B. E. 2009. "Obesity, Binge Eating, and Psychological Distress: The Moderating Role of Self-Concept Disturbance." *Current Psychiatry Reviews* 5(3): 175–181.

Blair, S. N. 2009. "Physical Inactivity: The Biggest Public Health Problem of the 21st Century." *British Journal of Sports Medicine* 43(1): 1–2.

Bramble, J., L. J. Cornelius, and G. Simpson. 2009. "Eating as a Cultural Expression of Caring among Afro-Caribbean and African American Women: Understanding the Cultural Dimensions of Obesity." *Journal of Health Care for the Poor and Uunderserved* 20(2S): 53–68.

Bruch, H. 1979. *Eating Disorders: Obesity, Anorexia Nervosa, and the Person Within.* Houston, TX: Basic Books.

Buscemi, J., B. M. Beech, and G. Relyea. 2011. "Predictors of Obesity in Latino Children: Acculturation as a Moderator of the Relationship between Food Insecurity and Body Mass Index Percentile." *Journal of Immigrant and Minority Health* 13(1): 149–154.

Caperchione, C. M., G. S. Kolt, and W. K. Mummery. 2009. "Physical Activity in Culturally and Linguistically Diverse Migrant Groups to Western Society: A Review of barriers, Enablers and Experiences." *Sports Medicine* 39(3): 167–177.

Cash, T. F., and K. L. Hicks. 1990. "Being Fat Versus Thinking Fat: Relationships with Body Image, Eating Behaviors, and Well-Being." *Cognitive Therapy and Research* 14(3): 327–341.

Cecchini, M., F. Sassi, J. A. Lauer, Y. Y. Lee, V. Guajardo-Barron, and D. Chisholm. 2010. "Tackling of Unhealthy Diets, Physical Inactivity, and Obesity: Health Effects and Cost-Effectiveness." *The Lancet* 376(9754): 1775–1784.

Centers for Disease Control and Prevention. 2004. *REACH 2010 Surveillance for Health Status in Minority Communities: United States, 1999–2002.* http://www.cdc.gov/mmwr/preview/mmwrhtml/ss5306a1.htm

Centers for Disease Control and Prevention. 2009. *Overweight and Obesity.* http://www.cdc.gov/obesity/childhood/index.html

Chandler-Laney, P. C., G. R. Hunter, J. D. Ard, J. L. Roy, D. W. Brock, and B. A. Gower. 2009. "Perception of Others' Body Size Influences Weight Loss and Regain for European American but Not African American Women." *Health Psychology* 28(4): 414–418.

Cline, K. and K. F. Ferraro. 2006. "Does Religion Increase the Prevalence and Incidence of Obesity in Adulthood?" *Journal for the Scientific Study of Religion* 45(2): 269–281.

Cohane, G. H. and H. G. Pope Jr. 2001. "Body Image in Boys: A Review of the Literature." *International Journal of Eating Disorders* 29(4): 373–379.

Collins, P. H. 2000. *Black Feminist Thought: Knowledge, Consciousness, and the Politics of Empowerment* (2nd ed.). New York: Routledge.

Consultation, W. E. 2004. "Appropriate Body-Mass Index for Asian Populations and Its Implications for Policy and Intervention Strategies." *Lancet* 363: 157–163.

Crago, M., C. M. Shisslak, and L. S. Estes. 1996. "Eating Disturbances among American Minority Groups: A Review." *International Journal of Eating Disorders* 19(3): 239–248.

Crespo, C. J., E. Smit, R. E. Andersen, O. Carter-Pokras, and B. E. Ainsworth. 2000. "Race/Ethnicity, Social Class and Their Relation to Physical Inactivity during Leisure Time: Results from the third National Health and Nutrition Examination Survey, 1988–1994." *American Journal of Preventive Medicine* 18(1): 46–53.

Croll, J., D. Neumark-Sztainer, M. Story, and M. Ireland. 2002. "Prevalence and Risk and Protective Factors Related to Disordered Eating Behaviors among Adolescents: Relationship to Gender and Ethnicity." *Journal of Adolescent Health* 31(2): 166–175.

D'Alonzo, K. T. and N. Fischetti, N. 2008. "Cultural Beliefs and Attitudes of Black and Hispanic College-Age Women toward Exercise." *Journal of Transcultural Nursing* 19(2): 175–183.

Daniels, S. R. 2009. "The Use of BMI in the Clinical Setting." *Pediatrics* 124(1S): S35–S41.

Daniels, S. R., M. S. Jacobson, B. W. McCrindle, R. H. Eckel, and B. M. H. Sanner. 2009. "American Heart Association Childhood Obesity Research Summit Executive Summary." *Circulation* 119(15): 2114–2123.

Dawson-Andoh, N. A., J. J. Gray, J. A. Soto, and S. Parker. 2011. "Body Shape and Size Depictions of African American Women in JET Magazine, 1953–2006." *Body Image* 8(1): 86–89.

Deckelbaum, R. J., and C. L. Williams. 2001. "Childhood Obesity: The Health Issue." *Obesity* 9: 239S–243S.

Dunkel, T. M., D. Davidson, and S. Qurashi. 2010. "Body Satisfaction and Pressure to be Thin in Younger and Older Muslim and Non-Muslim Women: The Role of Western and Non-Western Dress Preferences." *Body Image* 7(1): 56–65.

Eaton, D. K., L. Kann, S. Kinchen, S. Shanklin, J. Ross, J. Hawkins, and D. Chyen. 2008. "Youth Risk Behavior Surveillance—United States, 2007." *MMWR Surveillance Summaries* 57(4): 1–131.

Eisenberg, M. E., D. Neumark-Sztainer, and M. Story. 2003. "Associations of Weight-Based Teasing and Emotional Well-Being among Adolescents." *Archives of Pediatrics and Adolescent Medicine* 157(8): 733–738.

Epstein, L. H., R. A. Paluch, K. J. Coleman, D. Vito, and K. Anderson. 1996. "Determinants of Physical Activity in Obese Children Assessed by Accelerometer and Self-Report." *Medicine and Science in Sports and Exercise* 28(9): 1157–1164.

Erickson, S. J., A. Hahn-Smith, and J. E. Smith. 2009. "One Step Closer: Understanding the Complex Relationship between Weight and Self-Esteem in Ethnically Diverse Preadolescent Girls." *Journal of Applied Developmental Psychology* 30(2): 129–139.

Evans, R. K., R. Franco, M. Stern, E. P., Wickham, D. L. Bryan, J. E. Herrick, and J. H. Laver. 2009. "Evaluation of a 6-Month Multi-Disciplinary Healthy Weight Management Program Targeting Urban, Overweight Adolescents: Effects on

Physical Fitness, Physical Activity, and Blood Lipid Profiles." *International Journal of Pediatric Obesity* 4(3): 130–133.

Evenson, K. R., O. L. Sarmiento, M. L. Macon, K. W. Tawney, and A. S. Ammerman. 2002. "Environmental, Policy, and Cultural Factors Related to Physical Activity among Latina Immigrants." *Women and health* 36(2): 43–56.

Eyler, A. A., D. Matson-Koffman, D. R. Young, S. Wilcox, J. E. Wilbur, J. L. Thompson, and K. R. Evenson. 2003. "Quantitative Study of Correlates of Physical Activity in Women from Diverse Racial/Ethnic Groups: The Women's Cardiovascular Health Network Project Summary and Conclusions." *American Journal of Preventive Medicine* 25(3): 93–103.

Flegal, K. M., M. D. Carroll, B. K. Kit, and C. L. Ogden. 2012. "Prevalence of Obesity and Trends in the Distribution of Body Mass Index among U.S. Adults, 1999–2010." *The Journal of the American Medical Association* 307 (5): 491–497.

Flodmark, C. E., C. Marcus, and M. Britton. 2006. "Interventions to Prevent Obesity in Children and Adolescents: A Systematic Literature Review." *International Journal of Obesity* 30(4): 579–589.

Floyd, M. F., J. O. Spengler, J. E. Maddock, P. H. Gobster, and L. J. Suau. 2008. "Park-Based Physical Activity in Diverse Communities of Two U.S. Cities: An Observational Study." *American Journal of Preventive Medicine* 34(4): 299–305.

Franko, D. L., and J. B. E. George. 2009. "Overweight, Eating Behaviors, and Body Image in Ethnically Diverse Youth." In *Body Image, Eating Disorders, and Obesity in Youth: Assessment, Prevention, and Treatment,* edited by L. Smolak and J. K. Thompson, 97–112. Washington, D.C.: American Psychological Association.

Franko, D. L., and I. Herrera. 1997. "Body Image Differences in Guatemalan-American and White College Women." *Eating Disorders* 5(2): 119–127.

Freedman, D. S., W. H. Dietz, S. R. Srinivasan, and G. S. Berenson. 1999. "The Relation of Overweight to Cardiovascular Risk Factors among Children and Adolescents: The Bogalusa Heart Study." *Pediatrics* 103(6): 1175–1182.

Gluck, M. and A. Geliebter. 2002. "Body Image and Eating Behaviors in Orthodox and Secular Jewish Women." *The Journal of Gender-Specific Medicine* 5(1): 19–24.

Gluck, M. E. and A. Geliebter, A. 2002. "Racial/Ethnic Differences in Body Image and Eating Behaviors." *Eating Behaviors* 3(2): 143–151.

Goran, M. I., and K. Reynolds. 2005. "Interactive Multimedia for Promoting Physical Activity (IMPACT) in Children." *Obesity* 13(4): 762–771.

Goran, M. I., K. D. Reynolds, and C. H. Lindquist. 1999. "Role of Physical Activity in the Prevention of Obesity in Children." *International Journal of Obesity* 23: 18–33.

Gordon-Larsen, P., L. S. Adair, and B. M. Popkin. 2003. "The Relationship of Ethnicity, Socioeconomic Factors, and Overweight in U.S. Adolescents." *Obesity* 11(1): 121–129.

Gordon-Larsen, P., M. C. Nelson, and B. M. Popkin. 2004. "Longitudinal Physical Activity and Sedentary Behavior Trends: Adolescence to Adulthood." *American Journal of Preventive Medicine* 27(4): 277–283.

Grabe, S. and J. S. Hyde. 2006. "Ethnicity and Body Dissatisfaction among Women in the United States: A Meta-Analysis." *Psychological Bulletin* 132(4): 622.

Greendorfer, S. L. and M. E. Ewing. 1981. "Race and Gender Differences in Children." *Research Quarterly for Exercise and Sport* 52(3): 301–310.

Hallal, P. C., C. G. Victora, M. R. Azevedo, and J. C. K. Wells. 2006. "Adolescent Physical Activity and Health: A Systematic Review." *Sports Medicine* 36(12): 1019–1030.

Harrison, L. J., A. M. Lee, and D. Belcher. 1999. "Race and Gender Differences in Sport Participation as a Function of Self-Schema." *Journal of Sport and Social Issues* 23(3): 287–307.

Hofferth, S. L. and J. F. Sandberg. 2001. "How American Children Spend Their Time." *Journal of Marriage and Family* 63(2): 295–308.

Huizinga, M. M., L. A. Cooper, S. N. Bleich, J. M. Clark, and M. C. Beach. 2009. "Physician Respect for Patients with Obesity." *Journal of General Internal Medicine* 24(11): 1236–1239.

Hunter, H. L., R. G. Steele, and M. M. Steele. 2008. "Family-Based Treatment for Pediatric Overweight: Parental Weight Loss as a Predictor of Children's Treatment Success." *Children's Health Care* 37(2): 112–125.

James, D. 2009. "Cluster Analysis Defines Distinct Dietary Patterns for African-American Men and Women." *Journal of the American Dietetic Association* 109(2): 255–262.

Johnson, W. G., K. J. Rohan, and A. A. Kirk. 2002. "Prevalence and Correlates of Binge Eating in White and African American Adolescents." *Eating behaviors* 3(2): 179–189.

Kafatos, A., Y. Manios, I. Markatji, I. Giachetti, M. D. Vaz de Almeida, and L. M. Engstrom. 1999. "Regional, Demographic and National Influences on Attitudes and Beliefs with Regard to Physical Activity, Body Weight and Health in a Nationally Representative Sample in the European Union." *Public Health Nutrition* 2(1a): 87–96.

Keller, H., B. Lamm, M. Abels, R. Yovsi, J. Borke, H. Jensen, and A. J. Tomiyama. 2006. "Cultural Models, Socialization Goals, and Parenting Ethnotheories." *Journal of Cross-Cultural Psychology* 37(2): 155–172.

Kelly, N., C. Bulik, and S. Mazzeo. 2011. "An Exploration of Body Dissatisfaction and Perceptions of Black and White Girls Enrolled in an Intervention for Overweight Children." *Body Image* 8(4): 379–384.

Kim, Y., R. Schulz, and C. S. Carver. 2007. "Benefit Finding in the Cancer Caregiving Experience." *Psychosomatic Medicine* 69(3): 283–291.

Kington, R. S., and J. P. Smith. 1997. "Socioeconomic Status and Racial and Ethnic Differences in Functional Status Associated with Chronic Diseases." *American Journal of Public Health* 87(5): 805–810.

Krebs, N. F., and M. S. Jacobson. 2003. "Prevention of Pediatric Overweight and Obesity." *Pediatrics* 112(2): 424–430.

Kumanyika, S. K. 2008. "Environmental Influences on Childhood Obesity: Ethnic and Cultural Influences in Context." *Physiology and Behavior* 94(1): 61–70.

Kumanyika, S. and S. Grier. 2006. "Targeting Interventions for Ethnic Minority and Low-Income Populations." *The Future of Children* 16(1): 187–207.

Kurian, A. K. and K. M. Cardarelli. 2007. "Racial and Ethnic Differences in Cardiovascular Disease Risk Factors: A Systematic Review." *Ethnicity and Disease* 17(1): 143–152.

Lim, S., J. M. Zoellner, J. M. Lee, B. A. Burt, A. M. Sandretto, W. Sohn, and J. M. Lepkowski. 2009. "Obesity and Sugar-Sweetened Beverages in African-American Preschool Children: A Longitudinal Study." *Obesity* 17(6): 1262–1268.

Lin, H., O. I. Bermudez, and K. L. Tucker. 2003. "Dietary Patterns of Hispanic Elders are Associated with Acculturation and Obesity." *The Journal of Nutrition* 133(11): 3651–3657.

Lynch, W. C., D. P. Heil, E. Wagner, and M. D. Havens. 2007. "Ethnic Differences in BMI, Weight Concerns, and Eating Behaviors: Comparison of Native American, White, and Hispanic Adolescents." *Body Image* 4(2): 179–190.

Marcus, M. D. and M. A. Kalarchian. 2003. "Binge Eating in Children and Adolescents." *International Journal of Eating Disorders* 34(S1): S47–S57.

Marques, L., M. Alegria, A. E. Becker, C. Chen, A. Fang, A. Chosak, and J. B. Diniz. 2011. "Comparative Prevalence, Correlates of Impairment, and Service Utilization for Eating Disorders across U.S. Ethnic Groups: Implications for Reducing Ethnic Disparities in Health Care Access for Eating Disorders." *International Journal of Eating Disorders* 44(5): 412–420.

Marshall, S. J., D. A. Jones, B. E. Ainsworth, J. P. Reis, S. S. Levy, and C. A. Macera. 2007. "Race/Ethnicity, Social Class, and Leisure-Time Physical Inactivity." *Medicine and Science in Sports and Exercise* 39(1): 44.

Mazzeo, S. E., R. Saunders, and K. S. Mitchell. 2005. "Binge Eating Among African American and Caucasian Bariatric Surgery Candidates." *Eating behaviors* 6(3): 189–196.

Mintz, S. W. and C. M. Du Bois. 2002. "The Anthropology of Food and Eating." *Annual Review of Anthropology* 31: 99–119.

Mirza, N. M., E. R. Mackey, B. Armstrong, A. Jaramillo, and M. M. Palmer. 2011. "Correlates of Self-Worth and Body Size Dissatisfaction among Obese Latino Youth." *Body Image* 8(2): 173–178.

Mohler, B., and F. Earls. 2001. "Trends in Adolescent Suicide: Misclassification Bias?" *American Journal of Public Health,* 91: 150–153. doi:10.2105/AJPH.91.1.150

Monroe, K. R., J. H. Hankin, M. C., Pike, B. E. Henderson, D. O. Stram, S. Park, and L. N. Kolonel. 2003. "Correlation of Dietary Intake and Colorectal Cancer Incidence among Mexican-American Migrants: The Multiethnic Cohort Study." *Nutrition and Cancer* 45(2): 133–147.

Morland, K., S. Wing, and A. D. Roux. 2002. "The Contextual Effect of the Local Food Environment on Residents' Diets: The Atherosclerosis Risk in Communities Study." *Journal Information* 92(11): 1761–1768.

Mulasi-Pokhriyal, U., C. Smith, and L. Franzen-Castle 2012. "Investigating Dietary Acculturation and Intake among U.S.-born and Thailand/Laos-Born Hmong-American Children Aged 9–18 Years." *Public Health Nutrition* 2: 1–10.

Murcott, A. 1988. "Sociological and Social Anthropological Approaches to Food and Eating." *World Review of Nutrition and Dietetics* 55: 1–40.

National Heart, Lung, and Blood Institute. 1995. *Report of the Conference on Socioeconomic Status and Cardiovascular Health and Disease.* http://www.nhlbi.nih .gov/resources/docs/sesall.pdf

National Institute of Mental Heath Report: Eating Disorders. 2012. http://www .nimh.nih.gov/health/publications/eating-disorders/index.shtml

Nelson, M. C., D. Neumark-Stzainer, P. J. Hannan, J. R. Sirard, and M. Story. 2006. "Longitudinal and Secular Trends in Physical Activity and Sedentary Behavior During Adolescence." *Pediatrics* 118(6): e1627–e1634.

Neumark-Sztainer, D., J. Croll, M. Story, P. J. Hannan, S. A. French, and C. Perry. 2002. "Ethnic/Racial Differences in Weight-Related Concerns and Behaviors among Adolescent Girls and Boys: Findings from Project EAT." *Journal of Psychosomatic Research* 53(5): 963–974.

Nicdao, E. G., S. Hong, and D. T. Takeuchi. 2007. "Prevalence and Correlates of Eating Disorders among Asian Americans: Results from the National Latino and Asian American Study." *International Journal of Eating Disorders* 40(S3): S22–S26.

Nouri, M., L. G. Hill, and J. K. Orrell-Valente. 2011. "Media Exposure, Internalization of the Thin Ideal, and Body Dissatisfaction: Comparing Asian American and European American College Females." *Body Image* 8(4): 366–372.

O'Dea, J. A. 2005. "Prevention of Child Obesity: 'First, Do No Harm.'" *Health Education Research* 20(2): 259–265.

Odoms-Young, A. 2008. "Factors that Influence Body Image Representations of Black Muslim Women." *Social Science and Medicine* 66(12): 2573–2584.

Ogbu, J. U. 1985. "Research Currents: Cultural-Ecological Influences on Minority School Learning." *Language Arts,* 62(8): 860–869.

Ogden, C. L., M. D. Carroll, L. R. Curtin, M. M. Lamb, and K. M. Flegal. 2010. "Prevalence of High Body Mass Index in U.S. Children and Adolescents, 2007–2008." *The Journal of the American Medical Association* 303(3): 242–249.

Porter, J., M. Stern, S. Mazzeo, R. Evans, and J. Laver. (in press). "Relations among Teasing, Body Image, and Depression in Treatment Seeking Obese African American Adolescents." *Journal of Black Psychology.*

Price, J. H., S. M. Desmond, R. A. Krol, F. F. Snyder, and J. K. O'Connell. 1987. "Family Practice Physicians' Beliefs, Attitudes, and Practices Regarding Obesity." *American Journal of Preventive Medicine* 3: 339–345.

Puhl, R., and K. D. Brownell. 2001. "Bias, Discrimination, and Obesity." *Obesity Research* 9: 788–805.

Reilly, J. J., E. Methven, Z. C. McDowell, B. Hacking, D. Alexander, L. Stewart, and C. J. H. Kelnar. 2003. "Health Consequenecs of Obesity." *Archives of Disease Control* 88(9): 748–752.

Renzaho, A. 2012. Acculturation and Its Effects on the Nutrition and Physical Activity of African Migrant Children (unpublished dissertation). Deakin University, Australia.

Resnicow, K., R. Taylor, M. Baskin, and F. McCarty. 2005. "Results of Go Girls: A Weight Control Program for Overweight African-American Adolescent Females." *Obesity* 13(10): 1739–1748.

Rieger, E., S. W. Touyz, T. Swain, and P. J. V. Beumont. 2001. "Cross-Cultural Research on Anorexia Nervosa: Assumptions Regarding the Role of Body Weight." *International Journal of Eating Disorders* 29(2): 205–215.

Rinderknecht, K., and C. Smith. 2002. "Body-Image Perceptions among Urban Native American Youth." *Obesity* 10(5): 315–327.

Robinson, T. N., J. D. Killen, I. F. Litt, L. D. Hammer, D. M. Wilson, K. F. Haydel, and C. B. Taylor. 1996. "Ethnicity and Body Dissatisfaction: Are Hispanic and Asian Girls at Increased Risk for Eating Disorders?" *Journal of Adolescent Health* 19(6): 384–393.

Ruiz, S. Y., A. Pepper, and D. E. Wilfley. 2004. "Obesity and Body Image among Ethnically Diverse Children and Adolescents." In J.K. Thompson (Ed.). *Handbook of Eating Disorders and Obesity.* Hoboken: NJ: John Wiley and Sons, Inc.

Sallis, J. and J. Kerr. 2006. "Built Environment and Physical Activity." *President's Council on Physical Fitness and Sports Research Digest* 7(4): 1–8.

Sallis, J. F. and K. Glanz. 2009. "Physical Activity and Food Environments: Solutions to the Obesity Epidemic." *Milbank Quarterly* 87(1): 123–154.

Satia, J. A., R. E. Patterson, V. M. Taylor, C. L. Cheney, S. Shiu-Thornton, K. Chitnarong, and A. R. Kristal. 2000. "Use of Qualitative Methods to Study Diet, Acculturation, and Health in Chinese-American Women." *Journal of the American Dietetic Association* 100(8): 934–940.

Satia-Abouta, J., R. E. Patterson, M. L. Neuhouser, and J. Elder. 2002. "Dietary Acculturation: Applications to Nutrition Research and Dietetics." *Journal of the American Dietetic Association* 102(8): 1105–1118.

Schwartz, M. B. and K. D. Brownell. 2004. "Obesity and Body Image." *Body Image* 1(1): 43–56.

Schwartz, M. B. and K. E. Henderson. 2009. "Does Obesity Prevention Cause Eating Disorders?" *Journal of the American Academy of Child and Adolescent Psychiatry* 48(8): 784–786.

Schwarzer, R., A. Luszczynska, J. P. Ziegelmann, U. Scholz, and S. Lippke. 2008. "Social-Cognitive Predictors of Physical Exercise Adherence: Three Longitudinal Studies in Rehabilitation." *Health Psychology* 27(1S): S54–S63.

Seo, D. C. and J. Sa. 2010. "A Meta-Analysis of Obesity Interventions among U.S. Minority Children." *Journal of Adolescent Health* 46(4): 309–323.

Shaw, H., L. Ramirez, A. Trost, P. Randall, and E. Stice. 2004. "Body Image and Eating Disturbances across Ethnic Groups: More Similarities than Differences." *Psychology of Addictive Behaviors* 18(1): 12–18.

Smolak, L. and R. H. Striegel-Moore. 2001. "Challenging the Myth of the Golden Girl: Ethnicity and Eating Disorders." In *Disorders: Innovative Directions in Research and Practice,* edited by R. H. Striegel-Moore and L. Smolak, 215–232. Washington DC: American Psychological Association.

Sothern, M. S., H. Schumacher, T. Von Almen, L. K. Carlisle, and J. N. Udall. 2002. "Committed to Kids: an Integrated, 4-Level Team Approach to Weight Management in Adolescents." *Journal of the American Dietetic Association* 102(3S): S81–S85.

Stern, M., S. E. Mazzeo, J. Porter, C. Gerke, D. Bryan, and J. Laver. 2006. "Self-Esteem, Teasing and Quality of Life: African American Adolescent Girls Participating in a Family-Based Pediatric Overweight Intervention." *Journal of Clinical Psychology in Medical Settings* 13(3): 217–228.

Stice, E. 2002. "Risk and Maintenance Factors for Eating Pathology: A Meta-Analytic Review." *Psychological Bulletin* 128(5): 825.

Stice, E., W. S. Agras, and L. D. Hammer. 1999. "Risk Factors for the Emergence of Childhood Eating Disturbances: A Five-Year Prospective Study." *International Journal of Eating Disorders* 25(4): 375–387.

Story, M., N. E. Sherwood, J. H. Himes, M. Davis, D. R. Jacobs Jr., Y. Cartwright, and J. Rochon. 2003. "An After-School Obesity Prevention Program for African-American Girls: The Minnesota GEMS Pilot Study." *Ethnicity and Disease* 13(1): S54–S64.

Story, M., J. Stevens, J. Himes, E. Stone, B. Holy Rock, B. Ethelbah, and S. Davis. 2003. "Obesity in American-Indian Children: Prevalence, Consequences, and Prevention." *Preventive Medicine* 37: S3–S12.

Strauss, R. S. and J. Knight. 1999. "Influence of the Home Environment on the Development of Obesity in Children." *Pediatrics* 103(6): e85–e93.

Swanson, S. A., S. J. Crow, D. Le Grange, J. Swendsen, and K. R. Merikangas. 2011. "Prevalence and Correlates of Eating Disorders in Adolescents: Results from the National Comorbidity Survey Replication Adolescent Supplement." *Archives of General Psychiatry* 68(7): 714–723.

Taylor, W. C., A. K. Yancey, N. G. Murray, S. S. Cummings, S. A. Sharkey, C. Wert, and J. James. 2000. "Physical Activity among African American and Latino Middle School Girls: Consistent Beliefs, Expectations, and Experiences across Two Sites." *Women and Health* 30(2): 67–82.

Thompson, S. H., S. J. Corwin, and R. G. Sargent. 1997. "Ideal Body Size Beliefs and Weight Concerns of Fourth-Grade Children." *International Journal of Eating Disorders* 21(3): 279–284.

Thompson, S. H., R. G. Sargent, and K. A. Kemper. 1996. "Black and White Adolescent Males' Perceptions of Ideal Body Size." *Sex Roles* 34(5): 391–406.

Unger, J. B., K. Reynolds, S. Shakib, D. Spruijt-Metz, P. Sun, and C. A. Johnson. 2004. "Acculturation, Physical Activity, and Fast-Food Consumption among Asian-American and Hispanic Adolescents." *Journal of Community Health* 29(6): 467–481.

U.S. Department of Health and Human Services. 2001. *Mental Health: Culture, Race, and Ethnicity—A Supplement to Mental Health: A Report of the Surgeon General.* Rockville, MD: U.S. Department of Health and Human Services, Substance Abuse and Mental Health Services Administration, Center for Mental Health Services.

Wang, S., J. Quan, A. M. Kanaya, and A. Fernandez. 2011. "Asian Americans and Obesity in California: A Protective Effect of Biculturalism." *Journal of Immigrant and Minority Health* 13(2): 276–283.

Weiss, M. G. 1995. "Eating Disorders and Disordered Eating in Different Cultures." *Psychiatric Clinics of North America* 18(3): 537–553.

Whitaker, R. C., J. A. Wright, M. S. Pepe, K. D. Seidel, and W. H. Dietz. 1997. "Predicting Obesity in Young Adulthood from Childhood and Parental Obesity." *The New England Journal of Medicine 337*(13): 869–873.

Whitt-Glover, M. C., W. C. Taylor, M. F. Floyd, M. M. Yore, A. K. Yancey, and C. E. Matthews. 2009. "Disparities in Physical Activity and Sedentary Behaviors among U.S. Children and Adolescents: Prevalence, Correlates, and Intervention Implications." *Journal of Public Health Policy 30*: S309–S334.

Wickham, E. P., M. Stern, R. K. Evans, D. L. Bryan, W. B. Moskowitz, J. N. Clore, and J. H. Laver. 2009. "Prevalence of the Metabolic Syndrome among Obese Adolescents Enrolled in a Multidisciplinary Weight Management Program: Clinical Correlates and Response to Treatment." *Metabolic Syndrome and Related Disorders 7*(3): 179–186.

Wilfley, D. E., R. I. Stein, B. E. Saelens, D. S. Mockus, G. E. Matt, H. A. Hayden-Wade, and L. H. Epstein. 2007. "Efficacy of Maintenance Treatment Approaches for Childhood Overweight." *The Journal of the American Medical Association 298*(14): 1661–1673.

Williamson, D., P. D. Martin, M. White, R. Newton, H. Walden, E. York-Crowe, and D. Ryan. 2005. "Efficacy of an Internet-Based Behavioral Weight Loss Program for Overweight Adolescent African-American Girls." *Eating and Weight Disorders 10*(3): 193–203.

Williamson, D. A., H. M. Walden, M. A. White, E. York-Crowe, R. L. Newton, A. Alfonso, and D. Ryan. 2006. "Two-Year Internet-Based Randomized Controlled Trial for Weight Loss in African-American Girls." *Obesity 14*(7): 1231–1243.

Winkleby, M. A., H. C. Kraemer, D. K. Ahn, and A. N. Varady. 1998. "Ethnic and Socioeconomic Differences in Cardiovascular Disease Risk Factors." *The Journal of the American Medical Association 280*(4): 356–362.

Winkleby, M. A., T. N. Robinson, J. Sundquist, and H. C. Kraemer. 1999. "Ethnic Variation in Cardiovascular Disease Risk Factors among Children and Young Adults." *The Journal of the American Medical Association 281*(11): 1006–1013.

World Health Organization. 2005. *Nutrition in Adolescence: Issues and Challenges for the Health Sector: Issues in Adolescent Health and Development.* http://whqlibdoc.who.int/publications/2005/9241593660_eng.pdf

Xie, B., J. B. Unger, P. Gallaher, C. A. Johnson, Q. Wu, and C. P. Chou. 2010. "Overweight, Body Image, and Depression in Asian and Hispanic Adolescents." *American Journal of Health Behavior 34*(4): 476–488.

Zephier, E., J. Himes, and M. Story. 1999. "Prevalence of Overweight and Obesity in American Indian School Children and Adolescents in the Aberdeen Area: A population Study." *International Journal of Obesity and Related Metabolic Disorders: Journal of the International Association for the Study of Obesity 23S*: S28–S30.

CHAPTER TEN

Suicide across Cultures

Kristin M. Vespia and Kaitlyn J. Florer

Suicide is a mental health and public health crisis in the United States, one that appears to be worsening. Preliminary data for 2010 from National Vital Statistics indicate that suicide is the 10th leading cause of death across age groups in this country, accounting for 37,793 fatalities in that year alone (Murphy, Xu, and Kochanek 2012). Given this number reflects those deaths *officially* classified as suicide, it is likely an underestimate. In a recent analysis of national data from 2000–2009, Rockett and colleagues (2012) described an increase in suicide death rates such that it even eclipsed car accidents to rank as the leading cause of injury-related death.

Suicide does not discriminate. Although frequency may vary, it happens across racial and ethnic groups, genders, ages, spiritual belief systems, social classes, sexual orientations, and ability statuses. Nonetheless, there is a complex relationship between culture and self-harm. Authors point out that results from research examining the intersection of ethnicity and suicide are far from consistent—with large scale investigations suggesting everything from substantially higher risk for certain groups to a null relationship between racial and ethnic diversity and suicidal thoughts or actions (Perez-Rodriguez et al. 2008).

In this chapter we focus primarily on suicide across racial/ethnic minority groups within the United States and explore the myriad ways in which such diversity may, in fact, interact with suicidal behavior. Scholars have suggested, for example, that all of the following are influenced by cultural context: triggering events, risk and protective factors, understanding or interpretations of suicidal behavior, outward manifestations of suicidal ideation or intent, attitudes toward professional assistance, and sources sought for assistance (Goldston et al. 2008, Joe, Canetto, and Romer 2008).

With this context in mind we have organized the chapter around an exploration of suicidal behavior in major racial/ethnic minority groups in this country. The strategy permits an examination of within- and between-group differences, as well as a discussion of the unique cultural forces that may be in operation. This organization also allows for a description of culturally specific assessment and intervention strategies. There are some important caveats, however, to this approach. First, as we discuss between-group differences, we also acknowledge that racial/ethnic and other cultural groups are not singular entities. The group we refer to as American Indians or Native Americans, for example, consists of over 500 tribes speaking more than 200 different languages (Perez-Rodriguez et al. 2008). Furthermore, even individuals from very similar backgrounds may vary, for instance, in acculturation or the integration of race/ethnicity with other components of their identity (e.g., gender, age, or social class). Second, there are interventions and assessment principles we may recommend for multiple minority groups because of commonalities such as a shared history of discrimination, a view of mind and body as one, or a collectivist orientation. Lastly, research on the overall efficacy of typical crisis intervention strategies is not clear-cut, which means our understanding of the role of culture in suicide risk evaluation and treatment also remains incomplete (Choi, Rogers, and Werth 2009). We therefore work to point to the specific evidence supporting our statements, and we provide general recommendations and themes at the end of the chapter based on our analysis of the existing literature.

African Americans and Suicide

Incidence and Prevalence

African-American suicide rates are the lowest of all racial/ethnic groups (Heron 2012). According to the 2007 National Institute of Mental Health (NIMH) report, African Americans committed suicide at a rate of 5.1/100,000 compared to a rate of 13.5/100,000 for white Americans. Joe, Baser, Breeden, Neighbors, and Jackson (2006) indicated that African Americans had a lifetime prevalence of suicide ideation of 11.7 percent and a lifetime prevalence of attempts of 4.1 percent. Some may expect higher numbers for African Americans considering the group's historical and current issues with oppression and racism (Joe and Kaplan 2001). Others argue that they have this lower rate specifically because of an extreme inner strength that has resulted from the group's survival of racism and discrimination (Day-Vines 2007).

Suicide risk generally decreases after adolescence for African Americans. Across ages, it is the 16th leading cause of death (Heron 2012). By contrast, it is the third leading cause of death for 15–24 year olds, the sixth for those ages 25–34, and the eighth leading cause of death for 35–44 year old African Americans (Heron 2012). After age 44, suicide does not fall within the top ten mortality causes (Heron 2012). Authors of research reviews also note, however, that suicide rates have been rising dramatically for African Americans, especially among men in their teens and early adult years (Day-Vines 2007, Willis et al. 2002). The young men may be at higher risk due to societal changes such as increases in economic strains and declines in connections to others (e.g., to spiritual communities, which have served as a protective factor for many African Americans) (Chatters et al. 2011, Willis et al. 2002). Authors have also cited the misclassification of suicides for young African Americans as deaths from accidental or unknown causes as another possible explanation for the increase, which may have influenced accuracy and rate fluctuations over time (Joe and Kaplan 2001, Mohler and Earls 2001).

Within-Group Differences

Research on within-group differences has been limited, but we do know that African American women attempt suicide more often than men (4.9 percent vs. 3.1 percent, Joe et al. 2006), while men have completed suicide rates that are more than three times higher than those of women (American Association of Suicidology [AAS] 2010). As is true across many cultural groups, professionals often point to the more lethal means utilized by male attempters (Joe and Kaplan 2001) as one explanation for this gender difference.

In addition to these distinctions in rates of suicidal behaviors, there are gender differences related to protective and risk factors. For example, Griffen-Fennell and Williams (2006) hypothesized that one explanation for gender differences in suicide may be that African American women are more actively involved in church and rely on it more for social support, thus receiving a particular benefit from this literature-established protective factor. Motherhood may also serve as a protective factor for some African American women because it provides a reason for living, and reasons for living are associated with decreased suicidal ideation (Woods et al. 2013). Additional reasons for living for African American women, beyond spiritual well-being, include optimism and familial social support (West et al. 2011). Risks also differ across gender. For instance, in their review of past research on suicide in African American men, Joe and Kaplan (2001) highlighted socioeconomic variables, familial abuse and disruption, witnessing violence or knowing victims of it, and lack of connectedness with others as possible risks. On the other hand, when authors have reviewed literature related to risks for women, they have pointed to variables such as mental distress (especially PTSD symptoms), poor coping skills, weaker identification with one's racial/ethnic identity, and partner/spousal abuse, among other issues (Compton, Thompson, and Kaslow 2005).

Age is another area of within-group differences. As noted previously, African American suicide rates are higher in young people (Heron 2012). Furthermore, as was the case with gender, some risk factors also vary with age. Education, for instance, is particularly associated with suicide in adult African American men (Rowell et al. 2008). Rowell and colleagues systematically reviewed nine studies that examined suicide in African American males. Based on that existing literature, they noted that 25–44 year olds who had attended college had a higher risk of suicide completion, while 55–64 year-old men with a college degree had a lower risk. Another potential factor is marital status. When Luoma and Pearson (2002) examined national suicide statistics from 1991–1996, they discovered that widowed young African Americans had dramatically higher suicide rates when compared to their married counterparts. In the same study they noted that for older men divorce was more strongly linked to suicide than widowhood.

Risk Factors

The Centers for Disease Control (2010) provide a helpful overview of general risk factors for suicide across racial/ethnic groups on their website. Feeling hopeless or isolated and being prone to impulsive actions or aggression are examples of psychological risk factors. Prior experiences, such as those of loss, substance abuse, suicide attempts, mental illness diagnosis, or physical health concerns, are another set of risks. Personal and cultural attitudes are also included, such as a reluctance to seek assistance due to stigma or identification with a belief system that might tacitly endorse self-harm (e.g., suicide as an acceptable way to spare family shame). Furthermore, there are specific family-related factors (e.g., familial histories of suicide or child abuse). Finally, there are risks of a potential structural nature, such as the ease with which individuals can access firearms or other means of self-harm, the presence of financial or other obstacles to seeking professional services, and exposure to suicide clusters.

Focusing specifically on African Americans, social isolation is one example of an overall suicide risk factor that could be more detrimental to this group. The African American culture is more collectivist in nature, and social support networks are extremely important. Authors have described lack of social support and the experience of isolation as associated with a greater likelihood of attempting suicide (Compton et al. 2005, Utsey et al. 2007). As a second example, psychological distress is a suicide risk for African Americans, as is true for other groups (Kaslow et al. 2004). Some African Americans believe, however, that they are not susceptible to becoming depressed, for instance, because as a culture they have suffered worse in the past and should simply be strong enough to prevent depression (Day-Vines 2007). This attitude can be dangerous and promote ignoring symptoms instead of seeking help, which then becomes another risk factor. African Americans already appear less likely to seek services and are more apt to suffer from untreated mental illness (Snowden 2012) due to other factors, such as financial barriers (Willis et al. 2003).

The availability of lethal means, particularly firearms, is another risk factor that may be particularly salient for this group (Willis et al. 2003). A greater proportion of African American households contain a firearm (Willis et al. 2003). Although it is critical not to engage in stereotyping of African Americans as "violent," some authors do point to issues of violence and conflict. For example, they have suggested that those at risk for suicide in this group tend to have higher levels of physical aggression, anger, hostility, and impulsivity (Kaslow et al. 2004). They have further noted that past research points to conflict with law enforcement as associated with suicide for African Americans (Rowell et al. 2008). There is a positive correlation in the group between suicide rates and both threatening and witnessing violence (Rowell et al. 2008, Willis et al. 2003).

Finally, we can discuss risks for African Americans in terms of Emile Durkheim's sociological perspective on suicide, which states that such action is caused by individuals not experiencing a sense of "fit" with the society in which they live (Utsey et al. 2007). African Americans may feel that lack of fit as a result of racism and the distance it can create from the majority culture (Utsey et al., 2007). Davidson and Wingate (2011) pointed to one variable that may reflect such concerns with "belonging" in society: acculturative stress. They noted that past research found acculturative stress to be differentially associated with the link between depression and suicide for African Americans as opposed to European Americans. Ethnic identity is another factor to consider. Kaslow et al. (2004) conducted an empirical examination of suicide attempters versus non-attempters and discovered that African American suicide attempters had greater struggles with ethnic identity than non-attempters and, for example, had a lower sense of connection both with their own and other groups. Place of residence can be another variable in the sociological category. Willis et al. (2003) highlighted the repeated finding that African Americans living in northern or western states were at higher suicide risk than those in southern states. They further postulated that individuals from the South were better equipped to cope with blatant racism and had stronger ties to family and church (i.e., a stronger fit with society). Finally, having a disease such as HIV is associated with suicide risk (Rowell et al. 2008). Although there are certainly other possibilities, one potential explanation is that the stigma linked to HIV could create a sense of distance from society.

Protective Factors

Clearly, African Americans face numerous risks for self-harm, and that makes their comparatively low suicide rates a paradox. However, a multitude of cultural protective factors, along with the strength of those specific attributes, may explain such statistics (Davidson and Wingate, 2011).

Religion/Spirituality

Church and religion/spirituality have long been integral to African American culture and are key protective factors against suicide (Chatters et al. 2011, Davidson and Wingate 2011). Church can fill diverse roles for members (e.g., guidance, recreation, concrete educational or financial support); it is an outlet for expressing the group's cultural traditions (Early and Akers, 1993), and can be a significant social support mechanism (Chatters et al. 2011). Furthermore, church may serve as a protection due to exposure to religious doctrine that opposes suicide (Early and Akers 1993, Walker, Lester, and Joe 2006). In fact, Chatters and colleagues (2011) discovered a significant negative correlation between church attendance frequency and suicidal ideation and attempts, and between emotional bonds to church members and suicidal thoughts and actions. The researchers found that those who attended church every day or only a few times a year were at higher risk of suicide than those who attended services once per week. There are stipulations to religion as a protection against suicide. It is not simply a matter of going to services, but also the internalization of religion and one's individual relationship with God (Anglin, Gabriel, and Kaslow 2005, Davidson and Wingate 2011). Furthermore, the relationship between religiosity and suicide is not necessarily straightforward, as was seen with church attendance frequency. For example, Taylor, Chatters, and Joe (2011) discovered that although people who reported relying on God as a source of strength had fewer suicidal attempts and less ideation, individuals who expressed a belief in prayer during stressful times and those who read religious material actually had *higher* rates of suicidal thinking.

Psychological and Psychosocial Factors

Some additional protective factors for African Americans can be organized under the umbrella of psychological theories or psychosocial forces. For instance, one psychological viewpoint suggests that suicide is a result of internalizing anger; African American culture is consistent with open emotional expression, and not turning such feelings in on oneself (Utsey et al. 2007). If that theory holds, that outward expression of feelings should be healthier and buffer against self-harm. Hope theory, on the other hand, suggests that hope and its components of goals and motivation are important protective factors (Davidson and Wingate 2011). In a study with college student participants, Davidson and Wingate (2011) discovered that African Americans scored higher on measures of hope and goals than white students did, suggesting hope may serve as a protective factor for this racial/ethnic group. Turning to the psychosocial realm, family and social support (both of which are integral to African American culture) may function as protections against suicide. As a supporting example, Compton et al. (2005) conducted research on a community sample of African Americans and discovered links between suicide attempt risk and cohesion and adaptability in the family. Matlin et al. (2011) provided additional support in their research that identified both family and peer support as positively linked to reasons for living.

Assessment and Intervention Strategies

Assessment

Selecting culturally appropriate methods. Some scholars believe the assessment methods used for Caucasians are unlikely to suffice for African American clients and assert that context, including culture, must be considered in risk and other assessments (Day-Vines 2007). Professionals may look for existing measures that do have evidence for cross-cultural use. As an example, suicide risk is associated with depression, so detecting depression is extremely important. Joe et al. (2008) reported that the Beck Depression Inventory-II could be used with African Americans, making it potentially valuable in suicide risk assessment. Clinicians should consult tests' technical manuals to learn more about the representativeness of instruments' norm groups and to find out about any research supporting the use of specific measures with diverse groups.

Assessing risk and protective factors. Given the substantial number of risk and protective factors related to suicide for African Americans, learning more about those variables for individual clients will clearly be important. Common risks regardless of culture, such as client and peer drug use, should also be assessed (CDC 2010), along with those more specific to this cultural group, such as acculturative stress or ethnic identity. Furthermore, professionals should be aware of clients' risk-taking because some African Americans may attempt to harm themselves with reckless behavior (e.g., reckless driving, unprotected sex) since intentional suicide could violate cultural and spiritual norms (Day-Vines 2007). Clinicians should not simply focus on risks, however. Strengths and possible protections are also essential to evaluate. Religious or spiritual beliefs and practices are a particularly important topic for African Americans given their buffering potential (Day-Vines, 2007).

Prevention and Intervention

Perhaps because of the comparatively low suicide rates for this group, not enough is known about empirically supported prevention and intervention strategies for African Americans. Clearly, more research needs to be done. Many recommendations that do exist at this point are designed to address suicide risk factors, to decrease treatment barriers, and to promote protective factors that have been established in the literature.

Educating professionals and others. Education for therapists, clients, family members, friends, and the community are key to any prevention program (Utsey et al. 2007). For example, there is a myth that African Americans do not commit suicide because the group is immune due to strength from enduring hardships (Early and Akers 1993). African Americans also often dismiss this risk because suicide contradicts cultural values and is seen as a "white" problem (Early and Akers 1993). These are dangerous assumptions that could lead clinicians, friends and family, and even the client, to ignore warning signs and not intervene or seek help (Walker et al. 2006).

Implementing prevention screening programs at schools, particularly in urban settings where the risk for suicide is greater, is one potentially valuable suicide prevention method given the lack of awareness of suicide prevalence and risk among many African Americans (Brown and Grumet 2009). These screenings have detected young people at risk for suicide, even if family and friends miss the warning signs (Brown and Grumet 2009). School-based screenings and services are accepted and effective means of making contact with African American youth struggling with mental health concerns (Husky et al. 2012). Focusing prevention efforts on high-risk groups, such as adolescent and young adult males, is also important to address the increase in their rates of self-harm (AAS 2010, Day-Vines 2007, Heron 2012). Finally, educating African Americans about the benefits of using suicide prevention hotlines is an important intervention strategy because African Americans are less likely to use crisis lines when someone they know is suicidal (Larkin et al. 2011).

Addressing treatment barriers. African Americans as a group may be less likely to seek mental health care (Snowden 2012). Mental illness stigma is one obstacle to seeking treatment. African Americans are much less likely even to admit that they have ideas of suicide if they are aware of the stigma surrounding mental illnesses, and most are aware of this stigma (Thompson, Bazile, and Akbar 2004). Clinicians might use education, outreach efforts, clinical services located in trusted community locales (e.g., churches), among other strategies, to combat such stigma. A final method for addressing treatment obstacles is for therapists of all races/ethnicities to commit to honing cultural competence. Some African Americans have a distrust of Whites specifically and, depending on their Black racial identity, they may prefer a therapist from their own group (Nickerson, Helms, and Terrell 1994, Thompson et al. 2004). Professionals who work intentionally on cultural competence may develop a good reputation within the African American community that encourages service use.

Incorporating spiritual and family support when appropriate. Professionals should consider integrating the church and religion/spirituality in prevention and intervention methods given their centrality to African American culture. Churches provide not only religious guidance, but also educational, financial, and social support (Chatters et al. 2011, Early and Akers 1993). Thus, they could be good partners in education and prevention efforts, and professionals might consider collaborating with spiritual leaders when treating specific clients. Of course, another important asset available to clinicians is the family because kinship bonds are often very strong for African Americans. Therapists might consider the use of family therapy. In addition, education efforts aimed at the general community will be good investments if they result in family members who understand the risks of suicide and know how to seek help for their loved ones.

American Indians and Suicide

Incidence, Prevalence, and Within-Group Differences

High suicide rates among American Indians have been well documented for decades (Goldston et al. 2008). In fact, they have the highest percentage of total deaths by suicide (2.8 percent) among any major racial/ethnic group in the United States, making it their eighth leading cause of death compared to the rating of sixteenth, for example, for African-Americans (Heron 2012). One of the striking within-group differences among American Indians with regard to suicide rates relates to age. Suicide rates among youth are dramatically higher. Data from 2008 indicated that it was the second leading cause of death for American Indians ages 15 through 34, but it did not fall within the top ten for those ages 55 or older (Heron 2012). Given the particularly high suicide rates for young people, it is perhaps not surprising that they, and especially student groups, have been the focus of existing scholarship on suicide among American Indians (Perez-Rodriguez et al. 2008). More research is needed to develop a comprehensive understanding of self-harm within this population.

The gender pattern of suicidal actions is also noteworthy. As mentioned earlier, although females across cultural groups often have higher rates of attempting suicide, males typically have higher rates of completed suicide. For American Indians, however, suicide is actually the second leading cause of death for both males and females ages 15 through 24; it is not until ages 45 to 54 that one sees a separation in rank of more than one position for men (seventh leading cause of death) and women (tenth leading cause of death) (Heron 2012). Research reviews that report these gender differences, however, do not shed light on the reasons for them (e.g., Department of Health and Human Services 2001, Goldston et al. 2008). Gaps in the research literature also contribute to the lack of understanding of another potential within-group difference: place of residence. Much of the existing scholarship has focused on individuals living on or near reservations, but the majority of American Indians actually live in urban areas (Olson and Wahab 2006).

Risk Factors

Despite the lack of significant information about reasons for specific within-group differences in suicide among American Indians, authors have described any number of potential risk factors for this population. Some of these, such as having prior suicide attempts or a suicide in the family, are considered risks across racial/ethnic groups (Dorgan 2010).

There is a longer list of other risks, however, some of which are common to many groups and some of which have a unique relationship to American Indian culture. They include: high rates of substance use/abuse, and other mental disorders (i.e., depression, PTSD); significant present-day exposure to violence and other trauma; intergenerational or historical trauma; acculturative stress; loss of ethnic or spiritual identity; discrimination; living away from a reservation; an individualistic (versus collectivist) orientation; negative life events; and lack of accessible mental health services, as well as reluctance to use those services (Goodkind et al. 2010, LaFromboise, Albright, and Harris 2010, Hamilton and Rolf 2010, Middlebrook et al. 2001, Muehlenkamp et al. 2009, Olson and Wahab 2006, Perez-Rodriguez et al. 2008, Yoder et al. 2006). Finally, there is concern that American Indian youth may be more susceptible to contagion effects or suicide clusters, particularly when living on reservations (Hamilton and Rolf 2010, Goldston et al. 2008). Gone and Trimble (2012) point, for instance, to one two-month period in which there were nine completed and 88 attempted suicides on the Wind River reservation.

As another example of a culturally-specific risk, the Indian Health Service (IHS) provides care for the majority of individuals who live on reservations or near them, yet their programs are underfunded and rationing of such services occurs (Dorgan 2010, Olson and Wahab 2006). It can be difficult to access treatment, and whether through the IHS or community programs, American Indians may be distrustful of mental health professionals given a long history of exposure to institutional racism. In addition, they may prefer informal support networks or traditional healers. For example, in a study of American Indian college students, 57 percent of those who reported suicidal ideation indicated that they were not likely to seek help from a professional counselor (Scheel, Prieto, and Biermann 2011). There are also questions about the cultural appropriateness of existing interventions (Goodkind et al. 2010).

Moving to other culturally relevant suicide risk factors, American Indians are more likely to experience some type of trauma exposure, which may relate to the fact that they face higher poverty and unemployment rates than the general population (DHHS 2001, Lanier 2010). Beyond individual trauma, the history of Native peoples within the United States has clearly included violence, oppression, and systematic attempts at cultural destruction. The results over generations have been referred to using many different labels, including historical trauma; it has also been discussed as something that may feel like an injury to the soul or a spiritual wound (Goodkind et al. 2011). Information related to risks associated with cultural identity variables is less straightforward. Research reviews indicate that feeling pressure to acculturate or living in a tribal environment in which there is conflict about traditional values may be associated with increased suicide rates (Middlebrook et al. 2001, Olson and Wahab 2006). However, studies that have examined levels of acculturation or enculturation and its relationship to suicide risk have yielded mixed results (Scheel et al. 2011, Yoder et al. 2006).

Protective Factors

In addition to protective factors that exist across racial/ethnic groups, such as social and familial support, a number of buffering mechanisms exist with specific regard to American Indian cultures and suicidal ideation and action. LaFromboise and colleagues (2010) found in their study of 438 teens from more than 60 tribal nations that those who considered themselves bicultural were also less likely to experience a sense of hopelessness. Individuals in the study who resided on reservations also reported less hopelessness. Another investigation, this one of 1,456 tribal members of various ages, demonstrated that a cultural spiritual orientation was significantly associated with lower rates of suicide attempts (Garroutte et al. 2003). Based on their review of the existing literature, Muehlenkamp et al. (2009) also suggested that the existence of cultural continuity within the community, as well as individual knowledge and practice of cultural traditions, may serve to reduce suicide risk. Cultural factors are, therefore, often key components in existing suicide prevention programs for American Indians.

Assessment and Intervention Strategies

Assessment
Evaluating common risk factors. As was the case with African Americans, effective assessment of suicide risk with American Indian clients involves several components, one of which is assessing common risk factors for self-harm, such as depression. This assessment should be completed in a culturally respectful and competent manner. For example, American Indian cultures may not distinguish between mind and body in a dualistic fashion, and that can lead to experiencing psychological pain through physical symptoms (DHHS 2001). Clinicians cannot assume that interview questions or existing commercial measures of mood disorders will be as valid or reliable with this racial/ethnic group as with the majority group members upon whom they were likely normed (DHHS 2001).

In addition to assessing universal risk factors, professionals need to evaluate risks associated with suicide for American Indians specifically, such as individual trauma exposure and the experience of historical trauma. Clinicians may also wish to assess acculturation and enculturation and the client's understanding and level of agreement with cultural perspectives on mental illness, suicide, and mental health care. It will be important to know, for example, if the client believes that mental illness is primarily a spiritual issue, rather than a psychological one. Of course, that answer will impact who the individual approaches for assistance and openness to specific interventions.

Emphasizing areas of strength. Risk factors are not the only target of assessment. In fact, focusing on resilience and strengths can be equally if not more important (Stiffman et al. 2007). Time spent on evaluation likely will feel far less "negative" to the client if there is a more balanced approach to the process. Moreover, understanding the factors that protect the client and could prevent his or her suicide is critical to the effective prevention of self-harm. Thus, identifying and then promoting factors such as existing individual and family strengths, as well as sense of spirituality and community connection, may yield important dividends and serve to inject positivity and hope into sessions that can feel "heavy" when focused exclusively on topics of presenting problems, depression, and suicidal ideation or intent. To provide one specific example, Hodge and Limb (2010) assert the importance of evaluating spirituality with all Native clients, and they even review the strengths and weaknesses of five specific tools for doing so with a reading audience of clinicians in mind.

Avoiding stereotypes. Although knowing the relevant literature and common risk and protective factors is important, professionals must be cautious about allowing such knowledge to lead to stereotypes or assumptions (Goldston et al. 2008). For example, they should not assume that all American Indian teens will be suicide prone or likely to abuse substances. Within-group and individual differences always exist, and American Indians are not one cohesive cultural entity.

Using appropriate tools and strategies. Counselors should ask clinical interview questions that show an awareness of culture and/or use interview strategies that are culturally sensitive (e.g., asking about degree of identification with traditional values, openly acknowledging client-therapist cultural differences, and inquiring about client comfort before beginning an interview). Professionals should also be aware of possible different meanings of nonverbal behavior across cultures, such as understanding that lack of direct eye contact may be a sign of respect and/or adherence to cultural norms, not an indication of low self-esteem or depression (Sue and Sue 2013). Finally, clinicians should consider whether formal assessment instruments have been developed for and/or normed upon a sample that includes members of their client's culture. There are group-specific measures, such as the *American Indian Enculturation Scale,* that have been developed (Winderowd et al. 2006). Professionals could also consider instruments from clinical research with American Indians for potential clinical adaptation or use, e.g., *Awareness of Connectedness Scale* and *Reasons for Life* (Mohatt et al. 2011); *Suicidal Risk Questionnaire* (Westefeld, Cardin, and Deaton 1992, cited in Scheel et al. 2011).

Prevention and Intervention

Considering sociological explanations and interventions. There are some general principles to remember when working with those at risk for suicide in this group. For instance, authors have spoken about the importance of considering sociological, not just psychological or medical, explanations and interventions related to suicide (Lanier 2010, Wexler and Gone 2012). As an example, suicidal ideation may be experienced as an expression or reflection of a collective, not individual, pain (Wexler and Gone 2012). Therefore, community-level interventions may then be particularly appropriate; this is also true when one considers concerns related to suicide clusters with American Indian adolescents (Hamilton and Rolf 2010). Of course, for professionals to implement such recommendations it is also important to address underfunding of mental health resources, especially those for American Indian communities (Dorgan 2010).

Promoting collaboration and cultural competence. Other considerations for suicide prevention and intervention include making use of existing effective indigenous health resources and promoting cultural competence among mental health providers (Goodkind et al. 2010). As one example, clinicians may consult or collaborate with a shaman when providing treatment to an American Indian client who expresses such a preference. Professionals are also cautioned about overreliance on empirically supported treatments or ESTs (Goodkind et al. 2010, 2011). The research that has produced these interventions may not include American Indian clients, so the degree to which such techniques are appropriate when working with this population is unclear. Clinicians should investigate the diversity of research samples and consider cultural and individual appropriateness for their client before blindly applying such treatments. Gone and Trimble (2012) argue evidence-based practices can still be used, but they also discuss the importance of modifying them for cultural relevance and provide examples of doing so with certain cognitive interventions. Lastly, just as assessment efforts may be enhanced through a focus on strengths and resilience, the same may be true for prevention and intervention (Stiffman et al. 2007). For instance, professionals may not only work to decrease depressive symptoms but also encourage clients to increase their use of effective coping strategies, such as spending regular time each week exercising and maintaining healthy, supportive relationships.

Becoming aware of culturally-specific resources. Professionals should know about programs that have been developed specifically for use with American Indian clients. There are also web-based resources for professionals looking for information regarding suicide within this cultural group, along with potential intervention strategies. For example, the Department of Health and Human Services (http://aspe.hhs.gov/hsp/09/aian-suicidepreventionhotline/ index.shtml#Background), the Suicide Prevention Resource Center (http:// www.sprc.org/aian), and the Indian Health Service (http://www.ihs.gov/ NonMedicalPrograms/nspn/) all have specific sites devoted to the topic. In terms of the research literature regarding culturally-specific treatment, most programs seem to target adolescents or college students. These include the Zuni Life Skills Development Program for high school students (LaFromboise and Lewis 2008) and a suicide prevention model for college students based around the concept of the medicine wheel (Muehlenkamp et al. 2009, Gray and Muehlenkamp 2010). At least two critical reviews of suicide prevention programs for this cultural group have been published (Hamilton and Rolf 2010, Middlebrook et al. 2001). These reviews suggest that the programs do have beneficial effects, but they also point to challenges, such as lack of funding for treatment services (Hamilton and Rolf 2010) and to the importance of key elements: involving the community and infusing culture throughout the process of creating and implementing programs (Middlebrook et al. 2001).

Asian Americans and Suicide

Incidence, Prevalence, and Within-Group Differences

The lifetime prevalence of suicidal ideation has been estimated at 8.8 percent for Asian Americans; the corresponding rate of suicide attempts is 2.5 percent (Cheng et al. 2010). In 2008, suicide was responsible for 1.8 percent of deaths for Asian Americans or Pacific Islanders, making it the 10th leading cause of death (Heron 2012). There are not dramatic differences in these rankings between females and males, as is typical in many other racial/ethnic groups (Heron 2012, Goldston et al. 2008). Other within-group differences in suicide are striking. In terms of age, suicide is the second or third leading cause of death for individuals 15–34 (Heron 2012), and Asian American college students have reported higher levels of suicidal ideation and attempts than Caucasian peers (Chu, Hsieh, and Tokars 2011, Wong, Brownson, and Schwing 2011). Some authors have also argued that elderly Asian Americans are a high-risk group with especially elevated suicide rates, and this may be particularly true for older women (Sue et al. 2012) and Chinese men and women (Chu et al. 2011, Leong et al. 2007). Leong et al. (2007) point to intergenerational conflict caused by children's higher acculturation levels as one possible precipitating factor for suicide in older adults.

The other areas of substantial within-group variation in self-harm for Asian Americans are national origin and length of time since immigration. Some authors describe rates for South Asian adolescents as a source of particular concern (Goldston et al. 2008). Other research reviews suggest rates for Chinese, Japanese, and Filipino Americans may be lower than for majority group members, while rates for Native Hawaiians are substantially higher than their teenage peers (DHHS 2001). However, as mentioned previously, older Chinese adults have been mentioned as an at-risk group (Chu et al. 2011). Moreover, authors note immigrants who are labeled as "refugees" may be at higher risk for mental health concerns (DHHS 2001), but groups such as Laotians and Hmong have been understudied in terms of suicide when compared to Chinese or Japanese Americans (Leong et al. 2007), leaving unanswered questions.

There are actually two competing hypotheses regarding immigration status and well-being. One would suggest that immigrants should be at less risk for suicide because, by virtue of being able to come to a new country, they are likely emotionally and physiologically well; the other, of course, would argue that immigrants would be at greater risk because of the possibility of acculturative stress and economic, linguistic, and social challenges (Duldulao, Takeuchi, and Hong 2009). Recent lifetime prevalence estimates for Asians in the United States suggest that the highest suicide rates are for individuals who immigrated within the last 12 years (ideation = 15.48; attempts = 5.20), followed by those born in the United States (ideation = 13.52; attempts = 3.91), and, lastly, by those who arrived in this country 13 years ago or more (ideation = 6.10; attempts = 1.53) (Borges et al. 2012, 1180). These numbers reflect "Asians" in general and not specific ethnicities. In another investigation using a community sample of 2,095 Asian Americans from the National Latino and Asian-American Study (NLAAS), researchers did not find immigrants to be at significantly higher risk for suicide than those born in the United States (Duldulao et al. 2009), but they did not analyze data by length of time spent in the

United States as the previous authors did. Thus, clinician awareness of possible within-group differences based on time since immigration remains important and may point to different risk factors for suicide (e.g., migration trauma vs. intergenerational conflict).

Risk Factors

Asian Americans face a number of different suicide risk factors. Cheng and colleagues (2010) used data from the NLAAS study mentioned previously to examine correlates of suicidal ideation and attempts and found that risks included such factors as family conflict, sense of discrimination, and diagnosis of depressive or anxiety disorders. These results were supported by a more recent study using the same data set that used advanced statistical analyses to identify the best predictors of suicidal thoughts and actions (Kuroki and Tilley 2012). For suicidal ideation, for example, the authors discovered that the three strongest predictors were having a diagnosis of a depressive disorder, the presence of an anxiety disorder, and conflict in the family. Although these may appear to be generic risk factors that could apply to any cultural group, family conflict, for instance, may be a source of particular stress for Asian Americans given the collective orientation of the culture and the importance placed on a close family unit, as well as the deference expected within the hierarchical family relationships (Cheng et al. 2010, Sue and Sue 2013).

Authors have identified other risk factors for suicide, as well. Some of these include high level of enculturation or a strong sense of identification with one's original culture (Goldston et al. 2008), low levels of English fluency (Chu et al. 2011), acculturative stress (Goldston et al. 2008, Gomez, Miranda, and Polanco 2011), and seeing oneself as a target of discrimination (Cheng et al. 2010). In fact, Gomez and colleagues (2011) found that Asian participants in their study endorsed more acculturative stress than other racial/ethnic groups, as well as elevated rates of enduring recent discrimination. Wong et al. (2011) examined risk factors for suicidal thoughts within a national sample of 1,377 Asian American college students. The three most common were family problems, academic concerns, and financial pressures. In another investigation using a college student sample from one campus, seeing oneself as a burden was a significant predictor of suicidal thoughts (Wong et al. 2011). These latter findings are consistent with a collectivist orientation and the importance both of family and of saving face in the culture.

Suicide risk factors for Asian Americans may be exacerbated by the fact that they seek help for mental health concerns in general at lower rates than other racial/ethnic groups (Chu et al. 2011, DHHS 2001). Also using data from the NLAAS, researchers found that there was a positive relationship between suicide attempts and perceiving a need for and seeking assistance for Asian Americans (Chu et al. 2011). However, in the same investigation, those experiencing suicidal ideation were no more likely to see a need for help or seek it than those who had a diagnosable mental illness but no thoughts of suicide. Thus, it is possible that Asian Americans experience such thoughts differently or underestimate their significance (Chu et al 2011). One possible explanation is a cultural view of mind and body as one, which could contribute to experiencing symptoms of emotional distress physically and consulting medical rather than mental health professionals for assistance (Chu et al. 2011, Sue and Sue 2013). Researchers have also discovered that racial/ethnic minorities who pursue psychotherapy may be quite reluctant to volunteer information about suicidal thoughts unless a specific risk assessment is done by the clinician (Morrison and Downey 2000).

Protective Factors

Protective factors against suicide for Asian Americans are in many ways a mirror image of the risk factors, and many of them are associated with relationships and belongingness. Goldston et al. (2008) note in their research review that fluency with English, social support, and a focus on the present may serve as buffers against depression. Relying on data from the National Longitudinal Study of Adolescent Health, Wong and Maffini (2011) found that good relationships with family, school, and peers predicted fewer suicide attempts. Interestingly, however, they also discovered some differences across participants. For instance, family relationships did not provide statistically significant protection for some participants—often those who were more highly acculturated. Wong, Koo et al. (2011) discovered that both self-definitions focused on autonomy and those emphasizing bonds with others could serve as protective factors against suicidal ideation. They argued that these contrasting senses of self could each act to decrease a sense of burden on others, which is a risk for suicidal thoughts. Cheng and colleagues (2010) cited data suggesting a negative relationship between ethnic identity scores and suicide attempts. Using their national sample of college students, Wong et al. (2011) found that living with family or a partner had statistical associations with a decreased likelihood of morbid thinking. Those living with a family member also had significantly less suicidal ideation.

Assessment and Intervention Strategies

The intervention recommendations made for other racial/ethnic groups, such as considering sociological explanations and interventions for suicide, also hold for Asian American clients given the common collectivist orientation and the need to be mindful of cultural competence for all clients. Recommendations that have not been mentioned previously or are more unique to this group are described below.

Assessment

Choosing an appropriate language. One of the first considerations for suicide assessment with Asian American clients will be determining the language in which such assessment should occur if English is not their first or only language. Even if the client is fluent in English, he or she may not be most able to or most comfortable with describing symptoms or discussing highly personal topics in that language. If assessment within the client's native tongue is more appropriate and an interpreter is necessary, one should be employed. Given the nature of hierarchical familial relationships and concerns about losing face within the culture (Goldston et al., 2008), practitioners should use a professional interpreter, not a family member or friend who may have accompanied the client to the office.

Evaluating nonverbal messages. Clinicians must also be sensitive to nonverbal communication. In general, Asian cultures tend to use what is referred to as "high context communication" in which nonverbal messages are prioritized over verbal ones (Sue and Sue 2013). As a result, when considering responses to risk assessment questions, therapists must not only consider words, but also vocal volume and inflection, posture, and other cues. Because research suggests minority clients may be less likely to openly volunteer information about suicidal thoughts or behaviors, it is still very important for professionals to ask such questions directly. They simply also must be sensitive to the verbal and unspoken nature of responses. Professionals who are culturally sensitive to nonverbal communication also understand nonverbal behaviors may have different meanings across groups. As with American Indians, lack of eye contact from an Asian American client may signify respect for the therapist as an older person or authority figure.

Using appropriate assessment tools and questions. As was described with American Indian clients, professionals should only use assessment tools on individuals and groups for which they were intended (e.g., appropriate language and norms, established reliability/validity with the group), or, at the very least, be aware of the potential limitations and measurement errors that are inherent in not doing so. Adding to the information provided previously, clinicians should use multiple assessment methods, including multiple types of interview questions, and they should consider risk assessment an ongoing process (Granello 2010). Given the limitations of all assessment methods and tools, using more than one should result in more reliable findings. In the same way, therapists will achieve a more reliable and valid risk assessment by posing multiple inquiries and not just one standard suicide screening question. As an example, the therapist does not simply want to ask "Are you suicidal?" He or she may need to ask multiple questions to obtain a complete picture, such as ones regarding any history of thoughts of self-harm and more open-ended questions about feelings about life and death in general (Granello 2010). This strategy may be particularly important with clients who emphasize high context communication, who experience symptoms physically, and/or who experience a sense of shame or loss of face in admitting to strong emotions. Especially because of concerns they may have about expressing negative feelings or sharing unflattering information, authors have even suggested that professionals should provide additional information to Asian American clients about the importance of a comprehensive risk assessment, coupled with reassurances regarding confidentiality (Choi et al. 2009).

Finally, there are some formal instruments that may be worthy of consideration with Asian Americans. Choi and colleagues (2009) advocate for the use of the Collaborative Assessment and Management of Suicidality model (CAMS, e.g., Jobes 2000). CAMS attempts to understand the client's symptoms, particularly suicidal thoughts or actions, in an individualized context that considers his or her motivations for continuing to live and those for not doing so. Another possibility is the Positive and Negative Suicide Ideation Inventory (PANSI), which appears to hold a similar factor structure for African American, Asian American, Caucasian, and Latino/Hispanic individuals (Muehlenkamp et al. 2005).

Prevention and Intervention

The general recommendations for treatment for other culturally diverse clients would largely apply to this cultural group, such as considering recent developments in adapting evidence-based treatments for cultural appropriateness (Sue et al. 2012). Additional recommendations follow.

Involving family when appropriate. Therapists may find family involvement to be quite important in assisting Asian American clients (Goldston et al. 2008). Choi et al. (2009) indicate that individuals from this cultural group may be uncomfortable making treatment decisions without the involvement of family members, and relatives can provide support and help to recognize potential suicide risk factors and warning signs.

Educating others. Suicidal Asian Americans have shown a preference for nonprofessional assistance, so it is important for psychotherapeutic experts to educate those potential sources of help about suicide. This may include educating religious and spiritual leaders and even physicians and nurses, since medical staff may be the most sought source of professional help (Chu et al. 2011). Chu et al. 2011 also emphasize the importance of outreach within the overall Asian American community to address what to do if someone is suicidal, and they stress providing such outreach in languages other than English because lack of English fluency is a self-harm risk factor for this group.

Considering client beliefs about suicide. This strategy is likely appropriate for all clients, but Wong, Koo, et al. (2011) specifically assert that Asian American clients are likely to see the cause of suicidal thoughts as interpersonal difficulties, not mental illness. As a result they indicate that spending too much time in sessions discussing the ties between mental disorders and suicide may not be helpful. Clients may believe that time is spent more productively focusing on relationship concerns. This is simply one example. Other beliefs with potential implications for treatment include those about life after death and religious or other spiritual prohibitions to self-harm.

Hispanics/Latinos and Suicide

Incidence, Prevalence, and Within-Group Differences

There are a number of inconsistencies in suicide incidence and prevalence rates for this group. Perez-Rodriguez et al. (2008) note that there are investigations that have concluded suicide attempts are not as frequent for Hispanics/Latinos as they are for members of other cultural groups, but other studies have resulted in null findings in terms of the relationship between race or ethnicity and rates of suicidal thoughts or behaviors. Similarly, different researchers have arrived at contrasting conclusions in terms of variability in rates of self-harm among specific nationalities, although there is some agreement that the lifetime prevalence of attempts is higher among those from Puerto Rico and lower for Cuban Americans (Perez-Rodriguez et al. 2008).

The overall lifetime prevalence rates for suicidal ideation and suicide attempts for Hispanics/Latinos have been estimated at 11.35 percent and

5.11 percent respectively (Borges et al. 2012, 1178). Those numbers placed this group's level of ideation as higher only than Asians in the same study, but their level of attempts was the highest of any group in the investigation (Asians, blacks, Hispanics, and Whites were included). This high level of attempts was mentioned in earlier reviews of research, as well (DHHS 2001). By contrast, completed suicide was *not* among the ten leading causes of death for Hispanics in 2008 when looking across sexes and age groups, according to the Centers for Disease Control (Heron 2012).

Within-group differences are again important to consider. Although rates among the elderly are not as high, suicide is the third or fourth leading cause of death for those aged 15–34 (Heron 2012). Hispanic/ Latino males commit suicide in higher numbers than females of similar ages (Heron 2012). Research reviews suggest, however, that Hispanic/ Latina females attempt suicide in larger numbers and report more hopelessness, at least as teenagers, than do young men (Goldston et al. 2008). Multiple authors have commented on adolescent Latinas as a high-risk group for depression and suicide (Baumann, Kuhlberg, and Zayas 2010, Cespedes, and Huey 2008). Moreover, there are differences based on time of residence in the United States. Borges et al. (2012) reported the lowest rates of ideation and attempts for immigrants in this country for 13 or more years (5.59 and 2.62), higher rates for those who immigrated 12 or fewer years ago (13.55 and 5.28), and, finally, the highest numbers for individuals born in the United States (15.46 and 7.07; 1180). These findings may imply a role for acculturation in suicide risk or protection, but more research is needed on potential explanatory mechanisms (Borges et al. 2012).

Risk Factors

Because adolescents are a high-risk group for suicide for Hispanics/ Latinos, much of the research literature on risk and protective factors has focused upon them. For instance, one study of teenage Latinas concluded that family conflict presents a risk in terms of self-harm (Kuhlberg, Pena, and Zayas 2010). Another research team investigated peer relationships and found that friendship concerns were correlated with suicidal ideation for Mexican American girls in the 14–19 year-old range, but not for boys in the same sample (Winterrowd, Canetto, and Chavez 2010). As alluded to earlier, being born in the United States may actually be a risk factor for self-harm for Hispanics/Latinos (Goldston et al. 2008), as is having parents born in this country (Perez-Rodriguez et al. 2008).

Of course, the causal mechanisms responsible for such correlational findings are not completely clear. Goldston et al. (2008) asserted that the possible mismatch between an emphasis on collectivism and interdependence by family and simultaneous encouragement toward autonomy by teenage peers could be a suicide risk factor. Providing some support for this idea, Cespedes and Huey (2008) conducted a study with 130 Latino high school students and discovered that youth-reported differences between their own and their parents' gender role expectations were associated with depression.

Looking beyond a pure focus on adolescents, clinicians should consider that some Latino clients of any age may have immigrated to the United States under traumatic circumstances, and that trauma and acculturative stress in general could contribute to emotional difficulties (Goldston et al. 2008). In fact, in an investigation using 75 migrant farmers from Mexico as participants, Hovey and Magana (2002) found that acculturative stress was associated with higher depression levels. Additional variables correlated with depression in the same study included problematic family functioning, poor social support, and high education levels, among others.

Protective Factors

Identified protective factors for Hispanics/Latinos are largely relational, and studies of them have again focused on adolescents. Oquendo and colleagues (2005) discussed a sense of responsibility to family as one potential suicide deterrent. They also noted that this group, like African Americans, may have greater moral objections to self-harm, which in this case could be linked to a sense of belonging in a different kind of relationship—that with the Catholic Church. Baumann et al. (2010) conducted a study with mother-daughter pairs and discovered a sense of shared empathy and engagement may mitigate against teen suicide. This finding could be seen as related to the Latino value of familism (or familismo), which was identified in another study as a potential protection against self-harm for Hispanic/Latino teens (Kulberg, Pena, and Zayas 2010).

Assessment and Intervention Strategies

Assessment

Many, if not all, of the recommendations for culturally-sensitive assessment made previously also apply to Hispanics/Latinos. Conducting assessments in an appropriate language, being aware of nonverbal communication in this high context culture, and using multiple forms of assessment are all important. In addition, there are some specific measures that have been used in research with this group that could potentially be used or adapted for clinical use. For example, studies (e.g., Oquendo et al. 2005, Richardson-Vejlgaard et al. 2009) have employed the Reasons for Living Inventory (RFLI), which may help to identify protective factors against suicide for reinforcement by clinicians. Finally, decisions about the involvement of family in assessment efforts are important. Due to the potential role of family conflict and family cohesion in suicide risk and protection, some clients may not feel comfortable answering questions or pursuing treatment without family involvement. In other cases, where conflict is present, reassurances about confidentiality and making sure others are not present for evaluation sessions could be equally critical.

Prevention and Intervention

Again, the recommendations made for previous groups, such as attending to cultural competence, will hold here, as will the idea that culturally-specific treatments should be used when appropriate. However, Goldston and colleagues (2008) actually indicated at the time of their research review that there were no research-supported suicide prevention/intervention approaches for Hispanics or Latinos. It is possible to find information about treatment approaches for other concerns specifically designed for this group, such as a mentoring program called Club Amigas that matches Latina middle schoolers with college students of the same ethnicity (Kaplan et al. 2009). Other authors described the case study of a once-suicidal Latina client who was treated using an integration of cognitive-behavioral, multicultural, and feminist-oriented psychotherapies (Diaz-Martinez, Interian, and, Waters 2010). One case study is not enough to generalize, but the combination of these specific approaches, especially feminist and multicultural, is intriguing given the existence of traditional gender role expectations for many Hispanics/Latinos and the potential role of acculturation and acculturative stress in mental illness and suicide. Also, as with African Americans, Hispanic Americans are less likely to utilize suicide prevention hotlines (Larkin et al. 2011). Therefore, professionals could work to increase awareness and education about such resources and promote the creation of more culturally-competent suicide hotlines for individuals who speak languages other than English (Larkin et al. 2011).

Conclusions

Suicide is not merely an individual behavior. It occurs within larger family, community, economic, and sociocultural contexts. Rates of intentional self-harm and risks for and protections against suicide can be culturally specific, as can be assessment and intervention strategies. Much remains to be learned, however, about what is after all a very serious and high stakes public health issue. To close, then, we offer some themes that are important for health and mental health professionals to consider as they work with clients from across diverse cultural groups. We also suggest a research agenda that could continue to move the field forward.

Assessment Themes

- Be aware of cultural differences in verbal and nonverbal behaviors, including language barriers, and use translators when appropriate.
- Use culturally and linguistically appropriate instruments.
- Use multiple forms of assessment to increase accuracy.
- Ask directly and in different ways about suicidal thoughts and actions, and inquire about general feelings regarding hopelessness, life, and death. Consider verbal and nonverbal responses to the assessment.
- Evaluate ethnic identity, acculturation, and acculturative stress.
- Assess the impact of racism and discrimination (historical and current) on the client and potentially on the client-therapist dyad.
- Attend to the importance of trust and the relationship when conducting good assessment and include a careful review of informed consent and confidentiality.
- Involve others, such as family or spiritual or traditional healers, in the assessment process, as appropriate.
- Evaluate both strengths and weaknesses and both protective and risk factors.

Prevention/Intervention Themes

- Consider larger themes of evidence-based practice and cultural adaptations of research-supported interventions, not simply strict adherence to ESTs.
- Use strengths-based approaches and use cultural assets (e.g., ties to spirituality, family), rather than focusing solely on identifying and fixing problems.
- Understand the importance of cultural competence and commit to lifelong learning in that regard.
- Use culturally specific prevention and treatment approaches when appropriate for the client and his/her level of identification with the culture.
- Be aware that stigma against self-harm and/or mental illness can protect against suicide in some cases and actually reduce help-seeking behaviors in others.

- Be open to involving others in treatment (indigenous healers, family, spiritual leaders).
- Conduct outreach and increase flexibility of meeting spaces (e.g., a local church instead of an office) to address access to and stigma about treatment.

Research Themes

- Conduct more within-group research to enhance understanding of cultural influences on suicide.
- Implement more epidemiological studies.
- Work to identify explanatory mechanisms to enhance our understanding of correlational findings (e.g., relationship between length of time in the United States and suicide rates).
- Focus not only on high-risk groups (e.g., American Indian teenagers) but also on the population as a whole so that significant gaps are not present in our knowledge base.
- Continue to develop and test empirically supported assessment, prevention, and intervention strategies for suicide.
- Evaluate the reliability and validity of assessment tools within and across cultural groups.

References

American Association of Suicidology. 2010. "African American Suicide Fact Sheet." http://www.suicidology.org/resources/suicide-fact-sheets

Anglin, D. M., K. S. Gabriel, and N. J. Kaslow. 2005. "Suicide Acceptability and Religious Well-Being: A Comparative Analysis in African American Suicide Attempters and Non-Attempters." *Journal of Psychology and Theology* 33: 140–150. http://journals.biola.edu/jpt

Baumann, A. A., J. A. Kuhlberg, and L. H. Zayas. 2010. "Familism, Mother-Daughter Mutuality, and Suicide Attempts of Adolescent Latinas." *Journal of Family Psychology*, 24: 616–624. doi:10.1037/a0020584

Borges, G., R. Orozco, C. Rafful, D. Miller, and J. Breslau. 2012. "Suicidality, Ethnicity and Immigration in the USA." *Psychological Medicine* 42: 1175–1184. doi: 10.1017/S0033291711002340

Brown, M. M., and J. Grumet. 2009. "School-Based Suicide Prevention with African American Youth in an Urban Setting." *Professional Psychology: Research and Practice* 40: 111–117. doi:10.1037/a0012866

Centers for Disease Control and Prevention. 2010. *Suicide: Risk and Protective Factors.* http://www.cdc.gov/ViolencePrevention/suicide/riskprotectivefactors .html

Cespedes, Y. M. and S. J. Huey Jr. 2008. "Depression in Latino Adolescents: A Cultural Discrepancy Perspective." *Cultural Diversity and Ethnic Minority Psychology* 14: 168–172. doi:10.1037/1099-9809.14.2.168

Chatters, L. M., R. Taylor, K. D. Lincoln, A. Nguyen, and S. Joe. 2011. "Church-Based Social Support and Suicidality among African Americans and Black Caribbeans." *Archives of Suicide Research 15*: 337–353. doi:10.1080/13811118.2011.615703

Cheng, J. K. Y., T. L. Fancher, M. Ratanasen, K. R. Conner, P. R. Duberstein, S. Sue, and D. Takeuchi. 2010. "Lifetime Suicidal Ideation and Suicide Attempts in Asian Americans." *Asian American Journal of Psychology 1*: 18–30. doi:10.1037/a0018799

Choi, J. L., J. R. Rogers, and J. L. Werth Jr.. 2009. "Suicide Risk Assessment with Asian American College Students: A Culturally Informed Perspective." *The Counseling Psychologist 37*: 186–218. doi: 10.1177/0011000006292256

Chu, J. P., K. Hsieh, and D. Tokars. 2011. "Help-Seeking Tendencies in Asian Americans with Suicidal Ideation and Attempts." *Asian American Journal of Psychology 2*: 25–38. doi:10. 1037/a0023326

Compton, M. T., N. J. Thompson, and N. J. Kaslow. 2005. "Social Environment Factors Associated with Suicide Attempt among Low-Income African Americans: The Protective Role of Family Relationships and Social Support." *Social Psychiatry and Psychiatric Epidemiology 40*: 175–185. doi:10.1007/s00127-005-0865-6

Davidson, C. L., and L. R. Wingate. 2011. "Racial Disparities in Risk and Protective Factors for Suicide." *Journal of Black Psychology 37*: 499–516. doi:10.1177/0095798410397543

Day-Vines, N. L. 2007. "The Escalating Incidence of Suicide among African Americans: Implications for Counselors." *Journal of Counseling and Development 85*: 370–377. doi:10.1002/j.1556-6678.2007.tb00486.x

Diaz-Martinez, A. M., A. Interian, and D. M. Waters. 2010. "The Integration of CBT, Multicultural and Feminist Psychotherapies with Latinas." *Journal of Psychotherapy Integration 20*: 312–326. doi: 10.1037/a0020819

Dorgan, B. L. 2010. "The Tragedy of Native American Youth Suicide." *Psychological Services 7*: 213–218. doi:10.1037/a0020461

Duldulao, A., D. T. Takeuchi, and S. Hong. 2009. "Correlates of Suicidal Behaviors among Asian Americans." *Archives of Suicide Research 13*: 277–290. doi:10.1080/13811110903044567

Early, K. E., and R. L. Akers. 1993. "'It's a White Thing': An Exploration of Beliefs about Suicide in the African-American Community." *Deviant Behavior 14*: 277–296. http://www.tandf.co.uk/journals/tf/01639625.html

Garroutte, E. M., J. Goldberg, J. Beals, R. Herrell, S. M. Manson, and the AI-SUPERPFP Team. 2003. "Spirituality and Attempted Suicide among American Indians." *Social Science and Medicine 56*: 1571–1579.

Goldston, D. B., S. Molock, L. B. Whitbeck, J. L. Murakami, L. H. Zayas, and G. C. Nagayama Hall. 2008. "Cultural Considerations and Adolescent Suicide Prevention and Psychosocial Treatment." *American Psychol 63*: 14–31. doi:10.1037/0003-066X.63.1.14

Gomez, J., R. Miranda, and L. Polanco. 2011. "Acculturative Stress, Perceived Discrimination, and Vulnerability to Suicide Attempts among Emerging

Adults." *Journal of Youth and Adolescence 40*: 1465–1476. doi:10.1007/s10964–011-9688–9

Gone, J. P., and J. E. Trimble. 2012. "American Indian and Alaska Native Mental Health: Diverse Perspectives on Enduring Disparities." *Annual Review of Clinical Psychology 8*: 131–160. doi:10.1146/annurev-clinpsy-032511-143 127

Goodkind, J. R., K. Ross-Toledo, S. John, J. Hall, L. Ross, L. Freeland, and T. Becenti-Fundark. 2011. "Rebuilding Trust: a Community, Multiagency, State, and University Partnership to Improve Behavioral Healthcare for American Indian Youth, Their Families, and Communities." *Journal of Community Psychology 39*: 452–477. doi:10.1002/JC OP. 20446

Goodkind, J. R., K. Ross-Toledo, S. John, J. L., Hall, L. Freeland, D. Colletta, and C. Lee. 2010. "Promoting Healing and Restoring Trust: Policy Recommendations for Improving Behavioral Healthcare for American Indian/Alaska Native Adolescents." *American Journal of Community Psychology 46*: 386–394. doi: 10.1007/s10464-010-9347-4

Granello, D. 2010. "The Process of Suicide Risk Assessment: Twelve Core Principles." *Journal of Counseling and Development 88*: 363–370.

Gray, J. S., and J. J.Muehlenkamp. 2010. "Circle of Strength: A Case Description of Culturally Integrated Suicide Prevention." *Archives of Suicide Research 14*: 182–191. doi: 10.1080/13811111003704852

Griffin-Fennell, F. and M. Williams. 2006. "Examining the Complexities of Suicidal Behavior in the African American Community." *Journal of Black Psychology 32*: 303–319. doi:10.1177/0095798406290469

Hamilton, S. M. and K. A. Rolf. 2010. "Suicide in Adolescent American Indians: Preventative Social Work Programs." *Child and Adolescent Social Work Journal 27*: 283–290. doi: 10.1007/S10560-010-0204-y

Heron, M. 2012. *Deaths: Leading Causes for 2008. National Vital Statistics Reports.* Hyattsville, MD: National Center for Health Statistics. http://www.cdc.gov/nchs/data/nvsr/nvsr60/nvsr60_06.pdf

Hodge, D. R., and G. E. Limb. 2010. "A Native American Perspective on Spiritual Assessment: The Strengths and Limitations of a Complementary Set of Assessment Tools." *Health and Social Work 35*: 121–131. doi: 10.1093/hsw/35.2.121

Hovey, J. D., and C. G. Magana. 2002. "Exploring the Mental Health of Mexican Migrant Farmworkers in the Midwest: Psychosocial Predictors of Psychological Distress and Suggestions for Prevention and Treatment." *The Journal of Psychology 136*: 493–513.

Husky, M. M., D. A. Kanter, L. McGuire, and M. Olfson. 2012. "Mental Health Screening of African American Adolescents and Facilitated Access to Care." *Community Mental Health Journal 48*: 71–78: doi:http://dx.doi.org/10.1007/s10597-011-9413-x

Jobes, D. A. 2000. "Collaborating to Prevent Suicide: A Clinical-research Perspective." *Suicide and Life-Threatening Behavior, 30*: 8–17.

Joe, S., R. E. Baser, G. Breeden, H. W. Neighbors, and J. S. Jackson. 2006. "Prevalence of and Risk Factors for Lifetime Suicide Attempts among

Blacks in the United States." *JAMA: Journal of the American Medical Association* 296(17): 2112–2123. doi: http://dx.doi.org/10.1001/jama.296 .17.2112

Joe, S., S. S. Canetto, and D. Romer. 2008. "Advancing Prevention Research on the Role of Culture and Suicide Prevention." *Suicide and Life-Threatening Behavior* 38: 354–362.

Joe, S., and M. S. Kaplan. 2001. "Suicide among African American Men." *Suicide and Life-Threatening Behavior 31*: 106–121. doi: http://dx.doi.org/10.1521/suli .31.1.5.106.24223

Joe, S., M. E. Woolley, G. K. Brown, M. Ghahramanlou-Holloway, and A. T. Beck. 2008. "Psychometric Properties of the Beck Depression Inventory-II in Low-Income, African American Suicide Attempters." *Journal of Personality Assessment 90*: 521–523. doi:10.1080/00223890802248919

Kaplan, C. P., S. G. Turner, C. Piotrkowski, and E. Silber. 2009. "Club Amigas: A Promising Response to the Needs of Adolescent Latinas." *Child and Family Social Work 14*: 213–221. doi:10.1111/j.1365-2206. 2009.00625.x

Kaslow, N. J., A. Webb Price, S. Wyckoff, M. Bender Grall, A. Sherry, S. Young, and K. Bethea. 2004. "Person Factors Associated with Suicidal Behavior among African American Women and Men." *Cultural Diversity and Ethnic Minority Psychology 10*: 5–22. doi:10.1037/1099-9809.10.1.5

Kuhlberg, J. A., J. B. Pena, and L. H. Zayas. 2010. "Familism, Parent-Adolescent Conflict, Self-Esteem, Internalizing Behaviors and Suicide Attempts among Adolescents Latinas." *Child Psychiatry and Human Development 41*: 425–440. doi:10.1007/s10578-010-0179-0

Kuroki, Y. and J. L. Tilley. 2012. "Recursive Partitioning Analysis of Lifetime Suicidal Behaviors in Asian Americans." *Asian American Journal of Psychology 3*: 17–28. doi: 10.1037/a0026586

LaFromboise, T., K. Albright, and A. Harris. 2010. "Patterns of Hopelessness among American Indian Adolescents: Relationships by Level of Acculturation and Residence." *Cultural Diversity and Ethnic Minority Psychology 16*: 68–76. doi:10.1037/a0016181

LaFromboise, T., and H. A. Lewis. 2008. "The Zuni Life Skills Development Program: A School/Community-Based Suicide Prevention Intervention." *Suicide and Life-Threatening Behavior 38*: 343–353.

Lanier, C. 2010. "Structure, Culture, and Lethality: An Integrated Model Approach to American Indian Suicide and Homicide." *Homicide Studies 14*: 72–89. doi: 10.1177/1088767909352829

Larkin, G. L., H. Rivera, H. Xu, E. Rincon, and A. L. Beautrais. 2011. "Community Responses to a Suicidal Crisis: Implications for Suicide Prevention." *Suicide and Life-Threatening Behavior 41*: 79–86. doi:http://dx.doi.org/10.1111/j .1943-278X.2010.00013.x

Leong, F. T. L., M. M. Leach, C. Yeh, and D. Chou. 2007. "Suicide among Asian Americans: What Do We Know? What Do We Need to Know?" *Death Studies 31*: 417–434. doi:10. 1080/07481180701244561

Luoma, J. B., and J. L. Pearson. 2002. "Suicide and Marital Status in the United States, 1991–1996: Is Widowhood a Risk Factor?" *American Journal of Public Health* 92: 1518–1522. doi:10.2105/AJPH.92.9.1518

Matlin, S. L., S. D. Molock, and J. K. Tebes. 2011. "Suicidality and Depression among African American Adolescents: The Role of Family and Peer Support and Community Connectedness." *American Journal of Orthopsychiatry* 81: 108–117. doi:http://dx.doi.org/10.1111/j.1939-0025.2010.01078.x

Middlebrook, D. L., P. L. LeMaster, J. Beals, D. K. Novins, and S. M. Manson. 2001. "Suicide Prevention in American Indian and Alaska Native Communities: A Critical Review of Programs." *Suicide and Life-Threatening Behavior* 31: 132–149.

Mohatt, N. V., C. Fok, R. Burket, D. Henry, and J. Allen. 2011. "Assessment of Awareness of Connectedness as a Culturally-Based Protective Factor for Alaska Native Youth." *Cultural Diversity and Ethnic Minority Psychology* 17: 444–455. doi:10.1037/a0025456

Morrison, L. L., and D. L. Downey. 2000. "Racial Differences in Self Disclosure of Suicidal Ideation and Reasons for Living: Implications for Training." *Cultural Diversity and Ethnic Minority Psychology* 6: 374–386. doi:10.1037//1099-9809.6.4.374

Muehlenkamp, J. J., P. M. Gutierrez, A. Osman, and F. X. Barrios. 2005. "Validation of the Positive and Negative Suicide Ideation (PANSI) Inventory in a Diverse Sample of Young Adults." *Journal of Clinical Psychology* 61: 431–445. doi:10.1002/jclp.20051

Muehlenkamp, J. J., S. Marrone, J. S. Gray, and D. L. Brown. 2009. "A College Student Prevention Model for American Indian Students." *Professional Psychology: Research and Practice* 40: 134–140. doi:10.1037/a001.3253

Murphy, S. L., J. Q. Xu, and K. D. Kochanek. 2012. *Deaths: Preliminary Data for 2010. National Vital Statistics Reports* 60(4). Hyattsville, MD: National Center for Health Statistics.

National Institute of Mental Health. 2007. *Suicide Rates 2007: Suicides in the U.S. by Sex, Race, and Age in 2007.* http://www.nimh.nih.gov/statistics/4SR07.shtml

Nickerson, K. J., J. E. Helms, and F. Terrell. 1994. "Cultural Mistrust, Opinions about Mental Illness, and Black Students' Attitudes toward Seeking Psychological Help from White Counselors." *Journal of Counseling Psychology* 41: 378–385. doi:10.1037/0022-0167.41.3.378

Olson, L. M. and S. Wahab. 2006. "American Indians and Suicide: A Neglected Area of Research." *Trauma, Violence, and Abuse* 7: 19–33. doi:10.1177/1524838005283005

Oquendo, M.A., D. Dragatsi, J. Harkavy-Friedman, K. Dervic, D. Currier, A. K. Burke, and J. J. Mann. 2005. "Protective Factors against Suicidal Behavior in Latinos." *The Journal of Nervous and Mental Disease* 193: 438–443. doi:10.1097/01.nmd.0000168262.06163.31

Perez-Rodriguez, M. M., D. Baca-Garcia, M. A. Oquendo, and C. Blanco. 2008. "Ethnic Differences in Suicidal Ideation and Attempts." *Primary Psychiatry 15*: 44–53.

Richardson-Vejlgaard, R., L. Sher, M. A. Oquendo, D. Lizardi, and B. Stanley. 2009. "Moral Objections to Suicide and Suicidal Ideation among Mood Disordered Whites, Blacks, and Hispanics." *Journal of Psychiatric Research 43*: 360–365. doi: 10.1016/j.jpsychires.2008.03.008

Rockett, I. R. H., M. D. Regier, N. D. Kapusta, J. H. Coben, T. R. Miller, and G. S. Smith. 2012. "Leading Causes of Unintentional and Intentional Injury Mortality: United States, 2000–2009." *American Journal of Public Health 102*: e84-e92. doi:10.2105/AJPH.2012.300960

Rowell, K. L., B. L. Green, J. J. Guidry, and J. J. Eddy. 2008. "Factors Associated with Suicide among African American Adult Men: A Systematic Review of the Literature." *Journal of Men's Health 5*: 274–281. doi:10.1016/j.jomh. 2008.09.013

Scheel, K. R., L. R. Prieto, and J. Biermann. 2011. "American Indian College Student Suicide: Risk, Beliefs, and Help-Seeking Preferences." *Counseling Psychology Quarterly 24*: 277–289. doi:10.1080/09515070.2011.638444

Snowden, L. R. 2012. "Health and Mental Health Policies' Role in Better Understanding and Closing African American-White American Disparities in Treatment Access and Quality of Care." *American Psychologist 67*: 524–531. doi:10.1037/a0030054

Stiffman, A. R., E. Brown, S. Freedenthal, L. House, E. Ostmann, and M. S. Yu. 2007. "American Indian Youth: Personal, Familial, and Environmental Strengths." *Journal of Child and Family Studies 16*: 331–346. doi:10.1007/s10826-006-9089-y

Sue, S., J. K. Y. Cheng, C. S. Saad, and J. P. Chu. 2012. "Asian American Mental Health: A Call to Action." *American Psychologist 67*: 532–544. doi:10.1037/a0028900

Sue, D. W. and D. Sue. 2013. *Counseling the Culturally Diverse: Theory and Practice* (6th ed.). Hoboken, NJ: Wiley.

Taylor, R., L. M. Chatters, and S. Joe. 2011. "Religious Involvement and Suicidal Behavior among African Americans and Black Caribbeans." *Journal of Nervous and Mental Disease 199*: 478–486. doi:10.1097/NMD.0b013e318 22142c7

Thompson, V., A. Bazile, and M. Akbar. 2004. "African Americans' Perceptions of Psychotherapy and Psychotherapists." *Professional Psychology: Research and Practice 35*: 19–26. doi:10.1037/0735-7028.35.1.19

U.S. Department of Health and Human Services (DHHS). 2001. *Mental Health: Culture, Race, and Ethnicity—A Supplement to Mental Health: A Report of the Surgeon General*. Rockville, Maryland: U. S. Department of Health and Human Services.

Utsey, S. O., J. N. Hook, and P. Stanard. 2007. "A Re-Examination of Cultural Factors that Mitigate Risk and Promote Resilience in Relation to African American Suicide: A Review of the Literature and Recommendations for Future Research." *Death Studies 31*: 399–416. doi:10.1080/07481180701244553

Walker, R. L., D. Lester, and S. Joe. 2006. "Lay Theories of Suicide: An Examination of Culturally Relevant Suicide Beliefs and Attributions among African Americans and European Americans." *Journal of Black Psychology* 32: 320–334. doi:10.1177/0095798406290467

West, L. M., T. A. Davis, M. P. Thompson, and N. J. Kaslow. 2011. "'Let Me Count the Ways:' Fostering Reasons for Living Among Low-Income, Suicidal, African American Women." *Suicide and Life-Threatening Behavior* 41: 491–500. doi: http://dx.doi.org/10.1111/j.1943–278X.2011.00045.x

Westefeld, J. S., D. Cardin, and W. L. Deaton. 1992. "Development of the College Student Reasons for Living Inventory." *Suicide and Life-Threatening Behavior* 22: 442–452.

Wexler, L. M. and J. P. Gone. 2012. "Culturally Responsive Suicide Prevention in Indigenous Communities: Unexamined Assumptions and New Possibilities." *American Journal of Public Health* 102: 800–806. doi:10.2105/AJPH.2011.300432

Willis, L. A., D. W. Coombs, W. C. Cockerham, and S. L. Frison. 2002. "Ready to Die: A Postmodern Interpretation of the Increase of African American Adolescent Male Suicide." *Social Science and Medicine* 55(6): 907–920. doi: http://dx.doi.org/10.1016/S0277-9536(01)00235-0

Willis, L. A., D. W. Coombs, P. Drentea, and W. C. Cockerham. 2003. "Uncovering the Mystery: Factors of African American Suicide." *Suicide and Life-Threatening Behavior* 33: 412–429. doi:10.1521/suli.33.4.412.25230

Winderowd, C., D. Montgomery, G. Stumblingbear, D. Harless, and K. Hicks. 2006. "Development of the *American Indian Enculturation Scale* to Assist Counseling Practice." *American Indian and Alaskan Native Mental Health Research* 15: 1–14.

Winterrowd, E., S. S. Canetto, and E. L. Chavez. 2010. "Friendships in Suicidality among Mexican American Adolescent Girls and Boys." *Death Studies* 34: 641–660. doi: 10.1080/07481181003765527

Wong, Y. J., C. Brownson, and A. E Schwing,. 2011. "Risk and Protective Factors Associated with Asian American Students' Suicidal Ideation: A Multicampus, National Study." *Journal of College Student Development* 52: 396–408. doi: 10.1353/csd.2011.0057

Wong, Y. J., K. Koo, K. K. Tran, Y. Chiu, and Y. Mok. 2011. "Asian American College Students' Suicide Ideation: A Mixed-Methods Study." *Journal of Counseling Psychology* 58: 197–209. doi:10.1037/a0023040

Wong, Y. J., and C. S. Maffini. 2011. "Predictors of Asian American Adolescents' Suicide Attempts: A Latent Class Regression Analysis." *Journal of Youth and Adolescence* 40: 1453–1464. doi:10.1007s10964-011-9701-3

Woods, A. M., L. Zimmerman, E. Carlin, A. Hill, and N. J. Kaslow. 2013. "Motherhood, Reasons for Living, and Suicidality among African American Women." *Journal of Family Psychology* 27: 600–606. doi:http://dx.doi.org/10.1037/a0033592

Yoder, K. A., L. B. Whitbeck, D. R. Hoyt, and T. LaFromboise. 2006. "Suicidal Ideation among American Indian Youths." *Archives of Suicide Research* 10: 177–190. doi: 10.1080/13811110600558240

Afterword

There are clearly many different cultural approaches to health, and it is of great importance for health care workers and the administrations that support them to be culturally aware. Knowing about the different approaches to health can also help the lay consumer be better appraised of cultural differences which in turn can lead to a reduction in stereotyping or prejudicial attitudes towards behaviors that may be seen to be different from the norm. As the 24 chapters in these two volumes nicely illustrate, millions of Americans hold very different health beliefs from mainstream Western Biomedicine.

Chapter 1 in Volume I provides a summary of key recommendations for health care administrators and also provides perhaps the most critical reminder of why cultural awareness of differences is important. Many clinicians and health care workers may not have received the necessary instruction to be culturally competent but there are some easy ways to be prepared as demonstrated by the Purnell Model of cultural competence. There are other useful resources throughout the volumes for the interested reader that provide in-depth summaries of key characteristics of a variety of cultures and provide a single stop shop for learning about different cultural approaches.

In conclusion, it is important to acknowledge that many cultural variations exist within ethnic communities. Knowing how different cultural groups approach health and having a better understanding of how factors such as acculturation are important and can help clinicians, healthcare workers, and others with an interest in how lifestyle decisions are made, be more culturally competent. The efforts to increase cultural competency in the treatment of mental and physical health are promising but the wider health care arena and the general public need to pay attention to the causes of health disparities and the role played by multicultural approaches to health. We need a better connection between healthcare and the community so individuals can seek out treatments that best fit their cultural needs and the manifold health disparities can be reduced.

Regan A. R. Gurung

About the Editor and Contributors

EDITOR

Regan A. R. Gurung is Ben J. and Joyce Rosenberg Professor of Human Development and Psychology at the University of Wisconsin, Green Bay. Born and raised in Bombay, India, Dr. Gurung received a B.A. in psychology at Carleton College (MN), and a Masters and Ph.D. in social and personality psychology at the University of Washington (WA). He then spent three years at UCLA as a National Institute of Mental Health (NIMH) Research fellow.

He has received numerous local, state, and national grants for his health psychological and social psychological research on cultural differences in stress, social support, smoking cessation, body image and impression formation. He has published articles in a variety of scholarly journals including *Psychological Review* and *Personality and Social Psychology Bulletin,* and *Teaching of Psychology.* He has a textbook, *Health Psychology: A Cultural Approach,* relating culture, development, and health published with Cengage (now in its third edition) and is also the co-author/co-editor of ten other books. He has made over 100 presentations and given workshops nationally and internationally (e.g. Australia, India, Saudi Arabia, New Zealand).

Dr. Gurung is also a dedicated teacher and has strong interests in enhancing faculty development and student understanding. He was Co-Director of the University of Wisconsin System Teaching Scholars Program, has been a UWGB Teaching Fellow, a UW System Teaching Scholar, and is winner of the CASE Wisconsin Professor of the Year, the UW System Regents Teaching Award, the UW-Green Bay Founder's Award for Excellence in Teaching as well as the Founder's Award for Scholarship, UW Teaching-at-its-Best, Creative Teaching, and Featured Faculty Awards.

He has strong interests in teaching and pedagogy and has organized statewide and national teaching conferences, is a Fellow of the American

Psychological Association, the Association for Psychological Science and the Midwestern Psychological Association, and has served on the Div. 2 (Teaching of Psychology) Taskforce for Diversity, as Chair of the Div. 38 (Health Psychology) Education and Training Council, and as President of the Society for the Teaching of Psychology.

CONTRIBUTORS

Leticia Arellano-Morales, PhD, is a counseling psychologist. She is currently an Associate Professor within the Department of Psychology at the University of La Verne. Her research interests include Latina/o health and mental health, multicultural counseling competencies, multiracial feminism, and ethnic minority college students.

Sarah M. Bankoff, PhD, completed her undergraduate training at Dartmouth College, her doctorate in clinical psychology at Suffolk University in Boston, and is completing a postdoctoral fellowship with the Behavioral Medicine Service at the VA Boston Healthcare System. Her primary research interests include the study of psychosocial and physical health correlates and disparities in individuals with eating disorders and weight-related medical conditions, such as diabetes. She specifically aims to study eating behaviors and weight-related issues in veteran populations and in lesbian, gay, bisexual, and transgender individuals.

Amanda M. Brouwer, PhD, is an Assistant Professor of Psychology at Winona State University, Winona, MN. She studies how psychosocial concepts such as identity and self-efficacy influence health behavior enactment.

Chanté D. DeLoach, PsyD, is a licensed clinical psychologist in private practice and an Associate Professor of Clinical Psychology at The Chicago School of Professional Psychology. Her research and clinical interests center on issues of power, trauma, and resilience. A staunch advocate for using one's social capital, training, and privilege for the benefit of others, Dr. DeLoach has engaged in clinical and community work in numerous countries including Ethiopia, Zambia, Ecuador, Mexico, Brazil, and Haiti.

Sussie Eshun is a professor of Psychology at East Stroudsburg University and also a licensed psychologist in private practice. She graduated with a masters and doctorate in Clinical Psychology from SUNY at Stony Brook, New York. She enjoys teaching and mentoring and was recently honored with the *great teacher award* at her university. Her research interests include culture and mental health, mental health stigmatization, and perceptions about suicide.

Kaitlyn J. Florer received a bachelor of science degree in psychology at the University of Wisconsin-Green Bay. She is currently a graduate student in the counseling psychology program at Iowa State University. Research interests include mental illness stigma and multicultural counseling.

Donna Hodge graduated from the University of Michigan with a doctorate in community clinical psychology. She is a professor in the psychology department at East Stroudsburg University. Her research interests include factors that influence the mental health of minority groups, effects of stereotypic humor on self-perception and inaccurate affective perception. She has been the recipient of the Pennsylvania governor's *Outstanding African-American Professor Award.*

Katie E. Mosack, PhD, is Associate Professor of Health Psychology at the University of Wisconsin-Milwaukee. Dr. Mosack uses mixed methods to study the role of informal supporters in coping with chronic and life-threatening illness among marginalized populations.

John E. Pachankis is an Associate Professor in Chronic Disease Epidemiology and Social and Behavioral Sciences at the Yale School of Public Health. Dr. Pachankis's research, on the health of lesbian, gay, bisexual, and transgender (LGBT) individuals, seeks to identify the psychosocial (e.g., concealment, rejection sensitivity) and contextual (e.g., urban migration) processes underlying LGBT individuals' disproportionate experiences with adverse mental and physical health outcomes. His research combines social and clinical psychological methods and life course developmental models to inform investigations into stigma, LGBT mental health, and LGBT health intervention development.

David W. Pantalone is an Assistant Professor of Psychology at the University of Massachusetts, and a Behavioral Scientist at The Fenway Institute, both in Boston. His research centers on the "syndemic indicators" of childhood sexual abuse, partner abuse, mental health problems (depression, PTSD), and substance abuse—co-occurring factors that that affect sexual minority men's health and increase their risk for contracting HIV. Dr. Pantalone is an investigator on multiple NIH-funded behavioral intervention studies in this area that dually target improvements in mental health and decreases in health risk behaviors.

P.S.D.V. Prasadarao, PhD, is a Consultant Clinical Psychologist at the Waikato DHB and he is a honorary lecturer at the University of Waikato, Hamilton, New Zealand. He was formerly an Associate Professor at the National Institute of Mental Health and Neurosciences, Bangalore, India and at the USM Medical School, Malaysia. His areas of interest include cognitive behavior therapies, mental health of older persons, and, culture and mental health.

Rocío Rosales Meza earned her PhD in Counseling Psychology from the University of Missouri-Columbia. She is currently an Assistant Professor at the University of La Verne in the Psychology Department. Her research focuses on Latina/o mental health and Latina/os in higher education. Dr. Rosales Meza is Mexican, bilingual in Spanish and English, and is the first generation in her family to be born in the United States.

Brian A. Rood, MA, MPH, is a Doctoral Student in Clinical Psychology at Suffolk University in Boston. His research interests and experiences include HIV prevention and health promotion in lesbian, gay, bisexual, and transgender (LGBT) populations, and stigma, coping, and resilience among LGBT individuals living with HIV. His current research focuses on the psychological and physical health needs of transgender individuals, with an emphasis on the relations between external stressors (e.g., experiences of discrimination), internal stressors (e.g., identity concealment, internalized transphobia), and health outcomes.

Fyeqa Sheikh, PsyD, is currently a post-doctoral fellow at Hartgrove Hospital in Chicago, IL. Her research interests include culturally competent practice with South Asians and traumatic stress in children and adolescents. She was a participant in the Minority Fellowship Program through the American Psychological Association in 2010 based on her research on Pakistani women.

Marilyn Stern, PhD, is a professor in the Departments of Psychology, Pediatrics and Social & Behavioral Health at Virginia Commonwealth University. She also serves as the Director of Training in the American Psychological Association (APA) accredited Counseling Psychology program. Dr. Stern's primary professional focus has been in child health psychology, specifically in the areas of pediatric obesity and cancer. Dr. Stern is a fellow of APA (Divisions of Counseling, Pediatric and Health psychology), a Fulbright scholar (twice) and recipient of the Dorothy Booz Black Award for Outstanding Scholarship in Counseling Health Psychology.

Sujata R. Swaroop, Psy.D., is a postdoctoral fellow at the Trauma Center at Justice Resource Institute and the program coordinator of Project REACH, an anti–human trafficking program grant funded by the Office of Victims of Crime. She graduated from the Chicago School of Professional Psychology in 2013, with a concentration in international psychology and human rights. Dr. Swaroop specializes in clinical work, research, and advocacy with populations affected by political torture, war and displacement, gender-based violence, and intergenerational transmission of trauma. She received APA's 2011–2012 Division 12 Award in Distinguished Student Service for her dissertation research in northwestern Pakistan on trauma recovery following internal displacement.

Stephen K. Trapp, MS, M.Ed., is a doctoral student in Virginia Commonwealth University's Counseling Psychology program. His primary research focus is in health psychology, with special emphasis on the application of motivation and self-determination theories to patient health outcomes. Mr. Trapp's dissertation project focuses on the motivational factors associated with attrition in a multidisciplinary pediatric obesity intervention.

Kristin M. Vespia earned her PhD in counseling psychology. She is an Associate Professor of Psychology and Human Development at the University of Wisconsin-Green Bay, where she teaches undergraduate classes including multicultural counseling and psychology and culture. She has published in the areas of culture and mental illness, multicultural competence, college student mental health services, and the scholarship of teaching and learning.

Dean D. VonDras, PhD, teaches Adult Development and Aging, and Spirituality and Development at the University of Wisconsin-Green Bay. He is a gerontologist with special interests in the intertwining of health and psychological processes throughout adulthood. Dr. VonDras is a former Wisconsin Teaching Fellow and the founding Director of the Gerontology Center at the University of Wisconsin-Green Bay.

Angela R. Wendorf is a doctoral candidate in clinical psychology at the University of Wisconsin-Milwaukee, Milwaukee, Wisconsin. She uses mixed methods to study the patient experience of chronic illness and how psychological, contextual, and social factors influence treatment adherence, engagement in care and health outcomes among individuals living with HIV/AIDS.

Jacqueline Woods, MS, is a doctoral student in the Counseling Psychology program at Virginia Commonwealth University. Her research interests focus primarily on minority health disparities, specifically obesity in African American families. Ms. Woods received a diversity supplement from the NIH to fund her dissertation examining the role of the church community in supporting health behavior changes among African American caregivers of overweight children.

Index

Abu Bakr, 172

acculturation, 5, 37, 39, 42, 44–46, 51, 60, 62, 106, 115, 134, 181, 264, 265, 285; the "acculturation hypothesis," 72; bicultural acculturation, 46; and body image, 240–241; and eating disorders, 235; and poor diet choices, 233, 234; relation of to socioeconomic status (SES), 233; and the risk of suicide, 268, 274, 276. *See also* acculturative stress

acculturative stress, 96–97

African Americans, 4, 5, 38, 43, 47, 94, 95, 103, 106, 187, 232; binge eating among, 236; body image among African American women, 237; diagnosis of schizophrenia among, 39, 127; diets of, 234–235; and the "Driving While Black" cultural reference, 98–99; and "John Henryism," 102; obesity rates among African American women, 227; physical inactivity among, 231; sensitivity to African American cultural differences, 128; use of poor health behaviors as a coping mechanism among, 104–105; view of depression as a personal weakness, 123. *See also* African Americans, suicide among; mood/ anxiety disorders, among ethnic minorities

African Americans, suicide among: age as a factor in, 256; assessment of, 259–260; barriers to treatment of, 261; incidence and prevalence of, 254–255; prevention of, 260–261; psychological and psychosocial factors protecting against suicide, 259; rates of suicide among as the lowest of all racial/ethnic groups, 254; religion/spirituality as a protective factor against suicide, 258–259, 261; risk factors involved in, 256–258; and within-group differences, 255–256

Ahmed, R., 50

alcohol consumption/abuse, 45, 91, 104, 119, 149, 150, 201; among sexual minority men, 202; among sexual minority women, 204; among transgender individuals, 210

Alegria, M., 119

Allah, 171, 172–173, 174, 175, 177; connection and intimacy with, 178

allopathic medicine, 174, 175, 176, 178, 186

Altareb, B. Y., 174

American Indian Enculturation Scale, 266

American Psychological Association (APA), 41, 42–43, 51, 127

anorexia nervosa, 235–236

Arab Americans, 103

"Arab Spring," 170

Arole, R., 7

Asian Americans, 36–37, 45, 47, 95,
    103, 106, 187, 232; body image
    among, 238; negative attitudes of
    toward psychotherapy, 124; obesity
    rates among, 228. *See also* Asian
    Americans, suicide among; mood/
    anxiety disorders, among ethnic
    minorities
Asian Americans, suicide among:
    assessment of, 271–272; incidence
    and prevalence of, 267–269;
    prevention of, 272–273; protective
    factors working against suicide, 270;
    risk factors involved in, 269–270; and
    within-group differences, 268–269
Asians, 4, 10
Asnaani, A., 119
assimilation, 44, 45, 76, 124
Ayurveda, 18, 20

Baer, R. A., 145
Barzun, J., 137
Bates, B. R., 50
Bauman, A. A., 275
Beck Depression Inventory-II, 40,
    259–260
Berry, J. W., 44–45, 96
bicultural theory, 97
bipolar disorders, 116, 117, 122
Blevins, J., 18
Body Mass Index (BMI), 226, 230;
    among Asian Americans, 228
Bowen, K., 7
Brief Psychiatric Rating Scale (BPRS), 22
Brondolo, E., 96
Brown, C., 5
Brunder, J. S., 140
Buchan, L., 17
Buddhism, 18, 22, 154; and the *Eightfold
    Path,* 144; the four noble truths of,
    143–144; as an outgrowth of
    Hinduism, 143; seeking of the
    Atman (God) in, 143; use of
    meditation in, 144; use of
    mindfulness training, in, 144–145;
    values of, 145; views on organ
    transplantation, 148
bulimia nervosa, 235–236

cancer, 152, 203; among sexual minority
    women, 205, 206
Canino, G., 119
Cao, Z., 119
Cardemil, E. V., 81
Caribbean blacks, 119–120, 122, 125
Carpenter-Song, E., 5
Castillo, R. J., 38–39
Catholicism. *See* Roman Catholicism
Center for Epidemiologic Studies-
    Depression (CES-D) scale, 41
Centers for Disease Control, 256, 274
Cespedes, Y. M., 275
Chattapodhyay, S., 132
Chatters, L. M., 258, 259
Chavez, N., 94
Chen, C., 47
childhood obesity, 225–226; and body
    image, 236–239; and cultural eating
    behaviors, 233–235; and eating
    disorders, 235–236; gender
    differences in the prevalence of,
    227–228, 239; health risks
    associated with, 228–229; lower
    self-esteem among obese children,
    229; obese patients' communication
    with health providers, 229–230;
    obesity interventions, 241–242; and
    physical inactivity, 230–233;
    prevalence of all types of obesity in
    the United States, 226–228; and the
    role of acculturation in, 240–241;
    and the role of religion in,
    239–240
China: Chinese subcultures (*Han* and
    Kejia), 24; culture and mental health
    in, 22–24
Chinese Americans, 234, 268
Chinese medicine, 124
Christianity, 18, 148–150, 170; dietary
    restrictions practiced in, 149; and
    fasting, 149; and positive coping
    techniques, 151–152; positive
    health effects of ritual practices used
    in, 150–151; religious values of as
    an influence on health behavior,
    149–150; shared historical roots of
    with Judaism and Islam, 148–149

Chu, J. P., 273

Chun, C., 99

Clements-Nolle, K., 210

Cochran, S. D., 199

Cognitive Behavioral Therapy (CBT), 79

Cohane, G. H., 239

Collaborative Assessment and Management of Suicidality (CAMS) model, 272

collectivism, 42, 44, 46–47, 51, 92, 99, 128, 275; collectivist cultures, 93, 103, 146; horizontal collectivism (HC), 46; vertical collectivism (VC), 46

colonization, 169

Compton, M. T., 259

Confucianism, 22, 145–146; five key principles of, 146–147; view on organ transplantation, 148

Contrada, R. J., 94, 95

coping, 97, 106–107; and appraisal, 98; collective coping, 103–104; coping and the protective effects of culture, 105–106; culture and coping efficacy, 102; culture and coping goals, 99–101; culture and the coping process, 98–99; culture and coping resources, 102–105; culture and coping strategies, 101; types of coping strategies, 98, 101; use of poor health behaviors as a coping mechanism, 104–105

Corliss, H. L., 91

Corrigan, P., 4

Cuban Americans, 73

cuento therapy, 80

cultural adaptations, in the mental health field, 78–80; strengths of cultural adaptations, 79

cultural competence, 50, 52, 202, 210, 211, 261, 266–267, 271, 276; cross-cultural competence, 90, 106; in treating Latina/o mental health issues, 77–78

cultural conceptions, definition of, 6

cultural identity, 39, 50, 90, 98, 99, 106, 107, 232, 239, 264; and cultural dress, 93

culture, 7–8, 38; definition of, 89; and health belief systems, 24–25; influence of on mental health, 38–39; literature concerning the role of culture in mental illness, 8–9. *See also* stress, and culture

Curanderos, 125

De Coster, C., 167

depression, 54, 59, 76, 92, 111, 122, 125, 128, 199, 200, 203, 208, 209, 237, 259, 263, 274, 275; association of psychosocial concerns with, 209; clinical depression, 120; major depression, 117–118, 145, 199; postpartum depression, 8; as a result of witchcraft, 42. *See also* Beck Depression Inventory-II

Diagnostic and Statistical Manual of Mental Disorders, 4th edition (*DSM-IV*), 4, 38, 116, 195; Cultural Formation section of, 39

Diala, C., 4

Dichos therapy group, 80

discrimination, 15, 36, 44, 50, 72, 73, 100, 106, 115, 201, 208, 214, 254, 269; against Muslims, 170, 186; degree of discrimination among minority youths, 95–96; discrimination faced by Latina/os, 76, 77; five specific methods of discrimination, 94; institutional discrimination, 96; in the medical field, 124–125, 202; racial discrimination, 122, 205; and stress, 94–96

divination, 9, 11–12, 15

"Driving While Black" cultural reference, 98–99

Dube, A., 18

Durkheim, Emile, 257

eating disorders, 235–236

Ellison, C., 151

enculturation, 115, 264, 265, 269

equivalence, cultural, 49–50

Espiritismo, 125

ethnocentrism, 50

explanatory models, importance of in health care, 5–7

faith healing, 10–11
Falicov, J. C., 79
family, 14–15, 16–17, 146, 177, 227, 229, 235, 259, 261, 262, 265, 270; and the concept of *familismo* among Latina/os, 60–62, 70, 124; extended family, 39, 43, 61, 103–104, 124, 125; and the extension of the family system among Latina/os, 61; family conflicts, 7, 19, 67, 269, 274, 276; inclusive definition of among the LGBTQ community, 104; nuclear family, 109; role of in coping with stress, 103–104; and spirituality, 70, 72
Feinglass, J., 4
Feiser, J., 140
Filipino Americans, 268
Folkman, S., 97
Fong, A., 167
Foulks, E. F., 42

gender, 196; and body image, 239; gender expression and discrimination, 203; gender identity, 207; gender identity disorder (GID), 195, 207–208; gender stereotypes embedded in Confucianism, 147. *See also* sexual and gender minorities, health and wellness of
Generalized Anxiety Disorder, 118, 119
Ghali, W., 167
God, 138, 148–149, 175
Goldston, D. B., 275, 276
Gone, J. P., 266
grapefruit juice, and prescription drug blood levels, 128
Greden, J. F., 117
Green, B. A., 39–40
Greene, M. L., 95
Griffin-Fennell, F., 255
group identity, 104
Guidelines on Multicultural Education, Training, Research, Practice, and Organizational Change for

Psychologists (American Psychological Association), 127

health practitioners, personal biases of, 125; biases in diagnosis and treatment of mood disorders, 127–128
health psychology, 140
"Healthy People 2020" (U.S. Department of Health and Human Services), 202
Henry, J. D., 43
Hinduism, 19–20, 143, 144, 147, 148; and the caste system, 142; and the cultivation of positive health habits, 142; four major goals in life described by, 141; health and religion seen as one in, 143; and the idea of Karma, 142; ideological context/features of, 141, 142; and reincarnation, 142; techniques of used for positive health outcomes, 142
Hispanic American immigrants, 47, 48
Hispanics, 3, 36, 94, 120; body image within Hispanic culture, 237–238; obesity rates among, 227; stigma of mental health among, 123–124. *See also* Hispanics/Latinos, suicide among
Hispanics/Latinos, suicide among: assessment of, 275–276; incidence and prevalence of, 273–274; prevention of, 276; risk factors involved in, 274–275; and within-group differences, 274
HIV/AIDS, 9, 150, 152, 198, 199, 201, 208; and antiretroviral therapies (ARVs), 201–202; prevalence of among transgender individuals, 209
Hmong Americans, 234, 268
Hodge, D. R., 265
homelessness, among gay adolescents, 91
homophobia, internalized, 201, 203
Horne, S. G., 203
Hovey, J. D., 275
Huey, S. J., 275

India: culture and mental health in, 18–19; mental illness and temple healing in, 21–22; role of traditional healers in, 20–21

Indian Health Service (IHS), 263, 267

individualism, 42, 44, 46–47, 51, 92–93, 99, 101; horizontal individualism (HI), 46–47; individualistic cultures, 103; vertical individualism (VI), 46

integration, 44, 46, 68, 69, 120, 254

interventions, 16, 21, 70, 143, 254, 263, 277; clinical interventions, 182; faith-based interventions, 10, 192; lifestyle interventions, 230, 231; obesity interventions, 241–242; for suicide among African Americans, 260–261; for suicide among Asian Americans, 272–273; for suicide among Hispanics/Latinos, 276; for suicide among Native Americans, 266–267; wellness interventions, 153

Islam, 18, 148–150; derivation of the word "Islam" from *Aslama,* 171; dietary restrictions practiced in, 149; and fasting, 149; Five Pillars of, 173–174, 177; history and demographics of Islam immigrant populations in the United States, 168–171; and positive coping techniques, 151–152; positive health effects of ritual practices used in, 150–151; prophets of, 173; religious values of as an influence on health behavior, 149–150; shared historical roots of with Judaism and Christianity, 148–149; and *taqwa* (God-consciousness), 173; and *tawhid* (religious monotheism), 172, 174. *See also* Islam, approaches of to health and healing; Islamic psychology; Muslim Americans

Islam, approaches of to health and healing, 167–168, 174, 188–189; centrality of Allah to, 174; concepts of Islamic spiritual healing practices, 176–179; heath care utilization, 186–187; high value placed on allopathic medicine, 175, 186–187;

and *jinn* possession, 175–176; Muslim health and health-related paradigms, 174–176; prayer healing, 177–178; prophetic medicine, 174–175; traditional healing, 176; treatment of Muslim patients in the United States, 187–188; use of *fatwas* in healing, 175; use of witchcraft (*sihr*) in healing, 179

Islamic psychology, 179–180; approach of to psychotherapy, 183–184; case example (Murad), 184–185; case example (Samina), 180; discussion of the case of Murad, 185–186; discussion of the case of Samina, 180–181; and the four mental states that precede action, 182–183; goal of, 182, 184; holistic approach to, 181–182; and human nature, 181–183; stress of on balance between the worldly and spiritual worlds, 183

Jainism, 18

Japanese Americans, 268

Javaheri, F., 178

jinn possession, 17–18

Joag, K., 7

Joe, S., 255–256, 259

Jorm, F., 7

Judaism, 148–150; dietary restrictions practiced in, 149; and fasting, 149; and positive coping techniques, 151–152; positive health effects of ritual practices used in, 150–151; religious values of as an influence on health behavior, 149–150; shared historical roots of with Islam and Christianity, 148–149

Jung, C. J., 137

Kabat-Zinn, J., 144

Kaplan, M. S., 255–256

Kapur, R. L., 20, 21, 22

Kar, N., 11

Kaslow, N. J., 257

Kelly, E. W., 186

Kermode, M., 7
Khalili, S., 184
King, C. A., 117
Klienman, A., 24
Koo, K., 270, 273

LaFromboise, T., 264
Latina/os, 47, 94, 95, 103, 232, 234; binge eating among Latino females, 236; stigma of mental health among, 123–124. *See also* Hispanics/Latinos, suicide among; Latina/os, barriers to mental health care among; Latina/os, cultural focus on the mental health issues of; Latina/os, cultural values and beliefs of; mood/anxiety disorders, among ethnic minorities
Latina/os, barriers to mental health care among, 73; cost of mental health care as a barrier, 75; cultural barriers, 74–75; discrimination barriers, 76; gender as a barrier, 74; individual barriers, 74; organizational barriers, 75
Latina/os, cultural focus on the mental health issues of, 59–60, 81; and the "acculturation hypothesis," 72; complexity of cultural elements involved in the Latino view of mental illness, 69–70; and the cultural value of *familia,* 70; 80–81; culture-specific treatments (*Cuento* and *Dichos* therapies) for mental illness, 80–81; discrepancies among rates of mental illness among Latina/os, 71, 72–73; and the "immigrant or Latina/o paradox," 72–73; mental health and illness beliefs among Latina/os, 67–70; mental health care disparities among Latina/os, 71, 81; mental health profile for Latina/o mental health, 71–73; research on effective treatments for mental illness, 77; and the role of cultural competence in the treatment of mental illness, 77–78; and the role of spirits in mental illness, 67–68; and the stigma of mental health among Latina/os, 68–69
Latina/os, cultural values and beliefs of, 60–67; collectivist orientation of Latina/os, 61; *confianza* (sense of trust/intimacy), 64–65; *dignidad* (dignity), 64; and the extension of the family system, 61; *familismo,* 60–62, 70, 124; importance of Roman Catholicism in daily life, 65–66; maintenance of harmony within relationships through the use of *indirectas* (indirect messages), *bromas* (jokes), and *dichos* (parables/proverbs), 64; *personalismo* and valuing of relationships, 63–64; religious and spiritual beliefs, 65–67; *respeto* between parents and children, 62–63, 78
Lazarus, R. S., 97
Lee, S., 47
Levitt, H. M., 203
Lewis, K., 17
Lewis, R. J., 96
Lightfoot, E., 18
Limb, G. E., 265
low- and middle-income countries (LAMIC), 9
Lum, T., 18
Luoma, J. B., 256

Ma, G. X., 23
Maffini, C. S., 270
Magana, C. J., 275
Mal puesto, 38
Malcolm X, 170
manic episodes, 116
marginalization, 44, 101, 104, 106, 210
Martell, C. R., 212
Matlin, S. L., 259
Mays, V., 199
McNair, R., 92
Mead, Margaret, 138
meditation, 144–145, 148, 150, 151; mindfulness meditation, 151
mental health assessment, among minorities in the United States,

35–36, 51–52; assessment instruments, 39–41; and cultural equivalence, 59–50; demographics of, 36–37; and individualism/ collectivism, 46–47; language/ linguistic barriers to, 47–49; and non-verbal cues, 47–49; and past experiences of prejudice and perceptions about the health care system, 50; validity as a measurement of, 40–41. *See also* mental health assessment, key factors of

mental health assessment, key factors of, 41, 42; acculturation, 44–46; the individual's explanatory model of illness, 42–43

mental health models (universal), relevance of to the United States, 7–9

mental illness: definition of, 37–39; explanations of in the Third World, 6–7; influence of culture on, 121–122; international rates of, 8; literature concerning the role of culture in mental illness, 8–9; mental health stigmas among, 123; number of adults with severe mental illness in the United States, 2. *See also* India, culture and mental health in; India, mental illness and temple healing in; Latina/os, cultural focus on the mental health issues of

Mexican Americans, 117, 125; physical inactivity among, 231

Meyer, I. H., 199

mood/anxiety disorders, among ethnic minorities, 115–116, 264; anxiety disorder prevalence and incidence rates, 118–120; biases in treatment among ethnic minorities, 125–127; biases in treatment among health practitioners, 127–128; mood disorder prevalence and incidence rates, 116–118; reports of ethnic variations in mood disorders, 116–117

Muehlenkamp, J. J., 264

Muhammad the Prophet, 171, 171n1, 172

Mulvaney-Day, N., 119

Muslim Americans, 168, 176, 189, 239–240; health-seeking patterns of, 186; history and demographics of, 168–171; total number of in the United States, 169; variety of different ethnonational diasporas represented by, 169

Musto, R., 167

Nation of Islam, 170

National Alliance on Mental Illness (NAMI), 128

Native Americans, 37, 48; and acculturation, 45; belief in the link between mind-body-spirit in the treatment of disease, 126–127; body image among, 238–239; ghost sickness among, 38; obesity rates among, 227, 228; physical inactivity among, 231; substance abuse among, 263. *See also* mood/anxiety disorders, among ethnic minorities; Native Americans, suicide among

Native Americans, suicide among: assessment of, 264–266; incidence and prevalence of, 262; prevention of, 266–267; protective factors working against suicide, 264; risk factors involved in, 262–264; and within-group differences, 262

Nelson, J. M., 140

nervios, 69

Nguyen, T. A., 117

Nosek, B. A., 43

Noseworthy, T., 167

obesity: among adults, 227; among sexual minority women, 203, 205–206; prevalence of in the United States, 226–228. *See also* childhood obesity

Obsessive-Compulsive Disorder, 118

O'Dea, J. A., 230

Oquendo, M. A., 275

organ transplantation, view of in Eastern cultures, 148

Pahl, K., 95
Pantalone, D. W., 212
Paonil, W., 144
Pearson, J. L., 256
Perez-Rodriguez, M. M., 273
Perris, R. M., 43
phobias, 118
Polo, A., 119
Post-Traumatic Stress Disorder (PTSD), 118, 119, 120, 122, 256, 263
Powers, J., 140
psychology, 153, 179; community psychology, 150; ethnopolitical psychology, 80; Indian psychology, 19–20. *See also* health psychology; Islamic psychology
psychopathology, 11, 22, 35, 47, 120
psychopharmacology, 126
psychotherapy, 123, 125, 126, 179, 208, 270; Islamic psychotherapy, 183, 184; negative attitudes concerning, 124; traditional forms of, 80
Puerto Ricans, 80, 95, 125
Purnell Model for Cultural Competence, 285

Qian, M., 24
Quan, H., 167
Qur'an, 173, 174, 177, 178; diseases of the heart mentioned in, 182; use of in Islamic psychology, 180

racism, 76, 257; and the risk of hypertension, 96
Raguram, R., 21, 22
Rao, D., 4
Raub, J. S., 142
Reasons for Living Inventory (RFLI), 276
religion, and health, 137–138, 152–154; connection of all religions to an Ultimate Other, 152–153; and the holistic approach to wellness, 153; and the ideological contexts of religion, 140–141; interpretive challenges concerning, 139–140; religion as an aspect of cultural and psychological life, 138–139; religion/spirituality as a protective

factor against suicide among African Americans, 257–258. *See also specifically listed individual religions*; spirituality
Riolo, S., 117
Roberts, A. L., 120, 122
Rockett, I.R.H., 253
Roman Catholicism, 65–66
Rootwork, 38

Santería, 125
Santiago-Rivera, A. L., 62
Sarmiento, I. A., 81
schizophrenia, 5, 7, 15, 43; diagnosis of among African Americans, 39, 127; misdiagnosis of, 117; number of sufferers from worldwide, 8
science, and religion, 139
separation, 44; of mind and body, 174
Seventh-Day Adventist Church, 149
sex, 196; sexual identity, 197; sexual orientation, 197. *See also* sexual and gender minorities, health and wellness of
sex reassignment surgery (SRS), 208
sexual and gender minorities, health and wellness of, 195–197, 214; recommendations for health care providers concerning sexual and gender minorities, 211–214; the role of stigma in, 197–198, 200, 202; and stress, 91–92. *See also* sexual minority men's health disparities; sexual minority women's health disparities; transgender individual's health disparities
sexual minority men's health disparities, 199; and health care access/ utilization, 202–203; mental health, 199–201; physical health, 201–202
sexual minority women's health disparities, 203; and health care access/utilization, 206–207; mental health, 204–205; physical health, 205–206
sexually transmitted infections (STIs), 202, 209–210
Shapiro, L., 43

Shi'a Muslims, 172, 175
Sikhism, 18
Simmerlink, J., 18
Slavin, L. A., 97
Smith, H., 137, 139, 140, 146, 147
smoking. *See* tobacco use/smoking
Social Anxiety Disorder, 119, 199
social class, association of with physical inactivity, 232–233
somatization, 8, 76, 120
South African healers (*Sangomas*), 12
Spiritual Well-Being Scale, 151
spirituality, 18, 42, 44, 65, 66–67, 68, 73, 78, 139; and family, 70, 72; as the foundation of thought and action, 153–154; and health, 149, 150–151, 153, 177; importance of in African American culture as a protector against suicide, 258–259
Sringernyuang, L., 144
Stanford University Bipolar Clinic, 117
Stevenson, H. W., 47
stigmatization, 15, 122–123, 124, 204, 208, 229
Street, R. L., 49
stress, and culture, 89–91, 106–107; approaches to understanding stress, 90; discrimination and prejudice issues concerning, 94–96; and the pressure to conform to one's own cultural group, 94; and the role of cultural attitudes, values, and customs, 92–94; understanding minority status and stress, 91–92. *See also* acculturative stress; coping
Sub-Saharan Africa, mental health beliefs and practices in, 11–18; and African indigenous healing practices, 13–14; health education and health opportunities in, 12–13; in Kenya, 14; in Somalia, 16–17; and the spirits of deceased ancestors, 14; in Uganda, 14–16; in Zambia, 16
substance abuse, 59, 71, 72–73, 150, 199, 202, 208, 209, 256; among Native Americans, 263; among sexual minority women, 203, 205; among transgender individuals, 210

Sufism, 178
suicide, across different cultures, 253–254, 277; assessment themes of, 277; prevention and intervention themes of, 277–278; recent increase in suicide rates, 253. *See also* African Americans, suicide among; Asian Americans, suicide among; Collaborative Assessment and Management of Suicidality (CAMS) model; Hispanics/Latinos, suicide among; Native Americans, suicide among
Suicide Prevention Resource Center, 267
Sullivan, J., 199
Sunni Muslims, 172, 175

talisman, 10–11
Talmud, the, 137
Taoism, 22, 147–148; explanations of for physical and mental maladies, 147–148; and the practice of shamanism, 147; and Raja-style yoga, 147
Taylor, R., 259
Teachman, B. A., 43
tobacco use/smoking, 45, 91, 104, 149, 150, 201, 203, 205, 206, 230
Torres, M., 119
Torsch, V. L., 23
traditional healing practices, 10–11
transgender individual's health disparities, 207–208; and health care access/utilization, 210–211; mental health, 209; physical health, 209–210
Trimble, J. E., 266
Tuskegee Institute syphilis study, 124

United Kingdom, 10
United States, 1, 102; barriers to mental health in, 3–5; eating disorders among adolescent girls in, 235; emotional and behavioral disorders among children in, 2; Islamic immigrant populations in, 168–171; multicultural perspective of mental

United States, (continued)
health issues in, 1–3; number of adults with severe mental illness in, 2; prevalence of obesity in, 226–228; psychological distress among persons in, 2; racism in, 76; treatment of Muslim patients in, 187–188, 189; types of mental health treatment in, 2–3. *See also* mental health assessment, among minorities in the United States
U.S. Census Bureau, 48
U.S. Department of Health and Human Services, 267

vegetarianism, 143, 144, 149
Visual Analogue Scale (VAS), 48–49
von Hippel, C., 43

Wang, J., 167
Watts, A. W., 139
Way, M. L., 95
Whittaker, S., 17
Williams, M., 255
Willis, L. A., 258
witchcraft, 6, 7, 11–12, 13, 16, 121; as a cause of depression, 42; Islamic *sihr* witchcraft, 179
Wong, Y. J., 269, 270, 273
World Health Organization, 228, 235
World Health Organization Mental Health Atlas, 8

Xia, G., 24

yin/yang, concept of, 23–24
yoga, 142, 144; Raja-style yoga, 147

Zezuru people, 7
Zoroastrianism, 178
Zuni Life Skills Development Program, 267